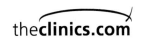

CLINICS IN
GERIATRIC MEDICINE

Movement Disorders

GUEST EDITORS
Roger L. Albin, MD, GRECC
Nancy R. Barbas, MD, MSW

November 2006 • Volume 22 • Number 4

SAUNDERS

An Imprint of Elsevier, Inc.
PHILADELPHIA   LONDON   TORONTO   MONTREAL   SYDNEY   TOKYO

W.B. SAUNDERS COMPANY
A Division of Elsevier Inc.

Elsevier, Inc. • 1600 John F. Kennedy Blvd., Suite 1800 • Philadelphia, PA 19103-2899

http://www.theclinics.com

CLINICS IN GERIATRIC MEDICINE	Volume 22, Number 4
November 2006	ISSN 0749-0690
Editor: Joanne Husovski	ISBN 1-4160-3797-7

Reprints. For copies of 100 or more of articles in this publication, please contact the Commercial Reprints Department, Elsevier Inc., 360 Park Avenue South, New York, New York 10010-1710 Tel.: (212) 633-3813; Fax: (212) 462-1935, e-mail: reprints@elsevier.com

The ideas and opinions expressed in the *Clinics in Geriatric Medicine* do not necessarily reflect those of the Publisher. The Publisher does not assume any responsibility for any injury and/or damage to persons or property arising out of or related to any use of the material contained in this periodical. The reader is advised to check the appropriate medical literature and the product information currently provided by the manufacturer of each drug to be administered to verify the dosage, the method and duration of administration, or contraindications. It is the responsibility of the treating physician or other health care professional, relying on independent experience and knowledge of the patient, to determine drug dosages and the best treatment for the patient. Mention of any product in this issue should not be construed as endorsement by the contributors, editors, or the Publisher of the product of manufacturers' claims.

Clinics in Geriatric Medicine (ISSN 0749-0690) is published quarterly by Elsevier Inc., 360 Park Avenue South, New York, NY 10010-1710. Months of issue are February, May, August, and November. Business and Editorial Offices: 1600 John F. Kennedy Blvd., Suite 1800, Philadelphia, PA 191023-2899. Customer Service Office: 6277 Sea Harbor Drive, Orlando, FL 32887-4800. Periodicals postage paid at New York, NY, and additional mailing offices. Subscription prices is $178.00 per year (US individuals), $297.00 per year (US institutions), $232.00 per year (Canadian individuals), $362.00 per year (Canadian institutions), $232.00 per year (foreign individuals) and $362.00 per year (foreign institutions). Foreign air speed delivery is included in all *Clinics* subscription prices. All prices are subject to change without notice. POSTMASTER: Send address changes to *Clinics in Geriatric Medicine*, Elsevier Periodicals Customer Service, 6277 Sea Harbor Drive, Orlando, FL 32887-4800. **Customer Service: 1-800-654-2452 (US). From outside of the US, call 1-407-345-4000.** E-mail: hhspcs@wbsaunder.com.

Clinics in Geriatric Medicine is covered in *Index Medicus, EMBASE/Excerpta Medica, Current Contents/ Clinical Medicine (CC/CM), and the Cumulative Index to Nursing & Allied Health Literature.*

Printed in the United States of America.

GUEST EDITORS

ROGER L. ALBIN, MD, GRECC, Chief, Neuroscience Research, Ann Arbor Veterans Administration Medical Center; and Professor, Department of Neurology, University of Michigan, Ann Arbor, Michigan

NANCY R. BARBAS, MD, MSW, Neurology Service, Ann Arbor Veterans Administration Medical Center; Department of Neurology, University of Michigan, Ann Arbor, Michigan

CONTRIBUTORS

ROGER L. ALBIN, MD, GRECC, Chief, Neuroscience Research, Ann Arbor Veterans Administration Medical Center; and Professor, Department of Neurology, University of Michigan, Ann Arbor, Michigan

NANCY R. BARBAS, MD, MSW, Neurology Service, Ann Arbor Veterans Administration Medical Center; Department of Neurology, University of Michigan, Ann Arbor, Michigan

NICOLAAS I. BOHNEN, MD, PhD, Associate Professor of Radiology and Neurology, Departments of Radiology and Neurology, University of Michigan, Ann Arbor, Michigan

RAKIÉ CHAM, PhD, Assistant Professor of Bioengineering, Department of Bioengineering, University of Pittsburgh, Pittsburgh, Pennsylvania

KELVIN L. CHOU, MD, Clinical Assistant Professor, Department of Clinical Neurosciences, Brown Medical School; and Associate Director, NeuroHealth Parkinson's Disease and Movement Disorders Center, Warwick, Rhode Island

ALBERTO J. ESPAY, MD, MSc, Assistant Professor, Department of Neurology, Movement Disorders Center, The Neuroscience Institute, University of Cincinnati College of Medicine, Cincinnati, Ohio

JOSEPH H. FRIEDMAN, MD, Clinical Professor, Department of Clinical Neurosciences, Brown Medical School; Director, NeuroHealth Parkinson's Disease and Movement Disorders Center, Warwick, Rhode Island

SID GILMAN, MD, FRCP, William J. Herdman Distinguished University Professor of Neurology, Department of Neurology, University of Michigan; Director, Michigan Alzheimer's Disease Research Center, Ann Arbor, Michigan

JOHN L. GOUDREAU, DO, PhD, Associate Professor, Department of Neurology and Department of Pharmacology and Toxicology, Michigan State University, East Lansing, Michigan

NINITH KARTHA, MD, Assistant Professor, Department of Neurology, University of Michigan Medical Center, Ann Arbor, Michigan

MATTHEW T. LORINCZ, MD, PhD, Assistant Professor, Department of Neurology, University of Michigan, Ann Arbor, Michigan

ELAN D. LOUIS, MD, MS, Associate Professor, Department of Neurology, G.H. Sergievsky Center; Associate Chairman for Academic Affairs and Faculty Development, Department of Neurology, College of Physicians and Surgeons, Columbia University, New York, New York

GEORGE T. MANDYBUR, MD, Assistant Professor, Department of Neurosurgery, Movement Disorders Center, The Neuroscience Institute and Mayfield Clinic, University of Cincinnati College of Medicine, Cincinnati, Ohio

SUSAN L. PERLMAN, MD, Clinical Professor of Neurology, Division of Neurogenetics, Department of Neurology, David Geffen School of Medicine at University of California, Los Angeles, Los Angeles, California

FREDY J. REVILLA, MD, Assistant Professor, Department of Neurology, and Director, Movement Disorders Center, The Neuroscience Institute, University of Cincinnati College of Medicine, Cincinnati, Ohio

MICHAEL A. WILLIAMS, MD, Associate Professor of Neurology and Neurosurgery, and Medical Director, Adult Hydrocephalus Program, The Johns Hopkins Hospital, Baltimore, Maryland

ROBIN K. WILSON, MD, PhD, Fellow, Adult Hydrocephalus Program, and Resident in Neurology, Department of Neurology, The Johns Hopkins Hospital, Baltimore, Maryland

CONTENTS

burden for the patient and family members. This article reviews the pathophysiology, risks, impact, major features, diagnosis, and treatment of these symptoms in Parkinson's disease.

Postural Control, Gait, and Dopamine Functions in Parkinsonian Movement Disorders

Nicolaas I. Bohnen and Rakié Cham

Balance impairments and falls, which are common in patients who have parkinsonian movement disorders, are a serious threat to the health of these individuals. However, the underlying mechanisms cannot be fully explained by presynaptic dopaminergic denervation, because balance impairment is least responsive to L-dopa therapy. This article reviews the latest clinically relevant literature relating postural control, gait, and dopamine in patients who have parkinsonian movement disorders.

Surgical Treatment of Movement Disorders

Alberto J. Espay, George T. Mandybur, and Fredy J. Revilla

A substantial body of evidence has accumulated regarding the efficacy and safety of neurosurgery for Parkinson's disease, essential tremor, and dystonia. Surgery for movement disorders (thalamotomy, pallidotomy, and subthalamic nucleotomy or subthalamotomy) was largely ablative (lesion-based). Given the safety and anatomy-preservation advantage, long-term electrical stimulation of these same targets (thalamus, globus pallidus, and subthalamic nucleus) is discussed as the treatment of choice. High-frequency deep brain stimulation procedures replicate the effects of ablative interventions, but do not require making a destructive brain lesion. This article outlines patient eligibility for surgery, targeting techniques, intraoperative findings, and potential complications and discusses the outcomes expected for each of the major interventions for which clinical trial data are available.

Parkinsonian Syndromes

Sid Gilman

The term *parkinsonian syndromes* refers to a group of disorders whose clinical features overlap those of idiopathic Parkinson's disease. The four major entities include three important neurodegenerations, multiple system atrophy, progressive supranuclear palsy, and corticobasal degeneration, and a lacunar cerebrovascular disorder, vascular parkinsonism. This article reviews the epidemiology, pathology, clinical features, diagnosis, and management of these disorders.

FORTHCOMING ISSUES

PREVIOUS ISSUES

CLINICS IN
GERIATRIC
MEDICINE

ELSEVIER
SAUNDERS

Clin Geriatr Med 22 (2006) xi–xii

Preface

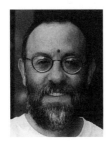 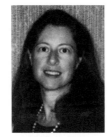

Roger L. Albin, MD, GRECC   Nancy R. Barbas, MD, MSW
Guest Editors

Common symptoms in the elderly include tremors, shaking, unsteadiness and imbalance, falls, difficulty initiating movements, and difficulty controlling undesirable movements. As our population ages, primary care physicians, geriatricians, neurologists, psychiatrists, and other health care specialists are increasingly confronted with the need to address these concerns. The elderly patient almost inevitably presents with multiple medical comorbidities, polypharmacy, and the normal changes in physiologic function that accompany aging. An important contributor to the morbidity of falls, tremors, and abnormal movements is that of movement disorders.

For this issue of the *Clinics in Geriatric Medicine*, we invited experts in their respective subspecialties to discuss the spectrum of movement disorders that affect the geriatric population. Parkinson's disease (PD) and Parkinsonian disorders are among the most common and most disabling of these diseases. The first half of this issue includes articles that address initial diagnosis and management of idiopathic PD, management of advancing PD, with its accompanying medication-induced complications, and the importance of recognition and treatment of nonmotor features of PD, including cognitive, affective, and psychiatric symptoms. The issue continues with an in-depth discussion of posture, gait, and dopamine function in Parkinsonian movement disorders and of the surgical interventions that are available for treating PD, as well as tremor and dystonias of non-PD etiology. Concluding the first half of this issue is a thorough review of non-PD Parkinsonian syndromes.

The second half of this issue contains reviews of additional types of important movement disorders or syndromes often seen with increased

doi:10.1016/j.cger.2006.06.013   *geriatric.theclinics.com*

frequency in elderly patients. The most common type of movement disorder in the elderly is an essential tremor. Chorea, ataxia, and dystonia are distinct movement disorders that can be recognized upon careful evaluation. Tremor, chorea, ataxia, or dystonia may be a sentinel feature of a primary neurology disorder or may present as a secondary manifestation of a number of medical, pharmaceutical, or toxic conditions, all discussed in the respective articles on these conditions. Finally, the important topics of tardive movement syndromes and normal pressure hydrocephalus are discussed.

The consequences of a movement disorder are numerous. Associated disabilities include reduced mobility and falls, interference with independence and emotional well-being, and cognitive and neuropsychiatric features, with their accompanying loss of personal autonomy. We hope that the discussions in this issue will help clinicians recognize, treat, and support their patients and their families who suffer from these disabling conditions. Although there is substantial work to be done on the development of future treatments, there is much that we can do now.

Roger L. Albin, MD, GRECC
Department of Neurology
University of Michigan
109 Zina Pitcher Place
Room 5031
Ann Arbor, MI 48109-2200, USA

E-mail address: ralbin@umich.edu

Nancy R. Barbas, MD, MSW
Department of Neurology
University of Michigan
1500 Medical Center Drive
Ann Arbor, MI 48109-0316, USA

E-mail address: nbarbas@med.umich.edu

ELSEVIER
SAUNDERS

CLINICS IN
GERIATRIC
MEDICINE

Clin Geriatr Med 22 (2006) 735–751

Parkinson's Disease: Background, Diagnosis, and Initial Management

Roger L. Albin, MD[a,b,*]

[a]Geriatrics Research, Education, and Clinical Center, Veterans Administration Medical
Center, Ann Arbor, MI 48109-0585, USA
[b]Department of Neurology, University of Michigan, 109 Zina Pitcher Place, Room 5031,
Ann Arbor, MI 48109-2200, USA

Parkinson's disease (PD) is a common neurodegenerative disorder associated with aging. After essential tremor (ET) (see article by Louis in this issue), it is the most common movement disorder of the elderly. PD is the most common disabling movement disorder. Parkinson [1] clearly identified PD as a distinct entity at the beginning of the nineteenth century, a period when classical and medieval medical concepts were giving way to careful empiricism in medical practice. Although Parkinson was ignorant of the pathology and pathophysiology of PD, he was an acute clinical observer, and his description of the cardinal features of PD remains valid: "Involuntary tremulous motion with lessened muscular power, in parts not in action and even when supported; and to pass from a walking to a running pace and of the hand failing to answer with exactness to the dictates of the will" [1].

The clinical features documented by Parkinson result from dopaminergic deficiency within the central nervous system. This fact and its clinical corollaries are the departure points for evaluation of patients with suspected PD. Dopamine deficiency, or blockade of dopamine effect, gives rise to a characteristic constellation of symptoms and findings that constitute the syndrome of parkinsonism. Clinical recognition of this syndrome allows differentiation of the etiologies underlying the syndrome. The basic neurobiology is that a small group of neurons within the rostral midbrain, substantia nigra pars compacta neurons, gives rise to a substantial projection to one of the major forebrain subcortical structures, the striatum. The primary neurotransmitter of the nigrostriatal projection is dopamine. The function of dopamine within the striatum is complex and understood incompletely,

The article was supported by NS15655, AG08671, and a Merit Review Grant.
* 5023 BSRB, 109 Zina Pitcher Place, Ann Arbor, MI 48109-2200, USA.
E-mail address: ralbin@umich.edu

doi:10.1016/j.cger.2006.06.003
geriatric.theclinics.com

but impairment of striatal dopaminergic neurotransmission causes a cascade of changes in the behavior of neurons projecting from the striatum to other brain regions. These "downstream" changes ultimately produce the clinical features of parkinsonism [2].

Syndrome of parkinsonism

Parkinsonism is defined conventionally by the presence of four cardinal features: tremor, rigidity, bradykinesia, and impaired postural stability. Tremor is a stereotyped, rhythmic involuntary movement. Tremor in parkinsonism typically involves the limbs and is a resting tremor, present with the limb relaxed and improving with use of the limb. Rigidity is an abnormality of muscle tone and refers to increased resistance to passive manipulation around a joint. In parkinsonism, two types of rigidity are encountered commonly: plastic or "lead pipe" rigidity and cogwheel rigidity. Plastic rigidity refers to a uniform increase in resistance to passive manipulation throughout the range of motion of the joint tested. Cogwheel rigidity, which may be the result of resting tremor superimposed on plastic rigidity, is characterized by a sense of the limb "catching," akin to operating a ratchet, during passive manipulation. Bradykinesia is slowed movement, which can be observed and documented in a variety of ways (see later). Postural instability refers to the impairment of mechanisms responsible for maintenance of upright posture during standing or walking. Determination of the presence or absence of features of parkinsonism is a clinical decision dependent on a careful history and examination. Imaging studies, clinical electrophysiologic studies, and blood tests play no role in the initial evaluation of patients with parkinsonism. Full-blown parkinsonism is a distinctive clinical syndrome and often obvious. With early, mild parkinsonism, however, the clinical features are often subtle, but thoughtful questions and a few simple examination maneuvers are revealing.

Patients with early parkinsonism complain of a limited range of symptoms. At onset of PD, asymmetric symptoms and findings are the rule. One hemibody or one limb is affected usually at onset. Tremor, usually in one arm or one leg, is a common early symptom. In asking about tremor, the clinician needs to distinguish under what circumstances the tremor is manifest. Is it present at rest (eg, when the patient is relaxed and watching television) or with use of the limb for some coordinated movement (eg, holding a book or newspaper, writing, holding a cup, or eating)? If present at rest, does it improve with use of the affected limb? For arm or hand tremors, is it present when the patient is walking but not when the arm or hand is used for coordinated activities? Patients often complain of hand clumsiness or incoordination, particularly for fine coordinated activities and particularly in one limb. The clinician should ask about buttoning, tying shoelaces, or applying makeup or fingernail polish. Some patients complain of clumsiness of one leg or foot. Parkinsonism is characterized by particular difficulties with initiation of movements. The clinician should ask about getting in and out of chairs or in and out of cars. Specific difficulties with these tasks and a history of slow initiation of gait, followed by relatively normal walking when gait is established suggest parkinsonism. It is particularly useful to ask about handwriting changes. If handwriting is altered, the clinician should ask if the letters have gotten larger or smaller. A history of letters becoming smaller or starting out with normal size letters that become increasingly small as writing continues is micrographia and almost pathognomonic for parkinsonism. Patients with parkinsonism often complain of being "weak," but formal examination of muscle power usually reveals normal strength. What patients are usually describing is bradykinesia. Normal motor performance of depends not only on muscle power per se, but also on appropriate speed of activation of relevant muscle groups. Patients with bradykinesia experience lower rates of force generation and a sense of "weakness." Additional questions to ask patients are if their voice, posture, or facial expression has changed. Voice alterations—generally diminished voice amplitude and speech clarity—are common, as is diminished facial expression (hypomimia) and a tendency to "stare" as blink rate decreases. Posture often becomes more stooped. Patients themselves often are not aware of changes in posture, voice, facial expression, or gait. It is useful to ask the patient's spouse or other family members about these phenomena. A subtle sign of parkinsonism is loss of associated movement of the affected arm when walking. Patients occasionally recognize loss of associated movements themselves, but more often it is noted by friends and family members.

Establishing a diagnosis of parkinsonism is a "show and tell" process. Perhaps the most useful aspect of the examination is watching the patient with suspected parkinsonism walk. In the author's clinic, physicians call patients from the waiting room and escort them to the examination room, largely to observe initiation of movement and gait informally. Important information is gleaned from watching the patient during the interview portion of the examination. Does the patient have diminished blink rate or hypomimia? Is the voice abnormal? Is there tremor of any body part? Is the tremor a resting tremor? Aspects of the formal neurologic examination that require careful attention are examination of eye movements, observation of initiation of movement, observation of posture and postural stability, evaluation of rapid movements, and formal observation of gait.

To examine eye movements, the clinician should ask the patient to track the tip of the clinician's finger slowly in all cardinal directions of gaze. These pursuit eye movements may be jerky instead of smooth. Parkinsonism is accompanied often by diminished efficiency of pursuit eye movements, requiring small accelerations of eye movement (saccades) to catch up with the moving fingertip. Gaze upward in the vertical plane may be reduced, although this may occur to some extent with normal aging.

The clinician should ask the patient to tap the index finger rapidly against the thumb, instructing the patient to make the movements as rapid and of greatest amplitude as possible. With parkinsonism, these movements are slower, often with diminished amplitude. Patients may start off with relatively rapid and large amplitude movements, only to experience slowing and amplitude decrement. One hand should be examined at a time; when both hands are used simultaneously, the slower hand may be entrained by the faster hand and give a misleading impression. To examine tone, the clinician should ask the patient to relax the arms and gently rotate the hand at the wrist or rotate the thumb. Plastic rigidity is felt as uniform resistance to passive manipulation throughout the range of movement of the joint. With cogwheeling, there is a repeated "catch" sensation. In some patients, abnormalities of tone can be brought out by performing "reinforcing" maneuvers with the contralateral limb. While examining tone at one wrist, the clinician should ask the patient to tap the contralateral palm on the thigh or mimic screwing in a light bulb.

To examine initiation of movement, the clinician should seat the patient in a regular chair and instruct the patient to cross the arms across the chest and then to arise. Because of bradykinesia, this task may be difficult. Some patients struggle to arise or bend forward rapidly to propel themselves out of the chair. After the patient is standing, assess posture.

To examine postural reflexes, the clinician should stand behind the patient and pull the patient sharply backward by the shoulders. The clinician should always warn the patient about what he or she is about to do, instruct the patient to move the feet if he or she starts to fall, and be prepared to catch the patient to prevent a fall. Individuals with normal postural reflexes take no more than 2 steps back to prevent a fall. Individuals with parkinsonism need to take many steps backward to maintain an upright position or actually fall.

To evaluate gait, the clinician should watch the patient walk for 10 to 15 yards and ask the patient to turn and walk toward the clinician. Stride length, base (distance between the feet), turning, and associated movements of the arms should be observed. A typical parkinsonian gait consists of a normal to narrow base, short steps, and slowed turns. Turning movements are often so-called en bloc turns, in which the normal fluid turn is replaced by a turn requiring two or more steps with the whole trunk held as a rigid object. An early, common feature of parkinsonism is loss of associated movements of the arms. Instead of swinging freely, the affected arms have reduced amplitude of movement and may be held close to the body in a fixed, partially flexed posture.

To assess tremor formally, the clinician should ask the patient to outstretch the arms in front and close his or her eyes. The hands should be observed for any tremor (postural tremor) with the arms in this fixed posture. To search for a tremor exacerbated by use of the arms (kinetic tremor), the clinician should ask the patient to drink a cup of water. For unclear reasons, tremor is often reduced when performing the usual test of limb coordination, the finger-nose-finger test. With a significant kinetic tremor, the tremor often becomes apparent or exacerbated as the cup nears the mouth.

Etiologies of parkinsonism

When the presence of parkinsonism is established, the next logical step is to establish the etiology of the parkinsonism. Four entities should be considered: drug-induced parkinsonism, parkinsonian syndromes, ET, and idiopathic PD.

Drug-induced parkinsonism results from use of pharmacologic agents that block dopamine effect or interfere with dopamine metabolism. The most common causes of drug-induced parkinsonism are dopamine antagonist antipsychotic medications. The risk of drug-induced parkinsonism is reduced significantly, but not obviated, with newer atypical antipsychotic agents. Another important group of drugs that can cause drug-induced parkinsonism are older (non–serotonin antagonist) dopamine antagonist antiemetics. Agents interfering with dopamine production or synaptic vesicular storage can cause drug-induced parkinsonism. These include α-methyl-para-tyrosine, α-methyldopa, and reserpine. A careful history is crucial for identifying drug-induced parkinsonism. If drug-induced parkinsonism is suspected, the suspected offending agent is withdrawn, and patients should improve. With dopamine antagonists or reserpine, improvements can occur within days to weeks after medication withdrawal, but there is sometimes a prolonged latency of months before marked improvement occurs.

It is sometimes difficult in elderly patients to differentiate drug-induced parkinsonism from drug-exacerbated parkinsonism. Are the clinical features of parkinsonism all due to an offending medication, or has the use of a dopamine antagonist or other agent exacerbated preexisting parkinsonism? The only way to differentiate these alternatives is to withdraw the possibly offending agent and wait. Complete recovery indicates drug-induced parkinsonism. Partial recovery is consistent with drug-exacerbated parkinsonism and the presence of an additional underlying cause of parkinsonism. Lack of recovery indicates the presence of another cause of parkinsonism. Because the effects of dopamine antagonists make take months to wear off, a definitive evaluation may require an observation period of months.

Parkinsonian syndromes, also called atypical parkinsonism or Parkinson's plus syndromes, are a family of neurodegenerative disorders that result from neuronal loss in different components of the basal ganglia, the brain system of which the dopaminergic midbrain neurons affected in PD are a part. For a detailed description of these disorders, see the article by Gilman in this issue. All of these disorders can be difficult to differentiate from PD early in the course of the illness. These disorders have distinctive clinical features, which may emerge only after the onset of parkinsonism. Important clinical clues that one of these disorders is present are symmetric onset of parkinsonism, absence of typical resting tremor, early autonomic dysfunction, prominent dystonia, significant early cognitive impairment, or prominent early falls. The most useful diagnostic maneuver is a treatment trial. Patients with PD should have a substantial response to dopamine replacement treatment; individuals with parkinsonian syndromes do not respond. Initial approaches to treatment are discussed subsequently. With serial follow-up by experienced clinicians, clinical differentiation of PD and parkinson's plus disorders is accurate. Clinicopathologic correlation data from the movement disorders service at the National Hospital for Neurology and Neurosurgery (NHNN) in London indicates high reliability of clinical diagnosis of PD by experienced clinicians [3]. In this study, the positive predictive value of a clinical diagnosis of PD was close to 100%. These results underscore the value of careful clinical evaluations. Although the parkinsonian syndromes are individually rare, in the aggregate they are uncommon as opposed to rare. At the NHNN movement disorders service, approximately 25% of patients with parkinsonism had a parkinsonian syndrome [3]. This proportion is inflated because NHNN is a tertiary referral center, but a reasonable estimate is that approximately 10% to 15% of patients seen initially for parkinsonism turn out to have a parkinsonian syndrome rather than PD.

ET is discussed at length by Louis in another article in this issue. ET is seen commonly in the elderly and is sometimes confused with PD. ET is a disorder whose primary manifestation is tremor; it lacks the rigidity, bradykinesia, and impairment of postural reflexes found in PD. The tremor is usually different from that found in PD. Typical ET is not a resting tremor, but rather present with fixed posture (postural tremor) or use of the affected limb (kinetic tremor). The distribution of tremor also is different in ET. At onset, most PD patients have unilateral resting tremor, and tremor may involve or start in the leg. ET tremor is typically a bilateral upper extremity tremor and only in rare variants involves the legs. ET often produces a characteristic head tremor—head nodding (no, no) or rotatory tremor—whereas PD patients may have a jaw, lip, or tongue tremor. ET patients sometimes exhibit a voice tremor, which is never seen in PD.

Simple examination maneuvers help characterize tremors. Observation during the interview or other parts of the examination is crucial. Is the tremor present when the affected limb is really relaxed? A postural tremor occasionally resembles a resting tremor because anxious patients may not be completely relaxed during formal examination. The finger digits should be observed. The tremor of PD is often a so-called pill-rolling tremor with flexion-extension of the fingers and thumb. Involvement of the thumb strongly suggests PD. Postural and kinetic tremor should be evaluated as described previously. If the patient has postural or kinetic upper extremity tremor, absence of resting tremor, and no other examination features of parkinsonism, ET is the diagnosis. The presence of a typical head tremor or voice tremor is helpful in establishing a diagnosis. Some patients may exhibit features of ET and PD. ET and PD are common problems in the elderly, and both may be present in elderly patients. Based on a relatively high rate of coincident ET and PD in clinic series studies, there was speculation that ET represented a risk factor for the development of PD, but it is more likely that individuals with coincident ET and PD are overrepresented in clinic series because of referral bias. There is no good evidence at present that ET is a risk factor for PD.

Having excluded drug-induced PD, parkinsonian syndromes, and ET as causes of a patient's symptoms, and having found typical features of PD, a clinical diagnosis of PD is likely. Formal diagnosis of PD requires the presence of at least two of the four cardinal features and significant response to dopamine replacement therapy [4,5]. PD is a progressive neurodegenerative disorder whose pathologic hallmark is loss of dopaminergic substantia nigra neurons with surviving neurons often containing a characteristic cytoplasmic inclusion body, the Lewy body (Fig. 1) [6]. At diagnosis, patients should be counseled that they have a progressive disease that will worsen over time. Individuals presenting with unilateral symptoms and findings inevitably develop contralateral symptoms and findings. The rate of decline varies, however, and is impossible to predict for individuals at time of diagnosis. Factors that seem to predict slower rate of progression are relatively young age at onset and tremor as an initial symptom [7]. Patients should be told that good treatment is available, but that this treatment is symptomatic and palliative and does not address the underlying causes of neurodegeneration.

Epidemiology, genetics, and pathogenesis of Parkinson's disease

PD is a common disorder. Reasonable estimates of prevalence average approximately 250 to 300 per 100,000 [8]. This gives an approximate total

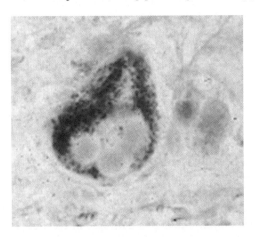

Fig. 1. Lewy bodies. Photomicrograph shows a neuron with three cytoplasmic Lewy bodies (PTAH-eosin stain). (Courtesy of Dr. Andrew Lieberman, University of Michigan.)

of 800,000 PD patients in the United States. This is likely a significant underestimate. Studies using rigorous identification methods indicate higher prevalence rates of 350 per 100,000. A study using large population-based databases in Ontario, a population comparable to the United States, and registry data from Nebraska indicate a PD prevalence of approximately 350 per 100,000, suggesting that there are approximately 1 million PD patients in the United States [9,10]. PD incidence rates are estimated at approximately 10 to 15 per 100,000. PD is primarily a disease of the aged with approximately 95% of incident cases occurring after age 60. After this age, incidence seems to increase exponentially. PD seems to be more prevalent among men than women and is suggested to be more prevalent among Americans of European than African descent. PD is associated with increased mortality compared with control populations, although some evidence indicates that modern treatment has improved the life expectancy of PD patients [11].

There is a large and confusing epidemiologic literature regarding possible environmental risk factors for PD. Briefly, only relatively weak associations have been reported, and in many cases, there are contradictory studies regarding proposed individual risk factors. One intriguing and relatively well-established association is the relationship between PD and a history of smoking [12]. Individuals with a history of smoking seem to have a lower risk of developing PD. This result has been replicated in several well-done studies and exhibits a dose-response relationship. Its significance is unknown. Does smoking itself offer some degree of neuroprotection or is a heightened susceptibility to tobacco addiction in some way a biomarker of a phenotype that resists neurodegeneration?

More recent work also has explored the possible role of genetic factors in the etiopathogenesis of PD. Studies using different methodologies have produced different results. Twin studies suggest low concordance rates for parkinsonism in typical, late-onset (>60 old years) PD, although with impressively increased concordance rates in earlier onset PD [13]. These results suggest that the small minority of early-onset PD cases have a largely genetic etiology, but that genetic factors play only a small role in typical PD. The largest of these studies features a relatively small number of twins, however, and concordance might increase with longer follow-up periods. Studies looking at relatives of individuals with PD have shown a higher prevalence of PD in first-degree relatives (parents, sibs) [14]. Most of these studies are clinic based and might have referral or ascertainment bias. Given the late onset of typical PD, it is likely that by the time patients become symptomatic, many first-degree relatives are deceased from other causes. Finding some evidence of genetic factors in a late-onset disease is suggestive. The DeCode Genetics group attempted to circumvent ascertainment problems with the unique genetics-disease-pedigree database in Iceland [15]. These data indicate substantially increased risk of PD in first-degree relatives of PD patients and support a genetic contribution to PD in Icelanders. This group subsequently has identified a possible locus that constitutes a risk factor for PD in this population. Whether these results are generalizable beyond the Icelandic population remains to be seen.

Defining genetic causes of PD has become a major focus of research [16]. Numerous pedigrees have been discovered in which clinically defined PD is inherited in typical mendelian patterns, either dominant or recessive. These inherited forms of PD usually are found in pedigrees whose probands have early-onset PD. Most of these clearly inherited forms of PD are rare, but mutations in the recessive PARK2 locus account for a significant number of early-onset cases of PD. Mutations in one recently discovered locus, PARK8, produce dominantly inherited PD and may contribute to a small but significant number of cases of typical late-onset PD. Some studies suggest that 1% of typical late-onset cases are due to mutations in this locus.

The real significance of ascertaining these unusual causes of PD is that they may cast light on the pathogenesis of more common sporadic PD. The first locus identified, PARK1, was found to have mutations of the α-synuclein gene. This protein is expressed highly in neurons and localized to presynaptic terminals. A possible link between sporadic PD and α-synuclein metabolism was established quickly when it was found that the major component of Lewy bodies is α-synuclein, suggesting that sporadic PD could result from abnormalities in the processing of this protein [17]. A major pathway for protein degradation is the ubiquitin-proteosome system. There are suggestions that α-synuclein mutations causing PD render this protein resistant to proteosomal degradation [18]. The PARK2 locus encodes the protein parkin, a key enzyme in the ubiquitin-proteosome pathway, and another candidate locus, PARK5, encoding ubiquitin terminal hydrolase L1, also functions in the ubiquitin-proteosome pathway. These findings suggest that sporadic PD could result from dysfunction of the ubiquitin-proteosome pathway. McNaught and colleagues [19] developed a new rodent model of PD, replicating key behavioral and histologic features of PD, with systemic administration of proteosome inhibitors.

Identification of other PD-causing loci has suggested a similar story centered on mitochondrial dysfunction [20]. PARK6, PARK7, and PARK8 are due to mutations in the proteins PINK1, DJ-1, and LRRK2. All these proteins are localized to mitochondria, supporting the hypothesis that mitochondrial dysfunction is a key feature of neurodegeneration in PD. Mitochondrial dysfunction has been suspected previously to be a crucial component of PD with postmortem studies showing selective deficits in complex I of the electron transport chain [21]. The proximate mechanism of action of the selective dopaminergic neuron neurotoxin, MPTP, is inhibition of complex I.

Relatively modest differences between individuals in proteosomal or mitochondrial function might predispose some individuals to the development of PD. It is possible that common polymorphisms in some of the loci identified as causing PD might play a role in the pathogenesis of typical PD.

Polymorphisms in loci yet to be identified also might constitute risk factors for PD.

Initial treatment of Parkinson's disease

As mentioned earlier, formal diagnosis of PD involves response to treatment. The decision to initiate therapy is not always straightforward, however. Individuals with initial symptoms of PD may not be experiencing significant disability. Treatment should be initiated only when patients are experiencing problems in their day-to-day lives. This situation can vary considerably from patient to patient, and the decision to initiate treatment requires thoughtful individualization of treatment. Several options exist for initial treatment. A few patients with prominent and bothersome tremor but minimal bradykinesia may benefit from initial treatment with anticholinergic agents, such as benztropine or trihexyphenidyl. These compounds are often effective for PD tremor, but have little effect on other features of PD, such as bradykinesia or rigidity. Anticholinergics should be used cautiously in patients in whom cognitive impairment is a concern. The author avoids these agents in any patient with a suggestion of impaired cognition and in frail, elderly patients. Amantadine has a modest but real effect in PD and is suitable for treatment of individuals with mild but still bothersome deficits. This agent is generally easy to use and tolerated well, but should be avoided in individuals with significant renal impairment. There is no "neuroprotective" therapy that slows or arrests progression of PD. There was a vogue of enthusiasm for using the selective monoamine oxidase B inhibitor selegiline in all newly diagnosed PD patients because some clinical trial data suggested that this agent might slow the progression of PD. Subsequent analyses undercut this claim, and most movement disorder specialists no longer recommend initial treatment with selegiline [22,23].

As PD progresses, all patients require dopamine replacement therapy. The major decision is whether to use a levodopa preparation or a dopamine agonist. These agents have markedly different mechanisms of action. Dopamine synthesis is a highly regulated process. The ultimate precursor for dopamine is tyrosine, and the major rate-limiting step for dopamine synthesis is tyrosine hydroxylase conversion of tyrosine to levodopa. Levodopa is the endogenous precursor of dopamine and is converted to dopamine by the aromatic acid decarboxylase (AADC), also called dopa decarboxylase. Tyrosine supplementation is useless because tyrosine hydroxylase enzyme activity is end product limited. Because dopamine does not cross the blood-brain barrier, direct supplementation with dopamine is impractical. Administration of pharmacologic amounts of levodopa results in increased synthesis of dopamine. This occurs in the remaining dopaminergic nigrostriatal neurons, but because virtually all cells contain AADC activities, dopamine is synthesized in nondopaminergic neurons and glia as well. In the remaining dopaminergic neurons, there is a simulacrum of the normal process of dopamine synthesis, vesicular storage, and release (Fig. 2). In nondopaminergic cells, these processes are unregulated, but contribute to increased extracellular striatal dopamine. An interesting implication is that a substantial component of dopamine action does not depend on tightly regulated synaptic release, but instead has a hormone-like action. Dopamine agonists bypass the whole machinery of dopamine synthesis and release to interact directly with dopamine receptors. There are five molecularly defined dopamine receptors, d1 through d5. Pharmacology defines two broad classes of dopamine receptors, D1-like (d1 and d5) and D2-like (d2, d3, d4). d1, d2, and d3 receptors are expressed at high levels in the striatum. Almost all dopamine agonists are primarily D2-like agonists, although apomorphine, which requires parenteral administration and has limited application in PD, is a full-spectrum agonist.

Other important differences between levodopa preparations and dopamine agonists are that levodopa has a short serum half-life (approximately 3–4 hours) and complex pharmacokinetics when administered orally. The principal advantage of dopamine agonists is their relatively long half-life and predictable pharmacokinetics.

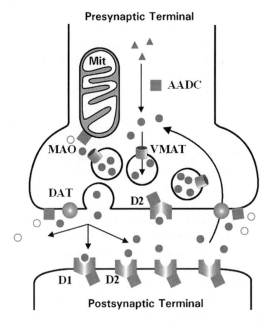

Fig. 2. The dopaminergic synapse and the synthesis pathway for dopamine from levodopa. *Triangles* represent levodopa, *solid circles* represent levodopa, and *open circles* represent dopamine metabolites. AADC, aromatic acid decarboxylase (dopa decarboxylase); D1 and D2, D1-like and D2-like receptors; DAT, dopamine transporter; MAO is monoamine oxidase; VAMT2, type 2 vesicular monoamine transporter (the protein responsible for pumping monoamine neurotransmitters into synaptic vesicles).

There has been some controversy regarding the initial choice of therapy. The background of this controversy is concern about the safety of levodopa. Potentially cytotoxic free radicals can be generated via normal catabolism of dopamine, and in some in vitro preparations, dopamine and levodopa are neurotoxic [24]. Administration of pharmacologic doses of levodopa was suggested to increase dopamine turnover and potentially accelerate neurodegeneration in PD. Solid evidence for this concept is slight, but it has had an impact on clinical practice with some clinicians withholding levodopa treatment as long as possible, sometimes to a ridiculous extent, and a search for alternative initial therapies [25]. A neurotoxic effect of levodopa is hard to reconcile with data indicating that levodopa treatment reduces the mortality rate of PD, a remarkable achievement for a palliative therapy [11].

Because of concerns about toxic effects of levodopa, the Parkinson Study Group conducted a major trial, ELLDOPA, addressing this issue [26]. Newly diagnosed PD subjects not yet requiring dopamine replacement therapy were randomly assigned to placebo or ascending doses of levodopa. These subjects were followed for 40 weeks and evaluated at the end of the study with standard clinical rating scales. Evaluations were performed while subjects were still on levodopa and after a 2-week washout period. Unexpectedly, the subjects treated with the highest doses of levodopa had the best performance after the washout period. Levodopa is known to have a so-called long duration therapeutic effect (see later), which could account for this result. Alternatively, levodopa might have a neuroprotective effect and slow progression of PD. Regardless, the ELLDOPA outcome mitigates concerns about the possible toxicity of levodopa.

Another argument for initial use of dopamine agonists is the suggestion that initial dopamine agonist use may retard the emergence of motor complications, specifically the involuntary movements called dyskinesias (see article by Goudreau), which often become troublesome after several years of treatment. This argument is based largely on experiments in animal models of PD in which the nigrostriatal projection is almost completely destroyed and levodopa is administered intermittently two to three times per day. Over a period of weeks, these animals develop heightened motor responses to levodopa [27]. Long-term, nonpulsatile levodopa administration mitigates the emergence of heightened motor responses. This influential set of experiments gave rise to speculation that long-term stimulation of dopamine receptors might delay the occurrence of dyskinesias, and that dopamine agonists might be preferable to levodopa preparations as initial therapy for this reason. This hypothesis was evaluated in the CALM-PD trial, a comparison of levodopa and the dopamine agonist pramipexole [28]. The results of this trial seemed to support the idea that initial dopamine agonist treatment would reduce the emergence of dyskinesias. Several factors complicated interpretation of CALM-PD, however, the most important of which was the fact that the levodopa-treated and pramipexole-treated arms of the study did not achieve equivalent levels of therapeutic effect [29]. The hypothesized advantages of initial treatment with dopamine agonists remain hypothetical. A Practice Parameter issued by the American Academy of Neurology emphasizes that levodopa preparations and dopamine agonists are reasonable choices for initial treatment of PD [30].

The CALM-PD study and similar trials offer some additional relevant comparative information about levodopa and dopamine agonist treatments. Levodopa is a more effective medication and has a lower incidence of side effects. Levodopa preparations also are less expensive than dopamine agonists. The author usually initiates treatment with a levodopa preparation. The major exception is relatively young patients with PD. If there is an advantage of initial treatment with dopamine agonists, it is likely to accrue to individuals who will be treated for many years. Patients with onset of PD before age 60 are the most likely to benefit from initial agonist therapy, if such benefits exist. Many of these patients end up on levodopa preparations anyway because of tolerability problems with dopamine agonists.

Introduction of levodopa is straightforward. The most appropriate preparation is the so-called 25/100. The first numeral indicates the milligrams of carbidopa, and the second numeral indicates the number of milligrams of levodopa. Carbidopa is an AADC inhibitor that does not pass the blood-brain barrier. Without carbidopa, most levodopa administered would be metabolized in peripheral tissues and never reach the brain. Because the area postrema–chemoreceptor trigger zone (the "vomit" center) of the brain is outside the blood-brain barrier, and because dopamine receptor activation in this region is powerfully emetic, administering levodopa without carbidopa or another AADC inhibitor can cause considerable nausea, a problem that plagued early trials with levodopa. Most individuals require about 75 to 100 mg of carbidopa per day to inhibit peripheral tissue AADCs. About 300 mg of levodopa is a good starting dose; hence carbidopa/levodopa 25/100 orally three times a day is usually a good starting dose. Carbidopa/levodopa preparations are available in conventional (immediate release) and extended release (CR or ER) preparations. For most initially treated patients, the extended-release formulations offer no advantage over the less expensive immediate-release preparations. The author usually recommends taking carbidopa/levodopa initially on a full stomach. Despite the presence of carbidopa, some individuals still experience nausea if carbidopa/levodopa is absorbed rapidly, and taking carbidopa/levodopa on a full stomach delays gastric emptying and slows absorption. The levodopa-related nausea is often a transient phenomenon that subsides after some weeks of treatment. In some patients with nausea, addition of supplemental carbidopa (Lodosyn) can be helpful. Some patients notice a rapid (within a few hours) response to carbidopa/levodopa treatment. Levodopa has an interesting pharmacology with a significant component of response owing to a "long duration" effect that builds up (and recedes) over a period of weeks [31]. The author counsels patients to wait 2 to 3 weeks before making a judgment as to whether or not levodopa is helping them.

Levodopa preparations are relatively easy drugs to use. There are virtually no concerns about drug interactions. The only real medical contraindication to use of levodopa is acute-angle glaucoma. There are anecdotal reports of malignant melanoma worsening after levodopa treatment, but more systematic reviews fail to show any causal relation. Levodopa preparations should not be withheld from patients with PD and melanoma. Levodopa preparations may produce several other side effects beyond the nausea described earlier. Some patients may experience sedation when taking levodopa preparations. This may be transient, but occasionally can be marked. Levodopa preparations may cause orthostatic hypotension leading to presyncopal symptoms and frank syncope; this happens most commonly in patients on antihypertensives, and adjustment of antihypertensive medications is useful in addressing this problem. Side effects related to stimulation of central nervous system dopamine receptors include hallucinations and dyskinesias. These side effects occur usually in patients who have taken levodopa preparations for years and are at least partly a result of disease progression. These phenomena are discussed at greater length in articles by Goudreau and Barbas. These side effects occasionally occur with initial treatment and resolve with reduction or cessation of levodopa treatment.

If a patient does not respond to initial treatment, the levodopa dose should be incremented gradually over weeks. The author usually aims for a maximum of $3 \times 25/100$ orally three times a day. If there is no response after 2 to 3 weeks on this dose, the levodopa should be tapered gradually. Levodopa should never be discontinued abruptly because this may precipitate a dangerous illness analogous to the neuroleptic malignant syndrome [32]. Nonresponse to levodopa should stimulate reconsideration of the diagnosis of PD. Assessment of response to levodopa is usually straightforward, but there are a couple of potential pitfalls. Patients with mild parkinsonism may not exhibit an evident response because of a virtual ceiling effect. Some patients with a good response may experience it over weeks, and their improvements in performance may occur slowly enough that they do not perceive the difference. In patients with an apparent nonresponse, it is prudent to ask them to monitor their status as levodopa is tapered. This may reveal an unexpected therapeutic response. Levodopa preparation dosing should be adjusted solely on the basis of clinical response. The best general principle is "enough is as good as a feast." It is difficult to make an individual clinically normal with levodopa; the goal should be a good level of function at the lowest dose possible.

Initiation of dopamine agonist therapy is more complicated. As mentioned earlier, these agents are more likely to cause complications, and introduction usually requires slower titration. There are several agonists on the market. The older compounds are bromocriptine and pergolide. These ergot derivatives are used rarely because of rare but potentially severe fibrotic complications, such as retroperitoneal and pulmonary fibrosis. More recently, there have been reports of cardiac valve fibrotic complications associated with pergolide use [33]. The more recently introduced dopamine agonists, pramipexole and ropinirole, are nonergot compounds and lack the risk of fibrotic complications. Pramipexole or ropinirole should be introduced at low doses according to the manufacturer's instructions and gradually incremented. Three-times-daily dosing schedules are customary. Side effects are due to their dopamine agonist properties and consequently similar to the side effects of levodopa preparations. Dopamine agonists are more likely to cause side effects, however, particularly sedation and hallucinations. In the author's experience, sedation secondary to dopamine agonists is not only more likely to occur, but also more likely to be a significant problem than with levodopa preparations. There also is concern that dopamine agonists may have unusual effects on sleep regulation. There have been reports of "sleep attacks" with dopamine agonists, with patients on these agents abruptly falling asleep [34]. With initiation of dopamine agonist therapy, the risk of sedation should be underscored, and driving risks should be mentioned specifically. Another rare but potentially serious complication associated with dopamine agonists is exacerbation or precipitation of serious compulsive behavior, such as compulsive gambling or sexual behavior [35]. This complication also may occur with levodopa preparations. Finally, dopamine agonists can be associated with lower extremity edema, which can be marked. As with levodopa preparations, dopamine agonists should be titrated upward based on clinical effectiveness, and the minimal dose needed to produce a good functional response should be employed. With disease progression, patients need additional increments of dopamine agonists. An alternative strategy is to add a low dose of a levodopa preparation (25/100 three times a day) because dopamine agonists seem to work best when given with levodopa, perhaps because dopamine agonists are primarily D2-like receptor agonists, and the addition of levodopa provides some D1-like receptor stimulation.

After the successful initiation of treatment, most patients notice a substantial improvement in their condition, with some achieving near-normal levels of function. This "honeymoon" period usually lasts at least 3 to 5 years and in patients with relatively slowly progressive PD can last considerably longer. The problems occurring with more advanced PD are described in subsequent articles by Goudreau and Barbas.

References

[1] Parkinson J. An essay on the shaking palsy. Whittingham & Rowland for Sherwood, Neely and Jones, 1817. Chicago: American Medical Association Press; 1936.
[2] Albin RL, Young AB, Penney JB. The functional anatomy of basal ganglia disorders. Trends Neurosci 1989;12:366–75.
[3] Hughes AJ, Daniel SE, Ben-Shlomo Y, et al. The accuracy of diagnosis of parkinsonian syndromes in a specialist movement disorder service. Brain 2002;125:861–70.
[4] Gibb WRG, Lees AJ. The relevance of the Lewy body to the pathogenesis of idiopathic Parkinson's disease. J Neurol Neurosurg Psychiatry 1988;51:745–52.

[5] Gelb GJ, Oliver E, Gilman S. Diagnostic criteria for Parkinson's disease. Arch Neurol 1999; 56:33–9.

[6] Oppenheimer DR. Diseases of the basal ganglia, cerebellum and motor neurons. In: Adams JH, Corsellis JA, Duchen LW, editors. Greenfield's neuropathology. 4th edition. New York: Wiley; 1984. p. 699–747.

[7] Suchowersky O, Reich S, Perlmutter J, et al. Practice parameter: diagnosis and prognosis of new onset Parkinson's disease. Neurology 2005;66:968–75.

[8] Mayeux R. Epidemiology of neurodegeneration. Annu Rev Neurosci 2003;26:81–104.

[9] Guttman M, Slaughter PM, Theriault M-E, et al. Burden of parkinsonism: a population-based study. Mov Disord 2002;18:313–9.

[10] Strickland D, Bertoni JM. Parkinson's prevalence estimated by a state registry. Mov Disord 2004;19:318–23.

[11] Uitti RJ, Ahlskog JE, Maraganore DM, et al. Levodopa therapy and survival in idiopathic Parkinson's disease: Olmsted County project. Neurology 1993;43:1918–26.

[12] Allam MF, Campbell MJ, Hofman A, et al. Smoking and Parkinson's disease: systemic review of prospective studies. Mov Disord 2004;19:614–21.

[13] Tanner CM, Ottman R, Goldman SM, et al. Parkinson disease in twins: an etiologic study. JAMA 1999;281:341–6.

[14] Marder K, Levy G, Louis ED, et al. Familial aggregation of early- and late-onset Parkinson's disease [erratum appears in Ann Neurol 2003;54:693]. Ann Neurol 2003;54:507–13.

[15] Sveinbjornsdottir S, Hicks AA, Jonsson T, et al. Familial aggregation of Parkinson's disease in Iceland. N Engl J Med 2000;343:1765–70.

[16] Gasser T. Genetics of Parkinson's disease. Curr Opin Neurol 2005;18:363–9.

[17] Spillantini MG, Crowther RA, Jakes R, et al. Alpha-Synuclein in filamentous inclusions of Lewy bodies from Parkinson's disease and dementia with Lewy bodies. Proc Natl Acad Sci U S A 1998;95:6469–73.

[18] Shimura H, Schlossmacher MG, Hattori N, et al. Ubiquitination of a new form of alpha-synuclein by parkin from human brain: implications for Parkinson's disease. Science 2001;293:263–9.

[19] McNaught KS, Perl DP, Brownell AL, et al. Systemic exposure to proteasome inhibitors causes a progressive model of Parkinson's disease. Ann Neurol 2004;56:149–62.

[20] Li C, Beal MF. Leucine-rich repeat kinase 2: a new player with a familiar theme for Parkinson's disease pathogenesis. Proc Natl Acad Sci U S A 2005;102:16535–6.

[21] Schapira AH, Cooper JM, Dexter D, et al. Mitochondrial complex I deficiency in Parkinson's disease. J Neurochem 1990;54:823–7.

[22] Stocchi F, Olanow CW. Neuroprotection in Parkinson's disease: clinical trials. Ann Neurol 2003;53:S87–97.

[23] Shoulson I. DATATOP: a decade of neuroprotective inquiry. Parkinson Study Group. Deprenyl And Tocopherol Antioxidate Therapy Of Parkinsonism. Ann Neurol 1998;44:S160–6.

[24] Agid Y. Levodopa: is toxicity a myth? Neurology 1998;50:858–63.

[25] Kurlan R. "Levodopa phobia": a new iatrogenic cause of disability in Parkinson disease. Neurology 2005;64:923–4.

[26] Parkinson Study Group. Levodopa and the progression of Parkinson's disease. N Engl J Med 2004;351:2498–508.

[27] Juncos JL, Engber TM, Raisman R, et al. Continuous and intermittent levodopa differentially affect basal ganglia function. Ann Neurol 2004;25:473–8.

[28] Parkinson Study Group. Pramipexole vs levodopa as initial treatment for Parkinson disease—a randomized controlled trial. JAMA 2000;284:1931–8.

[29] Albin RL, Frey KA. Initial agonist treatment of Parkinson disease: a critique. Neurology 2003;60:390–4.

[30] Miyasaki JM, Martin W, Suchowersky O, et al. Practice parameter: initiation of treatment for Parkinson's disease: an evidence-based review: report of the Quality Standards Subcommittee of the American Academy of Neurology. Neurology 2002;58:11–7.

[31] Chan PL, Nutt JG, Holford NH. Modeling the short- and long-duration responses to exogenous levodopa and to endogenous levodopa production in Parkinson's disease. J Pharmacokinet Pharmacodyn 2004;31:243–68.

[32] Kipps CM, Fung VS, Grattan-Smith P, et al. Movement disorder emergencies. Mov Disord 2005;20:322–34.

[33] Baseman DG, O'Suilleabhain PE, Reimold SC, et al. Pergolide use in Parkinson disease is associated with cardiac valve regurgitation. Neurology 2004;63:301–4.

[34] Frucht S, Rogers JD, Greene PE, et al. Falling asleep at the wheel: motor vehicle mishaps in persons taking pramipexole and ropinirole. Neurology 1999;52:1908–10.

[35] Dodd ML, Klos KJ, Bower JH, et al. Pathological gambling caused by drugs used to treat Parkinson disease. Arch Neurol 2005;62:1377–81.

ELSEVIER
SAUNDERS

CLINICS IN
GERIATRIC
MEDICINE

Clin Geriatr Med 22 (2006) 753–772

Medical Management of Advanced Parkinson's Disease

John L. Goudreau, DO, PhD*

*Department of Neurology and Department of Pharmacology and Toxicology,
Michigan State University, East Lansing, MI 48842, USA*

The management of advancing Parkinson's disease (PD) holds both challenge and rewards. Although treatment strategies are generally effective for patients who have early PD, the approach required to address the complexities of advancing disease dictates a deeper understanding of the natural history of PD and the nuances of pharmacotherapeutics. An informed physician, often in collaboration with a movement disorders specialist and allied health professionals, can truly enhance the quality of life for patients who have advanced PD. This article focuses on issues related to the diagnosis and treatment of complications associated with advancing PD. Complications include increased severity of motor symptoms in the absence of symptomatic treatments, treatment-related motor complications, medication-refractory motor symptoms, and nonmotor symptoms (Table 1). Evaluation and management of cognitive and psychiatric problems associated with advancing PD are discussed in other articles in this issue. Therapeutic strategies for commonly encountered motor and nonmotor complications of advancing PD are reviewed in the following sections, with an emphasis on practical decision making and management.

Progression and complications of advancing Parkinson's disease

Patients, often prompted by concerned family members, frequently return to their physician with concerns about progression of PD symptoms. Distinguishing true progression of disease from "pseudoprogression" (Table 2) is an important initial step in addressing this issue. PD is a slowly progressive disease, and it is unusual for symptoms to change appreciably over a few

---
* A217 Clinical Center, Department of Neurology, Michigan State University, East Lansing, MI 48821.
   E-mail address: john.goudreau@ht.msu.edu

0749-0690/06/$ - see front matter © 2006 Elsevier Inc. All rights reserved.
doi:10.1016/j.cger.2006.06.006   *geriatric.theclinics.com*

Table 1
Progression in Parkinson's disease

Feature	Example
Increase severity of off motor symptoms	Bradykinesia, rigidity, tremor
Treatment-related motor complications	Short-duration responses, dyskinesias, dose failure/delay
Medication-refractory axial motor symptoms	Freezing of gait, dysarthria, dysphagia
Nonmotor symptoms	Depression, anxiety, dementia, psychosis, autonomic dysfunction, sensory disturbance, pain, vision impairment, dyspnea, insomnia, fatigue

weeks' time [1]. In the setting of sudden worsening of symptoms, there is often a factor other than PD at play.

Pseudoprogression may arise out of several contexts. Not infrequently, patients and caregivers read extensively during the period after initial diagnosis and identify familiar symptoms and signs in well-meant listings of PD characteristics. In this setting, increased awareness produces a misleading impression of accumulating symptoms, which were previously present but unrecognized as manifestations of PD. Comorbid medical conditions that can contribute to motor dysfunction in PD are prevalent in the geriatric population and should be thoroughly investigated [2]. Addition of medications that interfere with the absorption, distribution, or metabolism of anti-PD medications should also be considered in the setting of sudden worsening of symptoms [3–5]. Occasionally, medications that are added to treat comorbid medical conditions have adverse side effects on the musculoskeletal system (eg, cholesterol-lowering agent–induced myopathy) or aggravate parkinsonism (eg, metaclopramide) [6,7]. Medication noncompliance, often occurring in the context of patients who have cognitive impairment, can sometimes manifest as disease progression [8].

Psychiatric disorders, especially affective mood disorders, can underlie a perception of worsening symptoms. Inadequate or inefficient sleep, along

Table 2
Other explanations for advancing Parkinson's disease

Explanation	Example or context
Increased awareness of symptoms	Insight from education about illness
Comorbid medical conditions	Osteoarthritis, congestive heart failure, diabetes
Other confounding neurologic conditions	Stroke, peripheral neuropathy, polymyositis
Drug–drug interactions	Pyridoxine (↓ levodopa), dopamine antagonists
Drugs that impair motor function	Cholesterol-lowering agents, metaclopramide
Change in levodopa formulation	Controlled release replacing immediate release
Medication noncompliance	Cognitive impairment, polypharmacy
Mood disorders	Depression, anxiety
Sleep disorders	Obstructive sleep apnea, restless legs syndrome

with attendant excessive daytime somnolence and fatigue, may also contribute to a sense of deteriorating motor function. Other common neurologic diseases may intervene to masquerade as progression of PD symptoms (eg, stroke, peripheral neuropathy, polymyositis), or they may indicate more aggressive forms of parkinsonism (eg, progressive supranuclear palsy, multiple system atrophy, frontotemporal dementia) [9].

True progression of PD symptoms occurs slowly, with a time course of several months or years [1]. Progression of motor symptoms encompasses worsening of symptoms during the medication off period, treatment-related motor complications, nonmotor complications, and the development of treatment-refractory symptoms (see Table 1). The rate of progression is variable; older age at symptom onset, akinetic-rigid symptomatology, comorbid depression, and dementia have all been identified as factors associated with increased rates of progression [10,11]. No therapies have been proved to slow progression at this juncture, though several are under development [12].

The initial management of PD is discussed elsewhere in this issue and typically consists of dopaminergic monotherapy with either carbidopa/levodopa or dopamine agonists. Occasionally, other nondopaminergic medications (amantadine, selegeline, rasagiline, anticholinergics) are employed to manage mild symptoms [13]. With progression, management will ultimately require the addition of carbidopa/levodopa for full control of motor symptoms of parkinsonism in the vast majority of patients [14]. Rational adjustments in dopaminergic drugs can mitigate many motor and some nonmotor complications while reducing treatment-induced side effects. However, some motor and most nonmotor symptoms do not improve with titration of dopaminergic drugs. Hence a broader approach is required for these refractory symptoms, incorporating both pharmacotherapeutic and nonmedication treatment strategies. Ultimately, the goal of managing the complications of advancing PD is preservation of patients' ability to function within the mainstream of their lives.

Treatment-related motor complications of advancing Parkinson's disease

Reduced medication response

The successful initial treatment of early PD (the "honeymoon" period), sometimes lasting as long as 10 years, is inevitably followed by the development of symptoms that are not adequately controlled by simple monotherapy approaches [15]. For example, patients find that, as PD progresses, the motor symptoms are no longer fully alleviated by dopamine agonist monotherapy or other medications with limited efficacy (eg, amantadine, selegeline, rasagiline, anticholinergics). Patients who are taking levodopa become acutely (and often selectively) aware of progression of motor symptoms in the medication off state as they begin to make the transition from long-duration to short-duration levodopa responses (Fig. 1). Side effects,

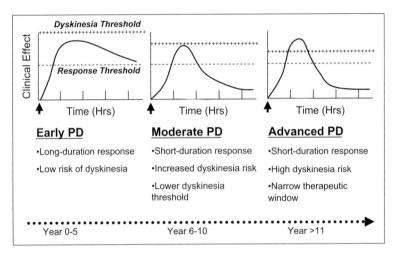

Fig. 1. Relationship of temporal response profiles for a single dose of carbidopa/levodopa (*arrow*). The clinical effect is represented as a solid curve and parallels the plasma concentrations of levodopa and hypothetical synaptic concentrations of dopamine. Thresholds for therapeutic benefit (- - - -) and dyskinesias (++++) and years following onset of motor symptoms (••••) are represented as lines.

especially medication-induced hyperkinetic disorders, hallucinations, fatigue, somnolence, and orthostatic hypotension, can all contribute to an overall sense of asthenia. Nonmotor symptoms and some treatment-resistant axial motor symptoms (eg, postural instability, dysarthria) are often vexing problems that accompany advancing PD. However, the cardinal features of PD rarely become completely resistant to symptomatic medications [16]. If patients have truly become refractory to appropriately titrated symptomatic medications within a few years of symptom onset, then concern arises about atypical forms of parkinsonism [9].

Dose failures and delayed on

Patients who have advancing PD may experience little or no response to an individual dose of levodopa (ie, a dose failure). Others may note a prolonged time to onset of therapeutic benefit (ie, delayed on) [17]. Both of these pharmacokinetic phenomena may be due to interference with levodopa absorption and penetration across the blood–brain barrier by dietary proteins, especially when doses of carbidopa/levodopa are taken close to protein-containing meals. The effects of dietary protein can be dramatic if the levodopa dose is close to the symptomatic response threshold. Dietary protein digestion liberates large-neutral amino acids, which compete with levodopa for transport across the blood–brain barrier and probably for entry into the neuron [17,18]; they may also compete with levodopa at the intestinal level, although this appears less important. Occasionally, delayed gastric emptying time can reduce intestinal medication absorption [19].

Medication noncompliance may also be an underlying factor in dose fail-ures: a scenario more likely in patients who are on complicated medication regimens or who have cognitive impairment [8].

An inadvertent change in the formulation of medication can contribute to a delayed or inadequate medication response. For example, controlled-release formulations of carbidopa/levodopa may be mistakenly provided in place of the immediate-release formulation. Controlled-release levodopa preparations were initially developed for patients with advanced PD who had short-duration responses to levodopa. Embedding levodopa in a poly-meric matrix extends the therapeutic benefit of controlled-release levodopa for as long as 1 hour but can significantly delay the onset of therapeutic ben-efit (as long as 2 hours) [20]. Although controlled-release levodopa is better absorbed when administered with food, competition with other dietary proteins for transport across the blood–brain barrier makes it difficult to predict the clinical response with respect to meals [21]. The reduced bioavail-ability and the slower release of the controlled-release formulation necessi-tate a 30% to 50% increase in the amount of levodopa administered with each dose to achieve plasma concentrations similar to those of immediate-release levodopa [20]. Therefore, it is understandable that a patient might experience a suboptimal response if immediate-release carbidopa/levodopa 25/100 tablets were inadvertently switched to the carbidopa/levodopa 25/100 controlled-release formulation.

Assessment of delayed responses to symptomatic medications begins with a careful review of medication intake. It is helpful to have patients or their caregivers describe the medication regimen, including the dose and time of each drug used to treat PD, in addition to the temporal relationship to meal-times. The potential for medication noncompliance becomes apparent when there is uncertainty about conveying the details of a daily medication rou-tine. Separating levodopa dosing from meals (1 hour prior or 2 hours after) is often all that is needed to resolve dose failures [17]. Levodopa intake may be increased (eg, 50 mg) for doses that cannot be isolated from mealtimes owing to frequency of administration [22]. Converting from the con-trolled-release to the immediate-release formulation of levodopa can im-prove bioavailability, while establishing a more rapid and predictable absorption pattern. When doses of symptomatic medications are close to the threshold of symptomatic improvement, an upward titration in dose can capture a more consistent and robust therapeutic benefit [15]. Finally, if there is absolutely no response to maximal doses of levodopa (>1000 mg daily or >300 mg three times a day) taken on an empty stomach, then it is likely that the patient has a condition other than idiopathic PD [9].

Short-duration responses

In concert with advancing PD, patients may develop medication re-sponses that are tightly time-locked to each levodopa dose, resulting in troublesome fluctuations in motor performance [18,23]. Motor fluctuations, also termed the short-duration responses, occur in approximately 40% of patients who are treated with levodopa for 4 to 6 years' duration [24]. In the mildest form, motor fluctuations manifest as the end of the dose's "wearing-off" effect, in which the beneficial response to each dose of levodopa declines before the next dose. Patients can also experience wearing off overnight or in the early morning. In the most severe form, the response may be dramatic, unpredictable, and sudden. This abrupt transition from a mobile to immobile state has been referred to as the "on-off" effect and is an intensely distressing event for patients who have advancing PD. Pronounced depletion of dopamine (DA) from presynaptic nigrostriatal terminals appears to be a prerequisite for the short-duration response [25–27], but postsynaptic changes, such as downregulation of postsynaptic DA receptors, may also be involved [28,29]. Motor fluctuations are not usually seen in early PD (ie, incidence of motor fluctuations is 3% in the first year of treatment, and this may reflect the time necessary for plastic changes to develop) [24]. Short-duration medication responses can complicate the symptomatic management of patients who have PD and usually require thoughtful medication changes.

Patients who are experiencing short-duration responses often report that their parkinsonism is "worse" and do not readily recognize the temporal relationship of motor fluctuations to their levodopa doses. Careful inquiry by the physician or dose-response daily diaries can be useful in identifying correlations between fluctuations and the timing of drug administration [30]. When uncertainty remains, direct monitoring of patients throughout a levodopa response cycle in the clinic may help resolve the issue. This monitoring can be accomplished by having the patient present to the physician's office in the morning (before breakfast), just before taking the first medication dose of the day; a brief motor examination for parkinsonism is then performed just before and serially after administration of medications. Careful documentation of the time to symptomatic onset, duration of beneficial effect, and temporal profile of adverse events can be invaluable in managing complicated patients.

Adjusting the dose interval to match levodopa response duration is the most direct method of treating short-duration responses and does not require adding a new class of medication. For example, when a patient reports the effect wearing off at 3 hours, levodopa may be administered every 3 hours or slightly less, so that the effects overlap. At times, however, the reductions in dose interval may not be acceptable to the patient because of the frequent need to take medication. Controlled-release levodopa was initially developed as a formulation to address the short-duration response and can prolong the response to levodopa by 60 to 90 minutes. If employed, the dose of the controlled-release formulation requires a 30% to 40% increase in levodopa to account for reduced bioavailability. Unfortunately, erratic absorption and variable clinical response can limit the utility of controlled-release levodopa in patients who have advanced PD. Other strategies could include addition of a catechol-*O*-methyltransferase inhibitor (tolcapone, entacapone), which may prolong the response duration by blocking the peripheral catabolism of levodopa and DA. Alternatively, adjunctive use of DA agonists, with their relatively long half-life, can be helpful in treating short-duration responses [31]. When these last two strategies are employed, a reduction in the dose of levodopa is often necessary to alleviate peak-dose dyskinesias.

Several strategies have been employed, with various degrees of success, to manage patients with brittle short-duration responses. Levodopa may be readily dissolved in water (1 mg/mL) and used as an oral or intragastric liquid preparation [32]. Ascorbic acid may be added to prolong stability in solution for as long as 24 hours, but it need not be added if the solution will be used within a few hours [33]. Dissolved in solution, levodopa is absorbed more rapidly than in tablets, and this approach is sometimes helpful in treating patients who have rapidly fluctuating motor responses and in "rescuing" patients who develop sudden-onset off states. Intravenous administration of levodopa has limited practical utility and has largely been restricted to clinical research centers [34]. Continuous duodenal delivery of levodopa and transdermal delivery systems for dopamine agonists are also under development for patients who have intractable motor complications [35,36].

"Freezing" refers to the inability to initiate movement, typically involving hesitancy in arising from a seated position, initiating gait, or turning. Transient freezing (<60 seconds) can occur at any time and is dependent on activity and environmental context. More prolonged freezing spells can occur as an off phase phenomenon or reflect suboptimum dosage of symptomatic medications. Abrupt development of the off state can result in profound freezing and is one of the most distressing events for patients who have PD. In this setting, one may administer a "rescue dose" of levodopa by crushing and dissolving the patient's established dose of levodopa in several ounces of liquid (eg, carbonated beverage or juice) and having the patient drink the entire amount. This method usually results in a rapid "on" response within approximately 20 minutes, although the symptomatic benefit of the "rescue dose" only persists for about 60 to 90 minutes [15]. Injection of subcutaneous apomorphine can also be helpful in this setting, but this requires careful titration in a physician's office, with blood pressure monitoring for hypotension and addition of scheduled doses of antiemetic medications (trimethobenzamide) to minimize the risk for nausea [37]. In rare cases, freezing can occur as a peak-dose effect (peak-dose freezing) and may require dose reduction of either levodopa or adjunctive medications (eg, agonists) [15].

Dyskinesias

Dyskinesias are dopaminergic treatment–induced hyperkinetic movements and represent a characteristic feature of advancing PD [38]. Dyskinesias typically present as involuntary chorea or stereotypic, repetitive movements involving the limbs, trunk, or head. Dystonia, myoclonus, involuntary respiratory movements, and punding (obsessive repetition of simple or complex motor tasks) have also been described as unusual manifestations of dyskinesias. Although dyskinesias are not bothersome to many patients, they can be severe enough to interfere with goal-directed voluntary movement and may be socially embarrassing. In this setting, dyskinesias can limit the dose of symptomatic therapy and complicate ongoing management of patients who have advancing PD.

Dyskinesias occur in approximately 40% of patients who receive levodopa treatment for 4 to 6 years [24]. The frequency of dyskinesias in patients who have young-onset PD, defined as PD symptom onset before age 40, is higher and approaches 100% by 5 years of levodopa treatment [39,40]. Although less frequent, dyskinesias can also occur with DA agonists and may be more sustained because of the longer duration of effect of agonists. Dyskinesias are uncommon in early PD, occurring in approximately 7% after 1 year of levodopa treatment, and do not occur in untreated patients [24]. In patients who have idiopathic PD, dyskinesias tend to reflect the duration of PD rather than the duration of levodopa treatment [24,41]. The correlation of dyskinesia frequency with PD duration probably reflects the severity of dopaminergic terminal loss, which is progressive. Dyskinesias have also been observed early in the treatment of patients inadvertently exposed to 1-methyl-4-phenyl-1,2,3,6-tetrahydropyridine who have an acute severe insult to the dopaminergic system. This finding further supports the concept that the degree of nigrostriatal DA terminal damage is an important substrate for levodopa-induced motor complications [42].

The most common form of levodopa-induced dyskinesia is peak-dose chorea or stereotypy. This type of dyskinesia occurs at the time of peak levodopa symptomatic effect and plasma levodopa concentrations. Many patients actually feel their best when their medication dosage is adjusted to the point at which subtle peak-dose dyskinesias are present, and they are often unaware of the involuntary movements [43]. When peak-dose dyskinesias become severe or dose-limiting, they can complicate the management of patients who have advanced PD.

If peak-dose dyskinesias require treatment, several options are possible (Table 3). A small (25- to 50-mg) reduction in the individual levodopa doses every 3 to 4 days, until dyskinesias abate, is often all that is necessary and may obviate the addition of a new class of drugs [22]. If dose reduction produces intolerable worsening of the other motor symptoms of PD, adjunctive treatment with DA agonists may be helpful, with subsequent reduction of levodopa once the agonist dosage is therapeutic. Discontinuation of adjunctive medications that potentiate the pharmacologic effects of levodopa (eg, selegeline, tolcapone, entacapone) in favor of monotherapy with levodopa is often helpful. Amantadine (200 to 400 mg/d in divided doses) has also been shown to reduce peak-dose dyskinesias [44–47]. Typical neuroleptic

Table 3
Treatment options for peak-dose dyskinesias

Strategy	Example
Decrease levodopa dose	Lower each dose of levodopa by 25 to 50 mg
Discontinue agents that potentiate levodopa	Entecapone, selegeline
Add dopamine agonist	Ropinirole, pramipexole
NMDA receptor antagonists	Amantadine, riluzole
Other agents	Clozapine, propranolol, buspirone, propranolol

dopamine D2 (D2) receptors can suppress dyskinesias but result in unacceptable exacerbation of parkinsonism [48,49]. Clozapine, an atypical neuroleptic, may reduce dyskinesias without worsening other motor features of PD but requires close monitoring for agranulocytosis [50]. Several other adjunctive medications have been reported to alleviate levodopa-induced dyskinesias with various degrees of success (eg, dextromethorphan, buspirone, sarizotan, idazoxan, riluzole, propranolol) [31,51–55].

Chorea or dystonia that occurs at the beginning and end of each dose cycle (biphasic dyskinesias) represents an uncommon pattern of dyskinesia that requires a different treatment approach from peak-dose dyskinesia [56]. In the dyskinesia-improvement-dyskinesia (D-I-D) response, an initial dyskinetic state occurs for approximately 10 to 30 minutes, just as the beneficial effects of levodopa begin, and a late dyskinetic period develops as the symptomatic benefit of levodopa begins to wear off. A satisfactory motor "on" response typically intervenes. Patients who have the D-I-D response improve with shortening of the dose interval, producing overlapping dose effects. In some who have biphasic dyskinesias, however, only four to five doses per day are tolerable; additional doses are associated with an adverse change in the pharmacodynamics, as Muenter and colleagues [56] described more than 25 years ago. Switching from controlled release to immediate release is usually necessary to facilitate careful dose and interval adjustments. Adjunctive use of a DA agonist may be helpful in some cases. Patients who have the D-I-D response usually experience unavoidable dyskinesias at the beginning and end of each day.

Functional neurosurgery and levodopa

Patients who have advancing PD may develop disabling motor complications that persist despite the medication treatment strategies outlined here. In select patients, particularly those in whom a previously satisfactory response to levodopa becomes limited by dyskinesias or fluctuations, functional neurosurgery may significantly improve motor function and quality of life [57,58]. Pallidotomy and deep brain stimulation of the pallidum and subthalamic nucleus are discussed in detail in the article in this issue by Revilla.

Medication treatment–refractory axial motor complications

Gait freezing

Freezing of gait (FOG) presents as sudden cessation of ongoing movement and the inability to initiate new movement. FOG is common, reported in as many as 50% of patients who have PD for more than 5 years; it often occurs in areas of transition (eg, doorways, stairs, turning) and can result in falls and injury [59]. No specific or proven treatment exists for FOG, although selegeline, L-threo-3,4-dihydroxyphenylserine, and transcranial magnetic stimulation have been reported to be effective in small or open-label clinical trials [59]. Nonpharmacologic therapies, such as the use of sensory cues, may be of some benefit when combined with a comprehensive physical and occupational therapy assessment and management program. Visual tools (eg, inverted walking sticks, visual laser-beam canes), auditory cues (eg, metronomes), and tactile cues (touching the lower limb) have all been proposed as strategies to "unlock" FOG and are reasonable to consider [60].

Postural changes

Progressive loss of postural corrective reflexes and dysregulation of axial antigravity muscle control represent a particularly disabling component of medication-refractory symptoms [61]. The risk for falling and the attendant injury-related morbidity are of paramount concern in managing patients who have advancing PD. Routine screening questions regarding balance issues and early institution of physical therapy and gait-assistive devices are essential components of patient care; overlooking them may lead to devastating consequences. Flexed posture and axial dystonia can contribute to balance problems by shifting the center of gravity. Camptocormia (severe anterior spinal flexion) and the "dropped head" syndrome, though more commonly seen in multiple systems atrophy, may be encountered in advanced PD as a particularly intractable and disabling feature [62]. As with other axial motor symptoms, there are no effective medications available to treat postural changes. Hence the importance of early and repeated physical and occupational therapy input for patients who have advancing PD cannot be overstated.

Dysarthria

Dysarthria affects the majority of patients who have advancing PD and can be particularly disabling and result in social isolation [63]. Although hypokinetic speech patterns are most common (hypophonic, monotone, and monopitch), patterns of ataxic speech with irregular breakdown in articulation and spastic speech (strained, raspy, hoarse) may also be observed. Speech therapy is frequently recommended, but with limited evidence from adequately performed clinical trials to support a single effective approach. The Lee Silverman Voice Therapy is the most widely practiced technique and involves exercises to increase vocal cord adduction and loudness [64]. Speech amplification devices and symbolic or alphanumeric artificial voice generators may be employed as strategies to maintain communication when other speech therapy modalities fail. Percutaneous laryngeal collagen augmentation has been reported as a beneficial surgical approach [65].

Dysphagia

Impaired triggering of swallowing mechanisms and bradykinetic oropharyngeal movements can produce dysphagia and sialorrhea, both significant and common complications of advancing PD [63]. A comprehensive dysphagia evaluation should be completed in all patients who report difficulty swallowing, choking, frequent coughing, or an episode of aspiration pneumonia. A speech therapist, often aided by a videofluoroscopic swallowing evaluation, can recommend physical maneuvers and changes in food consistencies to reduce the risk for aspiration and its attendant complications. In severe cases, percutaneous feeding tube placement may be considered [66]. Sialorrhea is another manifestation of disordered swallowing that frequently accompanies advancing PD. Cueing swallowing by using chewing gum, hard candies, and throat lozenges can provide a simple remedy. In more severe cases, sublingual anticholinergics (atropine, glycopyrrolate) and injection of botulinum toxin into salivary glands can reduce saliva production, but these approaches should be used with caution, because both can worsen dysphagia for solid foods [67].

Nonmotor complications of advancing Parkinson's disease

Nonmotor symptoms arising in the medication off state

A wide variety of nonmotor symptoms can occur as a manifestation of the levodopa off state [68]. These symptoms are reported to occur in 17% of patients who have motor fluctuations and often cause significant distress and disability for patients who have PD [69]. The clinical spectrum includes autonomic, sensory/pain, cognitive, and psychiatric symptoms, as listed in Table 4. Unexplained symptoms that occur in a time-locked fashion with the levodopa off state are suspicious for nonmotor manifestations of PD. Nonmotor symptoms often (75% of the time) respond to appropriate adjustment of levodopa dose and dose interval (described earlier) for achievement of optimum motor symptom control [69]. Recognition and treatment of these nonmotor manifestations of the levodopa off state can improve the patient's quality of life while obviating unnecessary tests and treatments.

Insomnia

Patients who have PD may experience significant insomnia, and this symptom, along with the resultant increased daytime somnolence, can be

Table 4
Nonmotor features of Parkinson's disease

Feature	Example
Sensory	Pain, paresthesia, restless legs syndrome, akithisia
Cognitive-psychiatric	Subcortical processing, depression, anxiety, panic attack, mania, moaning/screaming, compulsive behaviors, fatigue
Sleep	Insomnia, daytime somnolence
Autonomic	Tachycardia, hypotension, constipation, bloating, belching, dysphagia, sialorrhea, urinary frequency, urgency, incontinence, erectile dysfunction, pallor, sweating, skin temperature changes
Visual	Decreased acuity, diplopia, convergence insufficiency, dry eyes
Respiratory	Dyspnea, stridor, tachypnea
Other	Anosmia-hyposmia, seborrheic dermatitis

a source of significant disability [70]. Although many potential causes of insomnia exist in patients who have PD, re-emergence of uncontrolled nocturnal parkinsonism can be a significant factor after the effectiveness of daytime medication wanes. Nocturnal rigidity, immobility, tremor, and akathisia can contribute to insomnia, particularly in patients who have developed short-duration responses to levodopa [71]. Difficulty in initiating sleep due to poorly controlled parkinsonism should respond to an evening dose of immediate-release levodopa given at such a time as to achieve peak effects when the patient retires to bed. In addition, adding a bedtime dose of controlled-release levodopa may extend sleep; this is helpful to those who awaken several hours into the night because their levodopa effect has waned. In this particular setting, the delayed effect of controlled-release levodopa is advantageous. When patients awaken in an uncomfortable state with prominent parkinsonian symptoms, use of immediate-release levodopa is appropriate to obtain a rapid response [70]. Finally, if symptoms of restless legs syndrome are present, a dopamine agonist may be employed 1 hour before bedtime [70].

Evening and nighttime doses of levodopa should be equivalent to the optimum daytime dose to achieve the best sleep-sustaining effect. Overnight doses of levodopa can also serve to improve early morning functioning. Although nocturnal use of dopaminergic medications improves sleep in many patients, these drugs can disrupt normal sleep architecture [72]. However, from a practical point of view, those who have insomnia due to inadequate nocturnal dopaminergic coverage do experience gratifying responses to optimal nocturnal medication treatment. Rarely, bedtime doses of levodopa or dopamine agonists lead to insomnia, primarily when the medication induces significant dyskinesias.

Anxiety, akathisia, and panic

Anxiety and akathisia are common complaints of patients who have PD and may represent a manifestation of the levodopa off state [73]. These symptoms are frequently incorrectly attributed to levodopa overdosage when the opposite is the case. A correlation to levodopa dosing should be suspected when symptoms of anxiety wax and wane over the course of the day, worsening at the end of each levodopa cycle. At times, the anxiety may be profound and present as a panic attack. Akathisia during off-medication periods at night can mimic the symptoms of restless legs syndrome. Treatment of motor fluctuations, as described in the previous sections, should prove effective if these symptoms are occurring as a nonmotor facet of PD. In this setting, optimization of levodopa coverage works better than anxiolytic therapy.

Pain and paresthesias

Pain and uncomfortable sensory disturbances are frequent complaints of patients in the age group commonly affected by PD [69]. Although a variety of common comorbid conditions can produce these symptoms (eg, sciatica, peripheral neuropathy, osteoarthritis), they can also represent a nonmotor manifestation of undertreated PD. In one study, 46% of patients who had PD reported a complaint of pain, and in approximately two thirds of these cases, the pain correlated with motor fluctuations [74]. Descriptions of the pain range from superficial and burning to deep and boring. Even when the pain may be attributed to other causes, it can be exacerbated in the levodopa off state. A trial of levodopa dose or frequency adjustment may alleviate uncomfortable sensory symptoms and may obviate other diagnostic tests or treatment modalities.

Painful dystonia, in the absence of more typical choreiform dyskinesias, can occur at the end of a levodopa cycle or in the early morning and typically represents a wearing-off effect [15]. In this context, patients may complain of persistent pain, often associated with cramping, curling, or extension of the toes, in the affected extremity. Off-period painful dystonias respond to the strategies for short-duration responses described previously. Refractory dystonias sometimes diminish with anticholinergic therapy (eg, trihexyphenidyl, 2 mg, three times per day) or may be treated with localized botulinum toxin injections [38].

Dyspnea

Dyspnea is also a common complaint in patients who have PD and is often due to a comorbid primary pulmonary or cardiac condition [73]. Hence a full cardiac and pulmonary evaluation is recommended. A few significant exceptions exist, however. First, ergotamine-derived DA agonists (bromocriptine, pergolide, cabergoline) can induce inflammatory-fibrotic reactions that may lead to symptomatic pleuropulmonary fibrosis or constrictive pericarditis [75–78]. Although the fibrotic reactions to ergot-based agonists are rare, they may result in serious morbidity and always require discontinuation of the offending agent. Second, dyspnea may also be a nonmotor manifestation of the levodopa off state. This pattern usually becomes apparent when patients report resolution of dyspnea shortly after each dose of levodopa and reoccurrence at the end of each levodopa dose cycle. In this latter case, treatment is the same as that of any levodopa off-state symptom. In addition, dyspnea may be a persistent symptom in those who are generally undertreated with subtherapeutic levodopa doses, and respiratory symptoms may improve with upward titration in dose. Lastly, respiratory dyskinesias may present as dyspnea or hiccoughs and can be recognized with a video fluoroscopic examination of diaphragmatic movement during the peak of the levodopa dose cycle [38]. Respiratory dyskinesias, like other medication-induced hyperkinetic movements, may resolve with reduction in doses of symptomatic medications.

Nonmotor complications unrelated to dopaminergic therapies

Autonomic symptoms and complications

Symptoms related to autonomic dysfunction are frequently encountered in patients who have advancing PD. The pathologic changes associated with PD (ie, Lewy bodies) have been found in the central and peripheral autonomic systems, and there is evidence that autonomic symptoms can precede motor symptoms of PD [79,80]. Many of the autonomic symptoms described in patients who have PD are also prevalent in the aging population, making the link between autonomic symptoms and PD less clear. Because autonomic symptoms can often be related to comorbid medical problems and concomitant medications, a thorough evaluation for non-PD causes of dysautomonia should be pursued. Symptoms associated with autonomic dysfunction in PD do not typically improve with dopaminergic therapies and, in some instances, can be aggravated by drugs used to treat the motor features of PD.

Urinary urgency, frequency, nocturia, incontinence, and erectile dysfunction constitute some of the most common autonomic symptoms encountered in advancing PD [81]. Urologic consultation, combined with urodynamic studies, can help distinguish neurogenic detrusor–sphincter dyssynergy or bladder outlet obstruction as the cause of urinary symptoms and thus guide treatment. Anticholinergic agents, such as oxybutinin and tolterodine, can improve neurogenic bladder-related symptoms but can impair cognitive function in elderly patients. Alpha-adrenergic antagonists (doxazosin, tamsulosin) are most helpful in the setting of bladder outlet obstruction, but they can aggravate orthostatic hypotension. Evening fluid restriction and desmopressin may be helpful in managing nocturia but can cause electrolyte abnormalities and hypovolemia. Management of comorbid constipation, if present, can improve bladder symptoms by improving pelvic volume–pressure dynamics acting on intrinsic bladder contractile reflexes. Erectile dysfunction may respond to alprostadil (intracavernous or intraurethral) or to phosphodiesterase-5 inhibitors (eg, sildenafil, vardenafil, tadalafil), but patients should be screened for other medical contraindications to the use of this latter class of medications [82].

Orthostatic hypotension represents a feature of advancing PD, but it can also be induced or aggravated by dopaminergic medications used to treat extrapyramidal motor symptoms [83]. Screening for orthostatic hypotension (seated and standing blood pressure and heart rate) is an important component of routine office visits for patients who have PD and other neurodegenerative diseases. When necessary, patients and their caregivers may be instructed in proper techniques for home orthostatic blood pressure and heart rate monitoring to capture a longitudinal record of orthostatic cardiovascular changes. When symptomatic orthostatic hypotension is encountered, elimination of nonessential antihypertensive agents, especially diuretics and alpha-adrenergic antagonists, should be considered. Nonmedication strategies to increase intravascular fluid volume (eg, increased fluid and salt intake, positioning the bed in 30° reverse Trendelenberg) may be employed, as tolerated by the patient's cardiac output status. Waist-high compression hose may improve venous return sufficiently to improve standing blood pressure, but they are not well tolerated from a practical standpoint. If these nonmedication strategies do not improve orthostatic hypotension–related symptoms, then fludorcortisone or midodrine may be added. However, these require careful monitoring for electrolyte imbalances, fluid overload, and supine hypertension [83].

Constipation is another common autonomic symptom associated with PD at all stages, and it may even precede motor symptoms [84,85]. Dysregulation of the enteric nervous system can impair all aspects of gastrointestinal motility and result in dysphagia, gastroparesis, and impaired fecal evacuation. Severe constipation and gastroparesis, in addition to decreasing life quality, can impair the response to symptomatic medications like levodopa and aggravate urinary symptoms. Increased fluid intake, exercise, and dietary fiber content are useful initial strategies to address constipation. Stool softeners (eg, docusate sodium) may be used on a routine basis. Osmotic cathartics (eg, magnesium hydroxide or citrate, lactulose, polyethylene glycol) or enemas sometimes become necessary and may be incorporated into a routine bowel hygiene program for patients who have ongoing problems with constipation [84].

Other nonmotor symptoms

A wide variety of other symptoms may be encountered in the management of patients who have advancing PD [73]. Visual disturbance can result from retinal dysfunction, convergence insufficiency, or corneal dehydration [86]. Although ophthalmologic evaluation is recommended in most instances, instilling corneal hydrating preparations and reducing exposure to windy or dry environmental conditions may provide a simple solution to vision symptoms associated with the "dry eyes" syndrome [87]. Seborrheic dermatitis appears more frequently in patients who have PD and may be managed with frequent cleansing with soap to improve sebum removal. Antifungal preparations, topical corticosteroids, and keratolytics may be considered in severe cases [88]. Olfactory dysfunction has been reported in as many as 90% of patients who have PD, but no treatment is available thus far [89]. Finally, fatigue (with or without excessive somnolence) is a common and burdensome symptom that can respond to modafanil or amantadine once underlying medication side effects, sleep, and mood disorders have been addressed [70,90].

Summary

The management of advancing PD is a daunting task, complicated by dynamic medication responses, side effects, and treatment-refractory symptoms in an aging patient population. Motor and nonmotor complications of advancing PD also occur in the context of social and psychologic issues for patients and caregivers, adding another layer of complexity. Although new treatment approaches and modalities continue to be added to the therapeutic armamentarium for advancing PD, much work still needs to be done to address nonmotor and treatment-refractory complications. A thorough understanding of the natural history of advancing PD and in-depth knowledge of the pharmacology of antiparkinson medications are essential tools for the practical and successful management of this challenging group of patients. Careful assessment and rational treatment choices can significantly improve the lives of patients who have advancing PD.

References

[1] Poewe WH, Wenning GK. The natural history of Parkinson's disease. Neurology 1996; 47(6 Suppl 3):S146–52.
[2] Diederich NJ, Moore CG, Leurgans SE, et al. Parkinson disease with old-age onset: a comparative study with subjects with middle-age onset. Arch Neurol 2003;60(4):529–33.
[3] Bianchine JR, Shaw GM. Clinical pharmacokinetics of levodopa in Parkinson's disease. Clin Pharmacokinet 1976;1(5):313–38.
[4] Izzo AA, Ernst E. Interactions between herbal medicines and prescribed drugs: a systematic review. Drugs 2001;61(15):2163–75.
[5] Contin M, Riva R, Martinelli P, et al. Combined levodopa-anticholinergic therapy in the treatment of Parkinson's disease. Effect on levodopa bioavailability. Clin Neuropharmacol 1991;14(2):148–55.
[6] Bannwarth B. Drug-induced myopathies. Expert Opin Drug Saf 2002;1(1):65–70.
[7] Buchholz D, Kariya S. Metoclopramide-induced Parkinsonism. Arch Neurol 1983;40(8): 528–9.
[8] Grosset KA, Reid JL, Grosset DG. Medicine-taking behavior: implications of suboptimal compliance in Parkinson's disease. Mov Disord 2005;20(11):1397–404.
[9] Tolosa E, Wenning G, Poewe W. The diagnosis of Parkinson's disease. Lancet Neurol 2006; 5(1):75–86.
[10] Roos RA, Jongen JC, van der Velde EA. Clinical course of patients with idiopathic Parkinson's disease. Mov Disord 1996;11(3):236–42.

[11] Zetusky WJ, Jankovic J, Pirozzolo FJ. The heterogeneity of Parkinson's disease: clinical and prognostic implications. Neurology 1985;35(4):522–6.

[12] Ravina BM, Fagan SC, Hart RG, et al. Neuroprotective agents for clinical trials in Parkinson's disease: a systematic assessment. Neurology 2003;60(8):1234–40.

[13] Ahlskog JE. Parkinson's disease: medical and surgical treatment. Neurol Clin 2001;19(3): 579–605, vi.

[14] Ahlskog JE. Treatment of motor complications in advancing Parkinson's disease: which drugs and when? Formulary 2000;35:654–68.

[15] Ahlskog JE. Medical treatment of later-stage motor problems of Parkinson's disease. Mayo Clin Proc 1999;74:1239–54.

[16] Hely MA, Morris JG, Reid WG, et al. Sydney Multicenter Study of Parkinson's disease: non–L-dopa-responsive problems dominate at 15 years. Mov Disord 2005;20(2):190–9.

[17] Nutt JG. On-off phenomenon: relation to levodopa pharmacokinetics and pharmacodynamics. Ann Neurol 1987;22:535–40.

[18] Nutt JG, Woodward WR, Hammerstad JP, et al. The "on-off" phenomenon in Parkinson's disease: relation to levodopa absorption and transport. N Engl J Med 1984;310: 483–8.

[19] Djaldetti R, Baron J, Ziv I, et al. Gastric emptying in Parkinson's disease: patients with and without response fluctuations. Neurology 1996;46(4):1051–4.

[20] Ahlskog JE, Muenter MD, McManis PG, et al. Controlled-release Sinemet (CR-4): a double-blind crossover study in patients with fluctuating Parkinson's disease. Mayo Clin Proc 1988;63:876–86.

[21] Yeh KC, August TF, Bush DF, et al. Pharmacokinetics and bioavailability of Sinemet CR: a summary of human studies. Neurology 1989;39(Suppl 2):25–38.

[22] Nutt JG, Holford NH. The response to levodopa in Parkinson's disease: imposing pharmacological law and order. Ann Neurol 1996;39(5):561–73.

[23] Muenter MD, Tyce GM. L-dopa therapy of Parkinson's disease: plasma L-dopa concentration, therapeutic response, and side effects. Mayo Clin Proc 1971;46:231–9.

[24] Ahlskog JE, Muenter MD. Frequency of levodopa-related dyskinesias and motor fluctuations as estimated from the cumulative literature. Mov Disord 2001;16:448–58.

[25] Ballard PA, Tetrud JW, Langston JW. Permanent human parkinsonism due to 1-methyl-4-phenyl-1,2,3,6-tetrahydropyridine (MPTP): seven cases. Neurology 1985;35:949–56.

[26] Leenders KL, Palmer AJ, Quinn N, et al. Brain dopamine metabolism in patients with Parkinson's disease measured with positron emission tomography. J Neurol Neurosurg Psychiatry 1986;49:853–60.

[27] Papa SM, Engber TM, Kask AM, et al. Motor fluctuations in levodopa treated parkinsonian rats: relation to lesion extent and treatment duration. Brain Res 1994;662:69–74.

[28] Hwang WJ, Yao WJ, Wey SP, et al. Downregulation of striatal dopamine D2 receptors in advanced Parkinson's disease contributes to the development of motor fluctuation. Eur Neurol 2002;47(2):113–7.

[29] Barbato L, Stocchi F, Monge A, et al. The long-duration action of levodopa may be due to a postsynaptic effect. Clin Neuropharmacol 1997;20:394–401.

[30] Hauser RA, Deckers F, Lehert P. Parkinson's disease home diary: further validation and implications for clinical trials. Mov Disord 2004;19(12):1409–13.

[31] Goetz CG, Poewe W, Rascol O, et al. Evidence-based medical review update: pharmacological and surgical treatments of Parkinson's disease: 2001 to 2004. Mov Disord 2005;20(5): 523–39.

[32] Kurth MC, Tetrud JW, Irwin I, et al. Oral levodopa/carbidopa solution vs tablets in Parkinson's disease with severe fluctuations: a pilot study. Neurology 1993;43:1036–9.

[33] Pappert EJ, Buhrfiend C, Lipton JW, et al. The stability characteristics of levodopa solution. Mov Disord 1994;9:484.

[34] Quinn N, Parkes JD, Marsden CD. Control of on/off phenomenon by continuous intravenous infusion of levodopa. Neurology 1984;34:1131–6.

[35] Nilsson D, Nyholm D, Aquilonius SM. Duodenal levodopa infusion in Parkinson's disease—long-term experience. Acta Neurol Scand 2001;104(6):343–8.

[36] Waters C. Other pharmacological treatments for motor complications and dyskinesias. Mov Disord 2005;20(Suppl 11):S38–44.

[37] Dewey RB Jr, Hutton JT, LeWitt PA, et al. A randomized, double-blind, placebo-controlled trial of subcutaneously injected apomorphine for parkinsonian off-state events. Arch Neurol 2001;58(9):1385–92.

[38] Jankovic J. Motor fluctuations and dyskinesias in Parkinson's disease: clinical manifestations. Mov Disord 2005;20(Suppl 11):S11–6.

[39] Quinn N. Young onset Parkinson's disease. Mov Disord 1987;2:73–91.

[40] Schrag A, Ben-Shlomo Y, Brown R, et al. Young-onset Parkinson's disease revisited—clinical features, natural history, and mortality. Mov Disord 1998;13:885–94.

[41] Muenter MD, Ahlskog JE. Dopa dyskinesias and fluctuations are not related to dopa treatment duration. Ann Neurol 2000;48:464.

[42] Adler CH, Ahlskog JE, editors. Parkinson's disease and movement disorders. Diagnosis and treatment guidelines for the practicing physician. Totowa (NJ): Humana Press; 2000.

[43] Van Gerpen JA, Kumar N, Bower JH, et al. Levodopa-associated dyskinesia risk among Parkinson disease patients in Olmsted County, Minnesota, 1976–1990. Arch Neurol 2006; 63(2):205–9.

[44] Snow BJ, Macdonald L, McCauley D, et al. The effect of amantadine on levodopa-induced dyskinesias in Parkinson's disease: a double-blind, placebo-controlled study. Clin Neuropharmacol 2000;23:82–5.

[45] Verhagen Metman L, Del Dotto P, Blanchet PJ, et al. Blockade of glutamatergic transmission as treatment for dyskinesias and motor fluctuations in Parkinson's disease. Amino Acids 1998;14(1–3):75–82.

[46] Verhagen Metman L, Del Dotto P, van den Munckhof P, et al. Amantadine as treatment for dyskinesias and motor fluctuations in Parkinson's disease [see comments]. Neurology 1998;50(5):1323–6.

[47] Verhagen Metman L, Del Dotto P, LePoole K, et al. Amantadine for levodopa-induced dyskinesias. Arch Neurol 1999;56:1383–6.

[48] Klawans HL Jr, Weiner WJ. Attempted use of haloperidol in the treatment of L-dopa induced dyskinesias. J Neurol Neurosurg Psychiatry 1974;37(4):427–30.

[49] Tarsy D, Parkes JD, Marsden CD. Metoclopramide and pimozide in Parkinson's disease and levodopa-induced dyskinesias. J Neurol Neurosurg Psychiatry 1975;38(4):331–5.

[50] Bennett JP Jr, Landow ER, Dietrich S, et al. Suppression of dyskinesias in advanced Parkinson's disease: moderate daily clozapine doses provide long-term dyskinesia reduction. Mov Disord 1994;9(4):409–14.

[51] Verhagen Metman L, Del Dotto P, Natte R, et al. Dextromethorphan improves levodopa-induced dyskinesias in Parkinson's disease. Neurology 1998;51(1):203–6.

[52] Bonifati V, Fabrizio E, Cipriani R, et al. Buspirone in levodopa-induced dyskinesias. Clin Neuropharmacol 1994;17(1):73–82.

[53] Rascol O, Arnulf I, Peyro–Saint Paul H, et al. Idazoxan, an alpha-2 antagonist, and L-DOPA-induced dyskinesias in patients with Parkinson's disease. Mov Disord 2001; 16(4):708–13.

[54] Manson AJ, Iakovidou E, Lees AJ. Idazoxan is ineffective for levodopa-induced dyskinesias in Parkinson's disease. Mov Disord 2000;15(2):336–7.

[55] Carpentier AF, Bonnet AM, Vidailhet M, et al. Improvement of levodopa-induced dyskinesia by propranolol in Parkinson's disease. Neurology 1996;46(6):1548–51.

[56] Muenter MD, Sharpless NS, Tyce GM, et al. Patterns of dystonia ("I-D-I" and "D-I-D") in response to L-dopa therapy for Parkinson's disease. Mayo Clin Proc 1977;52:163–74.

[57] Deuschl G, Fogel W, Hahne M, et al. Deep-brain stimulation for Parkinson's disease. J Neurol 2002;249(Suppl 3):36–9.

[58] Vitek JL. Deep brain stimulation for Parkinson's disease. A critical re-evaluation of STN versus GPi DBS. Stereotact Funct Neurosurg 2002;78(3–4):119–31.

[59] Bloem BR, Hausdorff JM, Visser JE, et al. Falls and freezing of gait in Parkinson's disease: a review of two interconnected, episodic phenomena. Mov Disord 2004;19(8):871–84.

[60] Nieuwboer A, Feys P, de Weerdt W, et al. Is using a cue the clue to the treatment of freezing in Parkinson's disease? Physiother Res Int 1997;2(3):125–32 [discussion: 133–4].

[61] Michalowska M, Fiszer U, Krygowska-Wajs A, et al. Falls in Parkinson's disease. Causes and impact on patients' quality of life. Funct Neurol 2005;20(4):163–8.

[62] Azher SN, Jankovic J. Camptocormia: pathogenesis, classification, and response to therapy. Neurology 2005;65(3):355–9.

[63] Muller J, Wenning GK, Verny M, et al. Progression of dysarthria and dysphagia in postmortem-confirmed parkinsonian disorders. Arch Neurol 2001;58(2):259–64.

[64] Pinto S, Ozsancak C, Tripoliti E, et al. Treatments for dysarthria in Parkinson's disease. Lancet Neurol 2004;3(9):547–56.

[65] Kim SH, Kearney JJ, Atkins JP. Percutaneous laryngeal collagen augmentation for treatment of parkinsonian hypophonia. Otolaryngol Head Neck Surg 2002;126(6):653–6.

[66] Deane KH, Ellis-Hill C, Jones D, et al. Systematic review of paramedical therapies for Parkinson's disease. Mov Disord 2002;17(5):984–91.

[67] O'Sullivan JD, Bhatia KP, Lees AJ. Botulinum toxin A as treatment for drooling saliva in PD. Neurology 2000;55(4):606–7.

[68] Riley DE, Lang AE. The spectrum of levodopa-related fluctuations in Parkinson's disease. Neurology 1993;43:1459–64.

[69] Hillen ME, Sage JI. Nonmotor fluctuations in patients with Parkinson's disease. Neurology 1996;47:1180–3.

[70] Thorpy MJ, Adler CH. Parkinson's disease and sleep. Neurol Clin 2005;23(4):1187–208.

[71] Factor SA, McAlarney T, Sanchez-Ramos JR, et al. Sleep disorders and sleep effect in Parkinson's disease. Mov Disord 1990;5(4):280–5.

[72] Hogl BE, Gomez-Arevalo G, Garcia S, et al. A clinical, pharmacologic, and polysomnographic study of sleep benefit in Parkinson's disease. Neurology 1998;50(5):1332–9.

[73] Fahn S. Description of Parkinson's disease as a clinical syndrome. Ann N Y Acad Sci 2003; 991:1–14.

[74] Goetz C, Tanner CM, Levy M, et al. Pain in Parkinson's disease. Mov Disord 1986;1:45–9.

[75] Uitti RY, Ahlskog JE. Comparative review of dopamine receptor agonists in Parkinson's disease. CNS Drugs 1996;5:369–88.

[76] Mear J-Y, Barroche G, de Smet Y, et al. Pergolide in the treatment of Parkinson's disease. Neurology 1984;34:983–6.

[77] Ling LH, Ahlskog JE, Munger TM, et al. Constrictive pericarditis and pleuropulmonary disease linked to ergot dopamine agonist therapy (cabergoline) for Parkinson's disease. Mayo Clin Proc 1999;74:371–5.

[78] Pritchett AM, Morrison JF, Edwards WD, et al. Valvular heart disease in patients taking pergolide. Mayo Clin Proc 2002;77(12):1280–6.

[79] Braak H, Del Tredici K, Rub U, et al. Staging of brain pathology related to sporadic Parkinson's disease. Neurobiol Aging 2003;24(2):197–211.

[80] Ahlskog JE. Challenging conventional wisdom: the etiologic role of dopamine oxidative stress in Parkinson's disease. Mov Disord 2005;20(3):271–82.

[81] Singer C. Urinary dysfunction in Parkinson's disease. Clin Neurosci 1998;5(2):78–86.

[82] Bronner G, Royter V, Korczyn AD, et al. Sexual dysfunction in Parkinson's disease. J Sex Marital Ther 2004;30(2):95–105.

[83] Senard JM, Brefel-Courbon C, Rascol O, et al. Orthostatic hypotension in patients with Parkinson's disease: pathophysiology and management. Drugs Aging 2001;18(7):495–505.

[84] Jost WH. Gastrointestinal motility problems in patients with Parkinson's disease. Effects of antiparkinsonian treatment and guidelines for management. Drugs Aging 1997;10(4): 249–58.

[85] Abbott RD, Petrovitch H, White LR, et al. Frequency of bowel movements and the future risk of Parkinson's disease. Neurology 2001;57(3):456–62.

[86] Uc EY, Rizzo M, Anderson SW, et al. Visual dysfunction in Parkinson disease without dementia. Neurology 2005;65(12):1907–13.

[87] Rodnitzky RL. Visual dysfunction in Parkinson's disease. Clin Neurosci 1998;5(2):102–6.

[88] Fischer M, Gemende I, Marsch WC, et al. Skin function and skin disorders in Parkinson's disease. J Neural Transm 2001;108(2):205–13.

[89] Wszolek ZK, Markopoulou K. Olfactory dysfunction in Parkinson's disease. Clin Neurosci 1998;5(2):94–101.

[90] Aarsland D, Alves G, Larsen JP. Disorders of motivation, sexual conduct, and sleep in Parkinson's disease. Adv Neurol 2005;96:56–64.

ELSEVIER
SAUNDERS

CLINICS IN
GERIATRIC
MEDICINE

Clin Geriatr Med 22 (2006) 773–796

Cognitive, Affective, and Psychiatric Features of Parkinson's Disease

Nancy R. Barbas, MD, MSW[a,b,*]

[a]Department of Neurology, University of Michigan, 1920 Taubman Center 0316,
1500 Medical Center Drive, Ann Arbor, MI 48109-0316, USA
[b]Veterans Administration Medical Center, Ann Arbor,
MI 48109-0316, USA

Following the original description of the cardinal motor features of Parkinson's disease described by Parkinson in England in 1817, 50 years passed before Charcot in France credited him for his recognition of the syndrome [1]. It was around the same time that Charcot and others first mentioned in their writings observations of intellectual decline in patients with motor symptoms of PD. Most of these descriptions characterize the mental symptoms of PD as symptoms of advanced disease [2]. It has only been in the last 25 years that the pervasiveness of the cognitive, affective, and psychiatric features of PD has been recognized. Average frequency of dementia in PD was reported as 40% in one multistudy analysis [3], and prevalence rates range from 3% to 80%. Reports of frequency of depression range from 20% to 50% [4–6], and frequency of psychiatric symptoms of any type are reported at greater than 60% [7]. The variability in frequency rates reported for each of these features can be explained by numerous factors that influence survey results, including differences in symptom definition, absence of uniform clinical or pathologic diagnostic criteria, and evolution in application of diagnostic techniques.

The cognitive changes that accompany PD are now well acknowledged. Most common manifestations include executive, visuospatial, and memory impairments. Excellent reviews have been written on the topic [8–11].

This work was supported in part by Grant No. AG08671 (National Institutes of Health).

The author has had previous grant support within the last 5 years from Forest Pharmaceuticals, Inc., Glaxo, Smith, Kline Pharmaceuticals, Inc., and Elan Pharmaceuticals, Inc.

* Department of Neurology, University of Michigan, 1920 Taubman Center 0316, 1500 Medical Center Drive, Ann Arbor, MI 48109-0316, USA.

E-mail address: nbarbas@med.umich.edu

Cognitive changes may be subtle, but recognizable, even during the early stages of illness [12]. Frank dementia, defined as two or more cognitive deficits including memory impairment and at least one cognitive deficit of aphasia, apraxia, agnosia, or disturbed executive functioning, and which represent a decline to be sufficiently severe to interfere with occupational or social functioning, increases in frequency with stage of illness and age [13].

Affective changes also are common accompaniments of PD and manifest most frequently as depression, anxiety, and apathy. This topic also has been reviewed [14,15]. There seems to be a bimodal prevalence distribution of depression occurring in relationship with timing of diagnosis and with disease progression [16]. Although this distribution suggests the possibility that depression occurs as a reaction to illness, evidence supports the occurrence of an increased incidence of prediagnosis depression [17,18] and an increased frequency of depression in PD patients relative to patients with other chronic illness [19], although there is some controversy about this finding [20]. Depression seems to be an integral part of PD pathophysiology, although it is likely influenced further by reaction to illness and many other factors.

Psychoses in the form of visual hallucinations and paranoia are the most common features of psychiatric symptoms manifesting in PD patients. Numerous studies cite the relationship of psychiatric complications to administration of dopaminergic agents [21,22]. Reports also exist of a frequent occurrence of psychosis in patients not receiving these agents [23,24], including estimates of psychotic symptoms in PD in 5% of patients before the development of levodopa therapy [25]. This article presents an overview of current understanding of the pathophysiologic mechanisms underlying the cognitive and neuropsychiatric symptoms of PD; the risks associated with development of nonmotor symptoms; the consequences of these symptoms; and discussion of recognition, diagnosis, and treatment of these common and important aspects of PD.

Pathophysiology

As pointed out by Albin in another article in this issue, dopamine deficiency and lack of dopamine effects in the rostral midbrain, substantia nigra pars compacta, and their respective projections to subcortical striatal structures are likely responsible for the motor features of parkinsonism. The pathophysiologic basis of the cognitive, affective, and psychiatric features of PD is complex and not fully understood. Alterations in dopamine and other neurotransmitters involving subcortical projections and synaptic and neuronal changes involving limbic and cortical structures likely combine to result in these nonmotor symptoms.

A schema of parallel loops linking cortico-basal-ganglia-thalamo structures that use dopamine as their primary neurotransmitter illustrates the connections with extrastriatal structures [26]. In particular, the dorsolateral frontostriatal and orbitofrontal loops have been implicated. Impaired cognitive functioning believed analogous to frontal lobe dysfunction has been shown in animal studies [27–30], neuroimaging studies [31–34], and autopsy studies [35,36]. Although evidence strongly suggests a link between dopamine deficiency and impaired frontal lobe function, several factors should be borne in mind. Foremost is that dopamine levels fluctuate with disease severity, and altered dopamine levels affect specific brain regions differently, even within individual structures, such as the putamen and caudate nuclei and frontal lobes [37–40].

Others have linked dopamine depletion in the anterior cingulate loop of the cortico-basal-ganglia-thalamo loop involving the ventral striatum and mesocortical regions with alterations in mood and affect [40]. Neuroimaging studies have shown hypometabolism in frontal structures in depressed PD patients without dementia, with or without cognitive changes [41,42].

Explanations for the occurrence of psychosis in PD have been proposed most commonly in the setting of dopaminergic drug therapy. Upregulation of striatal dopamine receptors occurs after lesioning of the nigrostriatal pathway in animals or as a neurodegenerative event. There is thought to be an activation of receptors (denervation supersensitivity) when exposed to dopamine replacement, which may be partly responsible for psychotic symptoms [43]. Several hypotheses relating psychiatric symptoms in PD to denervation supersensitivity exist. There is evidence linking brainstem, striate, limbic, and cortical structures with dopamine as the primary neurotransmitter. Several models propose a system of interactions between dopaminergic, serotoninergic, and GABAergic neurons, which, when overstimulated or imbalanced, lead to hallucinations or other psychotic symptoms [44–47]. Variability in the occurrence of psychotic symptoms is likely due to numerous factors, including differences in cell loss of serotoninergic and cholinergic cells among PD patients [48,49].

Although evidence supports a role for dopamine in the cognitive and behavioral aspects of PD, other neurotransmitter systems also are implicated. Cell loss in the locus caeruleus and decrease in norepinephrine are more marked in demented PD patients relative to nondemented patients [50,51]. Numerous studies have identified decreased norepinephrine in PD patients in the neocortex and hippocampus, although these have not clearly identified a difference between demented and nondemented subjects [52]. Measuring a norepinephrine metabolite in nondemented PD patients, a correlation between decreased levels and poorer performance on several attentional tasks was observed [53].

PD patients also are deficient in serotonin as noted by decreased cells in the raphe nuclei and reduced concentrations in hippocampal and frontal regions and striatopallidal pathways [52,54]. Decrease in serotoninergic neurons and in serotonin metabolites in PD patients with depression compared with nondepressed patients has been observed [55,56]. Rapid depletion of the serotonin precursor tryptophan in the brain has resulted in learning and memory impairment, although this finding is not consistently replicated [57].

Connections between dopaminergic and serotoninergic brainstem and cortical systems have been implicated in symptoms of depression also [58,59].

Cholinergic deficit is consistently described in PD patients in numerous studies of patients with and without dementia. Cell loss is most severe in the basal nucleus of Meynert, a deep subcortical structure with projections to the cortex and hippocampus. Evidence correlating degree of cell loss with severity of cognitive impairment exists [52,60–65].

Based on evidence for multiple neurotransmitter deficits in PD and identification of links between a specific transmitter and identifiable cognitive or behavioral symptom, general associations can be drawn. Dopaminergic and cholinergic deficits are associated most with a frontal lobe dysexecutive syndrome, cholinergic deficits further add to impaired memory and attention, noradrenergic deficit also can be linked with attentional problems, and deficit in serotonin can be linked with depressed mood [66].

Examination of the pathologic substrate of nonmotor symptoms in PD has advanced tremendously in the past 15 years. Lewy bodies have long been recognized in the substantia nigra of PD patients [67]. With the development of immunostaining techniques with increased sensitivity for identifying aggregated ubiquitin and α-synuclein, Lewy bodies are now recognized in non-nigral brain regions [68–70]. Cortical Lewy bodies are now well recognized in PD patients, and their presence correlates with the presence of dementia [71–73]. Cortical Lewy bodies also are recognized in PD patients without dementia [71,74,75]. In a comparison of PD patients with and without dementia, one study found a 10-fold increase in neocortical and limbic Lewy body inclusions in dementia patients [76]. A correlation between the time of onset of dementia and presence of cortical Lewy bodies has not been established [76–78].

Deposition of amyloid β, the pathologic hallmark of Alzheimer's disease composing neuritic plaques, is commonly seen in postmortem brains of demented PD patients [74,79]. Studies conflict regarding an association between the amount of amyloid plaque deposition and the severity of dementia in PD patients with dementia [72,80–82].

Pathologically, there is significant overlap between diseases in which clinical features of parkinsonism and dementia coexist. PD with dementia (PDD), dementia with Lewy bodies (DLB), and Alzheimer's disease with extrapyramidal symptoms share many pathologic and clinical features, although they also have some distinguishing features. Excellent discussions of the distinguishing features of DLB and PDD have been published [9,72,83–86]. Guidelines for diagnosing DLB were revised more recently. Recommended criteria designate the use of the term *PDD* for dementia occurring at least 12 months after parkinsonian motor symptoms [87]. The most commonly identified pathologic marker associated with the cognitive and behavioral symptoms of PD is the cortical Lewy body. Likely, clinical heterogeneity is a function of additional contributions from variable changes in neurotransmitters, especially cholinergic deficits, and pathologies, including Lewy bodies and pathologies associated with Alzheimer's disease. Developments in the identification of the neurotransmitter and neuropathologic substrates for the cognitive, affective, and psychiatric symptoms associated with PD and related extrapyramidal syndromes are leading to improved diagnosis and treatment.

Risks

Although there are no definite predictors of which patient will develop nonmotor symptoms as an accompaniment of PD, numerous risk factors have been identified. The most well-documented factor for development of cognitive impairment is increased age [88–91]. There is only a weak association between nonmotor PD symptoms and age at onset of PD and with PD duration, so it is likely the increased occurrence of dementia in elderly PD patients reflects the increased prevalence of dementia-related pathology with aging in general [91–95]. Conflicting data exist regarding a possible association between PD dementia and presence of an apolipoprotein E H4 genotype, a known Alzheimer's disease risk factor [96]. A meta-analysis supports an increased risk for dementia in PD (odds ratio 1.6) when apolipoprotein E H4 is present, compared with apolipoprotein E H3 (odds ratio 0.54) or apolipoprotein E H2 (odds ratio 1.3) [97].

The degree of severity of motor symptoms and presence of dominant gait and postural symptoms compared with tremor has been associated with increased risk for development of cognitive symptoms [98–100]. Other risk factors for dementia are male sex and lower Folstein Mini Mental Status examination (MMSE) score at predementia baseline [91,92,94].

An increased risk for depression in PD has been associated with longer duration of PD diagnosis, a personal history of depression before PD, and symptoms referable to left hemispheric dysfunction at the time of initial presentation [101]. Severity of extrapyramidal motor symptoms has not been correlated with depression [102,103], although studies have identified an association between onset of motor symptoms and anxiety. Presence of anxiety is not increased presymptomatically, but is correlated with on-off motor fluctuations and poor medication response. Anxiety may be a reaction to the discomfort and fear of motor dyscontrol and is less clearly a result of underlying PD pathology [25,104]. It is a common accompaniment of PD with or without depression.

Determination of risk factors for occurrence of psychotic features in PD patients is complicated because of the known association between administration of dopaminergic medications and hallucinations [105]. Other identified risk factors include older age, duration of PD, ocular and visual disturbances, and sleep disturbances [106–110], although not all studies control for dopaminergic medication usage.

Risk factor determination is complicated further by difficulty in clinically distinguishing between PDD and DLB. The strong association between the presence of hallucinations in nonmedicated DLB patients has been suggested as a criterion for distinguishing PDD from DLB [111]. The occurrence of delusions and hallucinations is found with increased frequency when comparing patients with PD without dementia (7%/14%), PDD (29%/54%), and DLB (57%/76%) [112]. Although the presence of hallucinations and temporal onset of dementia versus motor symptoms may be helpful for distinguishing between PDD and DLB, the common occurrence of dementia, hallucinations, motor changes, neurospychiatric symptoms, and fluctuations in both conditions continue to make clinical distinctions difficult.

Lastly, significant relationships have been observed between the presence of dementia, depression, and psychosis in PD patients. Correlations have been made between dementia and depression [113,114], dementia and confusional states and hallucinations [90–92,94,115], and depression and psychosis [94].

Impact of nonmotor symptoms

Dementia associated with PD seems to be associated with shortened life span. Although this association is difficult to quantify among individuals with advanced age, the mortality hazard ratio for patients with PD is twice that compared with individuals without PD [116–118]. Among a group of PD patients without dementia who were followed for a mean period of 3 years, dementia developed in approximately half of the patients who died compared with approximately one quarter among longer term survivors [117]. Depression also is associated with an increased mortality hazard ratio of 2.66 [119] and with decreased quality of life [120].

Nursing home placement is increased among PD patients with dementia. A particularly strong predictor of nursing home placement is the presence of psychosis and hallucinations [116,121,122]. The occurrence of psychosis also imparts a greater impact on quality of life and caregiver burden than motor symptoms alone [22,123]. Caregiver burden, as reflected in depression scales, also is increased in spouses of depressed PD patients [124,125].

The cost of cognitive and psychiatric symptoms and their sequelae in PD patients is unknown. Extrapolating from figures estimating that PD costs $27 billion annually for the 1 million Americans affected, and the prevalence of neuropsychiatric symptoms and their huge impact on patients and caregivers, one can only surmise that the contribution is tremendous [126].

Symptom recognition and diagnosis

Recognition of cognitive impairments and other nonmotor symptoms of PD can be challenging to the clinician, but with an awareness of risk factors and specific features, clinical recognition and accuracy in diagnosis can be accomplished. Patients themselves may be unaware of their deficits and unable to bring them to the attention of their physician. Patients who have noted memory or other cognitive difficulties may attribute them to normal aging. It is common for patients, when asked, to respond that "all my friends" are experiencing similar forgetfulness. Patients may hide their concerns out of embarrassment or, in the case of hallucinations, out of worry that they will be viewed as "crazy." It is common for a spouse, adult child, or other caregiver to observe cognitive or behavior changes in a loved one, but they, too, may find it difficult to discuss their observations and threaten the patient's autonomy. Conversely, a patient's family may intervene on behalf of the patient and offer information that can be extremely helpful for the patient's care. The physician can overcome these barriers by recognizing the frequency of symptom occurrence in the PD population, by actively making inquiries of the patient, by requesting patient permission to involve family members and caregivers in their assessment, and by administering some screening tests or questionnaires.

The cognitive deficit most characteristically associated with PD is a dysexecutive syndrome [8,127–129]. Tasks generally implicated in executive functioning include attention, inhibition, planning, and task management [130]. Patients or observers may describe difficulty in completing tasks that previously were easily performed. Often activities that require sequencing of multiple steps and planning are abandoned. The interviewer can inquire about meal planning and preparation, completion of simple household chores or repairs, hobbies, and job-related activities. Careful attention must be paid to distinguishing a change in abilities in these areas owing to motor-induced limitations versus cognitive changes, and, if possible, inquiries should be made about activities that make fewer demands on motor skills.

Visuospatial skills are commonly and prominently affected in PD [131–133]; it is unclear whether this is due to a disruption in visual processing or an extension of impaired executive functioning [8]. Patients may complain of poor vision in the absence of abnormalities on ophthalmologic examination. The patient's description of visual problems is often vague and nonspecific. Patients may report that they are no longer able to read, or they may have difficulty completing a reading task. Navigation abilities may become impaired. Patients or their families may speak of the patient getting lost while driving or of inability interpreting a map. Poor driving may be observed by family members with descriptions suggesting inability to stay within lanes or bumping curbs when turning corners, or there may be a history of motor vehicle accidents. There may be difficulty navigating through rooms in new, or even familiar, environments.

Memory may be impaired or relatively spared [134]. The pattern is usually one of poor retrieval. Patients may complain of poor memory for recent events, although family members may comment that cueing is helpful. A patient often recognizes families' descriptions of an event and may even be able to fill in some details when prompted. This differs from the memory impairment seen in patients with Alzheimer's disease, in which memory generally does not improve with cues. The memory deficits observed in PD patients seem related to impaired retrieval and working memory, in contrast to encoding problems. Additionally, memory impairment in PD is more severe for visual than verbal material [8,66].

A fluctuating pattern of alertness and cognition is commonly observed in PD patients, and fluctuating attention and alertness is considered a core feature for diagnosing DLB [135]. Families often report periods of poor alertness and confusion interspersed with periods of lucidity, consistent with premorbid abilities. Duration of fluctuations varies between and within individuals and may be described as days to weeks. Families also describe excessive daytime sleeping. The assessment of fluctuating alertness and daytime sleepiness is complicated by known sedating effects of dopaminergic drugs, and there is likely a dose-dependent relationship. The patient and family should be asked about changes in alertness in relation to medication administration or in relation to changes in medication doses.

Cognitive changes resulting in apraxia, agnosia, or aphasia usually are not prominently seen. Speech production problems that may be present and are thought to be reflective of the motor symptoms of PD include reduced rate, volume, prosody, and articulation. This may be confused with or coupled with slowed cognitive processing or bradyphrenia, believed by some to be overrepresented in PD patients [136]. Bradyphrenia also is a common hallmark of depression. The patient or family description of slowed speech should be interpreted in the context of other accompanying symptoms.

In assessing depression, the patient and family members should be queried about expressions of sadness, pessimistic thinking, loss of interest or engagement in previously enjoyed activities, shortened temper or irritability, and difficulty concentrating because these are characteristics most commonly identified with PD depression [15,102]. The patient should be asked about suicidal ideation, although suicide is not thought to be common among PD patients [137]. It is worthwhile to ask about sleep disturbances and poor appetite, although their presence may reflect either depression or PD accompaniments. Affirmative responses should be considered in context. Anxiety may be present with or without depression. Anxiety may manifest as generalized anxiety disorders, panic disorders, agoraphobia, or social phobias [7,138].

Psychosis, usually hallucinations, in the setting of antiparkinson treatment administration is well recognized, whereas psychosis in PD patients not on treatment remains controversial. Along with fluctuations in cognition, hallucinations are recognized as a cardinal feature of DLB, and their presence is included among chief criteria for a DLB diagnosis. Whether treatment dependent or occurring independently, it is valuable to ask patients whether they have experienced a visual or auditory hallucination or an unusual perception that is not observed by others (lacks external stimulus). In PD, visual hallucinations are estimated to occur approximately two to three times more frequently than auditory hallucinations, and all hallucinations are more likely to occur as disease advances, especially in the presence of dementia [21,139]. It is common for patients to maintain insight regarding hallucinations, and when asked, patients might describe in detail vivid hallucinations of people, often familiar, or animals. Poor reality testing also is commonly present, and family members should be queried about patient's unusual behaviors or perceptions. Paranoid delusions or delusions of other sorts are the second most common type of psychotic symptom occurring in PD. They often involve false beliefs of spousal infidelity or jealousy or persecution concerns [140].

A thorough, detailed history is crucial for recognizing cognitive and affective features accompanying PD and can be refined further by use of clinical screening or assessment tools that can be easy to administer. The sensitivity and specificity of most of the commonly used tools for assessing mental status are not always optimal when applied in the setting of PD. A full description of individual measurements tools is beyond the scope of this article, but a brief discussion of some of those most commonly used is included. The Folstein MMSE is often thought of as the "gold standard" of screening tests because its reliability and validity have been extensively examined [141]. A maximum of 30 possible points can be scored, with 16 achievable primarily on the basis of orientation or memory questions. Only one task, the three-part command, requires performance using sequencing. Executive function tasks, that are most prominently affected in PD, especially early in the course of cognitive decline, are minimally reflected in the MMSE, and a patient's score may be an inaccurate representation of their losses [142]. It can be helpful to supplement MMSE testing with measurements that address executive function, such as asking the patient to create a representation of a clock and time (Clock Drawing Test) or asking the patient to connect sequentially letters of the alphabet alternating with numerals (Weschler Trails B subtest). Verbal fluency, believed to test semantic memory, which relies on intact executive function, can be tested by asking the patient to list items beginning with a specified letter of the alphabet within 1 minute. This ability may be impaired (naming <12 items), whereas categorical naming (eg, animals) is relatively preserved. Another scale that assesses executive function and memory performance is the SCale for Outcomes of PArkinson's disease-COGnition (SCOPA-COG) [143]. Several easily administered depression scales exist for use in the office setting, including the Geriatrics Depression Scale of Yesavage, which is a self-rating questionnaire; the Cornell Scale for Depression in Dementia; the Beck Depression Inventory; and the depression component of the Hospital Anxiety and Depression Scale.

Many formal neuropsychologic and neuropsychiatric test batteries exist that contain measures of multiple aspects of cognition or mood, including memory, verbal function, visuospatial abilities, judgment and reasoning, attention, processing speed, and presence of affective symptoms. Some of these batteries have been developed specifically to address dementia diagnosis, such as the Consortium to Establish a Registry for Alzheimer's Disease (CERAD) and the University of California Alzheimer's Disease Research

Center (UCSD-ADRC) test battery. Scales that address depression appropriate for use in the PD population, such as the Hamilton Depression Rating Scale, are also available. In general, referring a patient for formal neuropsychometric test evaluation can result in further delineating an individual's areas of strength and weakness, but it should be borne in mind that the utility of the tests is often weakened by absence of age-adjusted norms, medical conditions and sensory impairments may have an impact on testing, and estimates of an individual's starting intellectual abilities are difficult to establish. There is a large volume of literature reporting attempts to correlate specific patterns of cognitive or mood alterations with specific diagnoses. Although many of these are excellent investigations and informative for providing a general description of characteristic findings clustered among diseases, large areas of overlap remain, and profiles applicable for making definite diagnosis remain elusive.

When the presence of cognitive decline, mood disorder, or psychosis has been established or is strongly suspected, a specific diagnosis should be sought. Evaluation for possible contributing factors should be undertaken, and reversible problems should be addressed. Medical conditions, including conditions that might contribute to vascular pathology and hormonal or metabolic imbalances such as thyroid, renal, or liver disease, should be assessed. Deficiency states, such as low cobalamin (vitamin B_{12}), should be considered. Evaluation of testosterone level should be undertaken because deficiency states in men with PD have been associated with depression. Infectious etiologies for delirium or confusion should be sought. Adverse effects of medications or polypharmacy should be sought. A history of substance abuse or illicit drug use should be considered. One of the greatest challenges facing the clinician is assessing the contribution that anti-Parkinson's drugs make on a patient's cognitive, mood, or psychiatric symptoms. Lastly, neuroimaging of the cranial fossae should be undertaken to rule out structural abnormalities [144]. Guidelines for initial assessment of PD dementia, depression, or psychosis are summarized in Table 1.

Clinically distinguishing PDD from other degenerative dementing illnesses is challenging. Recognition of a patient's clinical features and familiarity with disease-associated features is essential. Many conditions have notable features of parkinsonism and cognitive and psychiatric symptoms. Most common among them are Alzheimer's disease, DLB, and vascular dementia. Temporal onset of symptoms is used as one of the main distinguishing features. In Alzheimer's disease and DLB, memory impairment precedes parkinsonism. In DLB, dementia is accompanied by at least two core features of fluctuating cognition, recurrent visual hallucinations, or spontaneous parkinsonism. Vascular dementia is diagnosed in patients whose cognitive symptoms appear temporally related to the occurrence of a stroke as assessed by history, clinical examination, or brain imaging [145]. Behavior or language disorders are the usual initial developments in frontotemporal dementias, although several subtypes exist [146]. The syndrome of

Table 1
Initial assessment of Parkinson's disease dementia, depression, and psychosis

Assessment	Evaluating for
Medical	Infection, thyroid, renal, liver disease, testosterone deficiency
Pharmacologic	Drug reaction or interaction (eg, anticholinergics, dopaminergics, sedatives, β-blockers)
Neurologic	Focal finding or concurrent symptoms suggesting other primary central nervous system disease and for correctable sensory deficits
Nutritional	Vitamin B_{12} deficiency, general malnutrition
Substance use	Alcohol, substances of abuse
Brain imaging (CT, MRI)	Mass, infection, ischemia, hemorrhage, normal-pressure hydrocephalus, subdural fluid collection

parkinsonism and dementia (dementia pugilistica) can occur after head injury. Progressive supranuclear palsy, multiple system atrophy, and other diseases that have been delineated as parkinsonian syndromes are discussed in the article by Gilman and are usually differentiated from PDD by characteristic findings. With thorough clinical assessment, reversible causes for cognitive or psychiatric symptoms can be identified and corrected, and a clinical diagnosis can be ascertained that can aid in directing treatment and management.

Drug treatments

Medical management of PDD can be especially challenging, often requiring establishment of a balance between optimal motor control and cognitive, affective, and psychiatric symptom control. It is common for a gain in one area to be accompanied by a loss in another [147]. Patients and their families need to be thoroughly educated when prescribing drugs regarding potential benefits, risks, and complications. They should be advised that individual responses vary. Appropriate expectations should be presented, acknowledging the absence of treatments that provide cures or complete remissions or that modify the underlying disease pathology. Identifying patient and family priorities can be extremely useful. The practitioner should bear in mind that the progressive nature of PD is likely to result in changing priorities, and these should be reviewed regularly.

Cognitive impairment and dementia

Based on marked cholinergic deficits present in PDD and DLB, treatments aimed at improving cholinergic function have been evaluated for the treatment of cognitive and behavioral symptoms. There are currently four Food and Drug Administration–approved acetylcholinesterase inhibitors for treatment of Alzheimer's disease: tacrine, donepezil, rivastigmine, and galantamine. Rivastigimine gained US Federal Drug Administration approval for the treatment of PD dementia in June, 2006.

Approval based on a single study of PD patients receiving rivastigmine versus placebo. Outcome scales used included the Alzheimer's Disease Assessment (ADAS-Cog), the Clinician's Global Impression of Change (CGIC) scale, and secondary measures including the Neuropsychiatric Inventory (NPI), MMSE, Activities of Daily Living (ADL) scale verbal fluency, clock drawing, and Cognitive Drug Research attentional scales. A total of 541 patients were randomly assigned to receive placebo or rivastigmine titrated up weekly in 1.5-mg increments to a maximum of 12 mg daily. A mean dose of 8.7 mg/d was achieved, and patients received 24 weeks of treatment on stable dose. Significant differences in change from baseline were present for the rivastigmine-treated group on ADAS-Cog scale and all secondary outcomes. Adverse events resulting in dropout occurred in 17% of the treated group versus 8% in the placebo group. The most common adverse events were nausea and vomiting. The Unified Parkinson's Disease Rating Scale (UPDRS) motor scores did not differ between groups [149].

Donepezil was studied in 14 patients with mild-to-moderate dementia in a crossover design trial of 10 weeks per study arm. During the treatment phase, donepezil was initiated at 5 mg/d during weeks 1 through 6 and increased to 10 mg/d weeks 7 through 10. Donepezil treatment was associated with significant improvements in MMSE and Caregiver Interview Based Impression of Change scores relative to placebo. There were no group differences in Neuropsychiatric Inventory (NPI) scores or Unified Parkinsons Disease Rating Scale UPDRS [148].

DLB patients with mild-to-moderate stage dementia were studied in a double-blind, placebo-controlled trial of rivastigmine. A total of 120 patients received treatment titrated up to a maximum of 12 mg/d (mean dose 9.4 mg/d) or placebo for 20 weeks. Primary outcome measures were subscales of the NPI evaluating delusions, hallucinations, apathy, and depression. Secondary outcome measures included MMSE, CGIC, and a computerized cognitive assessment battery. Significantly more (63%) patients receiving rivastigmine than placebo (30%) reached at least 30% improvement on NPI scores. Only the computer-based cognitive measure was found to be associated with significant cognitive improvement in the treatment group, with other cognitive measures nonsignificant compared with placebo. The most common side effects were nausea, vomiting, anorexia, and somnolence, occurring more frequently among the treatment group (92%) compared with the placebo group (75%). Motor scores on the UPDRS were similar between groups [150].

Numerous open-label studies, case-control studies, and case reports assessing the impact of acetylcholinesterase inhibitors in PDD or DLB have shown positive trends on cognitive performance and behavioral and psychotic symptoms. Most studies that have evaluated drug effects on motor function have not shown motor deterioration [9,151].

Overall, although generalization to all drugs within the class is not clearly established, acetylcholinesterase inhibitors are useful in the treatment of dementia with PD and DLB. Safety is well established. Although gastrointestinal side effects are common, it is less common for them to lead to drug discontinuation. When prescribed, patients and families should be advised that expected treatment effects are delay in progression of cognitive decline, similar to results seen in treatment of Alzheimer's disease. There are currently no medications with established efficiency for treating the mild cognitive impairments in PD.

Research into disease mechanisms continues. Developments in pharmacogenetics in rivastigmine-treated DLB patients have disclosed heterogeneity in enzyme activity, in performance on neuropsychologic tests, and in response to cholinesterase inhibitor medications depending on butyrylcholinesterase allelic expression on chromosome 3. Developments such as this may aid in future ability to identify a group of patients more likely to respond to treatment [152].

The effects of dopamine on cognition also have been studied, with mixed results. Studies evaluating dopaminergic effects on executive functioning have resulted in improvements, no change, or deterioration. Most likely, the influence of dopamine depends on stage of illness and type of motor impairment, specifically axial-gait disturbance versus the more dopamine-responsive akinetic-rigid form. A role for the use of memantine, an N-methyl-D-aspartate receptor antagonist used in the treatment of moderate-to-severe Alzheimer's disease, has not been established for PDD or DLB patients.

Depression

There are few evidence-based studies for treating depression in PDD or DLB. The tricyclic antidepressant (TCA), nortriptyline, was evaluated in a randomized, double-blind crossover study of 22 levodopa-treated patients for a duration of 8 weeks per study arm. Based on an author-designed rating scale, there was a significant reduction in median depression scores while on treatment. Motor rating scales showed no significant difference between nortriptyline treatment and placebo [153]. Orthostatic hypotension was the major treatment-related adverse event identified in this study. The tricyclic antidepressants have well-established antimuscarinic, antiadrenergic, antihistaminergic, and antiserotoninergic activity. Sedation, memory impairment, and confusional states including hallucinosis and delirium are common side effects. Orthostatic hypotension has been reported in 10% of patients treated for major depression. Although rare, cardiac arrhythmias, most notably bundle blocks, have been reported in patients with pre-existing cardiac disease [154].

Selective serotonin reuptake inhibitors (SSRIs) have been studied only in open-label trials, which have been predominantly positive in improving symptoms of depression in PD, with little effect on motor symptoms [155–158]. Generally identified adverse effects of SSRIs include sleep disorders and gastrointestinal complications. There is a lower incidence of anticholinergic-related events and cardiac arrhythmias compared with tricyclic antidepressant medications. The combination of SSRIs with the monoamine oxidase (MAO)-B inhibitor, deprenyl, has posed theoretical concern about a possible so-called serotonin syndrome, characterized as tremor, myoclonus, mental status changes, diarrhea, hyperpyrexia, diaphoresis, and hyperreflexia. The incidence of this occurrence was found to be low, 0.24%, in one well-conducted survey [159].

A single randomized controlled trial of MAO-A and MAO-B inhibitors used in combination versus an MAO-A inhibitor used alone showed significant improvement in depression in the group receiving combination therapy. Use of MAO-A inhibitors concurrently with tricyclic antidepressants or SSRIs is associated with high incidence of severe serotonin syndrome, including fatalities, and should be avoided.

Little is known about effects of the newer antidepressant medications in PD patients. Based on the few small or open trials reporting use of antidepressant drugs in this population, data on their use in depressed non-PD patients, and safety profiles in non-PD patients, the following recommendations can be made: (1) SSRIs are likely safe, although effectiveness is not clearly established; (2) nortriptyline is likely effective, although other tricyclic antidepressants have not been studied, and safety concerns exist; and (3) the use of MAO-As with SSRIs, tricyclic antidepressants, or levodopa poses unacceptable risks [154].

Psychosis

The approach to the medical management of psychotic symptoms first should address minimizing or eliminating drugs that may be an inciting factor. All of the antiparkinsonian drugs have been associated with psychotic side effects [160,161]. Concurrent development of psychiatric symptoms on initiation of a drug should alert the physician to a causal relationship. Elimination of antiparkinsonian drugs based on a risk-to-benefit evaluation model has been proposed [162]. The model suggests withdrawing or reducing, in order from first to last, anticholinergics, deprenyl, amantadine, dopaminergic agonists, catechol *O*-methyltransferase inhibitors, controlled-release levodopa, and standard levodopa. The presence of polypharmacy and of centrally acting drugs should be assessed.

In the setting of continuing psychiatric symptoms that are troubling to the patient or patient's family, the judicious use of antipsychotic medication can be considered. In a patient whose symptoms are mild and who maintains insight, nonpharmacologic interventions, such as education, may be sufficient. Frequently, when more disturbing symptoms are present, families choose control of psychotic symptoms at the risks of worsening the patient's movement disorder. Additionally, judicious use of antipsychotic medication may improve tolerance for increased doses of levodopa or dopamine agonist drugs to improve motor function.

Classic neuroleptics, including haloperidol and phenothiazines, have been strongly linked to worsened motor function, confusion, neuroleptic malignant syndrome, and mortality, especially in patients with PD, PDD, and DLB [163,164], likely owing to their strong affinity to dopamine D2 receptors [14].

Among atypical antipsychotic medications, only clozapine and olanzapine have been studied in randomized, placebo-controlled trials in PD or DLB patients. In a trial of 60 PD patients, those receiving clozapine showed significant improvement on psychosis rating scales for the CGIC for psychosis, UPDRS scales, Brief Psychiatric Rating Scale (BPRS), modified BPRS (controlling for PD confounders), and Scale for Assessment of Positive symptoms (SAPs), without deterioration of motor function. During the 4-week study, three patients in the treatment group dropped out, one each for reversible leukopenia, myocardial infarction, and sedation. One additional patient developed leukopenia during a 3-month extension. Also, six deaths occurred, none related to leukopenia [165]. A second study of 60 patients found significant improvement on the CGIC and Positive Subscale of the Positive and Negative Syndrome Scale at the end of 4 weeks, without worsening of motor symptoms [166].

In a 6-week trial comparing clozapine with olanzapine, 28 patients were evaluated using the SAPs scale for psychiatric symptoms and SAPs visual hallucination item, BPRS, ADL scale, and UPDRS. Fifteen patients completed this 9-week trial because the study was prematurely stopped owing to the development of worsened motor symptoms in the olanzapine group. The clozapine group showed statistically significant improvement over baseline in SAPs and visual hallucination SAPs subtest and in BPRS, without motor deterioration [167].

Clozapine used in treatment of patients with primary psychiatric disease has been associated with leukopenia, sometimes fatal, and myocarditis and cardiomyopathy. In PD patients, leukopenia occurs infrequently, and cardiac abnormalities associated with PD have not been reported [161].

Little is known about the efficacy of quetiapine, risperidone, and other newer antipsychotic medications in PD, PDD, and DLB. Quetiapine is pharmacologically similar to clozapine. Several small open-label series of PD or DLB patients have shown efficacy treating psychosis [168,169], although mild worsening of motor symptoms also is reported [168].

Food and Drug Administration warnings regarding increased risk of death and hyperglycemia for patients taking all atypical antipsychotic medications is of concern. The benefit-to-risk balance must be taken into consideration and discussed with patients and families.

There is a role for use of atypical antipsychotic medications in the treatment of psychosis in the setting of PD. If using clozapine, blood count must be monitored weekly. Quetiapine also may be a good option because leukopenia is not a risk, although efficacy is less established. Finally, all patients should be fully informed regarding increased risk of death. Treatment should be initiated with low doses. Required doses are typically one tenth or less than doses used for treatment of schizophrenia. Dose adjustment should proceed slowly, and patients should be monitored closely for worsened confusion or motor symptoms or hallucinations.

The benefits of the cholinesterase inhibitor, rivastigmine, for treatment of psychosis in DLB, studied in a small double-blind placebo-controlled trial, has been discussed in the section on treatment of cognitive symptoms. Small case studies and open-label trials with donepezil and rivastigmine have reported similar results [151,170]. Table 2 summarizes medications used in the treatment of PD dementia, depression, and psychosis and studied in evidence-based trials.

Nonpharmacologic treatments

In addition to drug therapy, nonpharmacologic intervention should be customized for individual patients. Programs for cognitive rehabilitation,

Table 2
Medications used in the treatment of Parkinson's disease dementia, depression, and psychosis[a]

Symptom	Medication	Usual starting dose	Usual therapeutic dose	Common side effects for medication class
Dementia	Donepezil[b]	5 mg daily	10 mg daily	AchI
	Rivastigmine[b,d]	1.5 mg twice daily	3–6 mg twice daily	Insomnia, dizziness, nausea, vomiting, anorexia, diarrhea
Depression	Sertraline[c]	25–50 mg daily	25–200 mg daily	SSRI
	Paroxetine[c]	10–20 mg daily	10–40 mg daily	Somnolence, dizziness,
	Citalopram[c]	12.5–25 CR mg daily	12.5–50 mg daily	tremor, nausea, diarrhea, sweating, ejaculatory dysfunction, xerostomia
	Nortriptyline[b,e]	10–25 mg daily	10–50 mg daily	TCA Somnolence, confusion, dizziness, headache, nausea, constipation, weight gain, hypotension, blurred vision, xerostomia, rare cardiac arrhythmia
Psychosis	Clozapine[b]	2.5 mg daily	10–50 mg daily	Atypical antipsychotic
	Quetiapine[c]	12.5 mg daily	12.5–150 mg daily	Clozapine only Agranulocytosis, myocarditis Both Somnolence, dizziness, headache, constipation

[a] Evidence-based only.
[b] Level I, placebo-control, double-blind, randomized trials.
[c] Level II, III, not fitting Level I criteria or case series.
[d] FDA approved for this indication.
[e] Side effects often serious.

Table 3
Nonpharmacologic treatment of Parkinson's disease dementia, depression, psychosis

Treatment	Target audience
Education about disease	Patient, family
Education about treatments	Patient, family
Cognitive rehabilitation	Patient with mild cognitive impairment or early dementia
Psychological/psychiatric counseling	Patient with preserved insight Caregiver for psychological support
Electroconvulsive therapy	Patient with medication-refractory depression
Community resource referral	Patient, family
Home health assessment	Patient, family

for patients in less advanced stages of dementia, may improve cognitive abilities and improve functional status [171–173]. The use of electroconvulsive therapy in PD patients with depression has been studied in open-label and case-control trials with improvements favoring treatment, although the common complication of delirium is described [161]. Traditional psychotherapy, behavioral therapy, or counseling may be an option for nondemented or mildly demented, depressed PD patients.

Patient and caregiver education can improve quality of life. Coping strategies can be improved with knowledge of disease processes, natural history, prognosis, treatment options, and possible treatment complications. Caregivers may benefit from referral for psychological support. Educational and respite services can be accessed through community resources, such as the Parkinson's Foundation or Alzheimer's Association. Home assessments to evaluate needs and institute environmental changes to accommodate needs of PD patients often prove beneficial. Nonpharmacologic treatments of PD dementia, depression, and psychosis are summarized in Table 3.

Summary

Cognitive, affective, and psychiatric symptoms in PD are common and associated with significant morbidity and stress for patients and their families. It is important for the clinician to recognize and address these symptoms. Careful use of pharmacologic and nonpharmacologic strategies can improve quality of life.

References

[1] Louis ED. The shaking palsy, the first forty-five years: a journey through the British literature. Mov Disord 1997;12:1068–72.
[2] Fenelon G, Goetz CG, Karenberg A. Hallucinations in Parkinson disease in the prelevodopa era. Neurology 2006;66:93–8.
[3] Cummings JL, Darkins A, Mendez M, et al. Alzheimer's disease and Parkinson's disease: comparison of speech and language alterations. Neurology 1988;38:680–4.

[4] Dooneief G, Bello J, Todak G, et al. A prospective controlled study of magnetic resonance imaging of the brain in gay men and parenteral drug users with human immunodeficiency virus infection. Arch Neurol 1992;49:38–43.

[5] Mayeux R, Stern Y, Rosen J, et al. Depression, intellectual impairment, and Parkinson disease. Neurology 1981;31:645–50.

[6] Tandberg E, Larsen JP, Aarsland D, et al. The occurrence of depression in Parkinson's disease: a community-based study. Arch Neurol 1996;53:175–9.

[7] Aarsland D, Larsen JP, Lim NG, et al. Range of neuropsychiatric disturbances in patients with Parkinson's disease. J Neurol Neurosurg Psychiatry 1999;67:492–6.

[8] Bosboom JL, Stoffers D, Wolters E. Cognitive dysfunction and dementia in Parkinson's disease. J Neural Transm 2004;111:1303–15.

[9] Elmer L. Cognitive issues in Parkinson's disease. Neurol Clin 2004;22:S91–106.

[10] Emre M. What causes mental dysfunction in Parkinson's disease? Mov Disord 2003; 18(Suppl 6):S63–71.

[11] Lauterbach EC. The neuropsychiatry of Parkinson's disease. Minerva Med 2005;96: 155–73.

[12] Muslimovic D, Post B, Speelman JD, et al. Cognitive profile of patients with newly diagnosed Parkinson disease. Neurology 2005;65:1239–45.

[13] American Psychiatric Association. Diagnostic and statistical manual of mental disorders. 4th edition. Washington (DC): American Psychiatric Association; 1994.

[14] Schrag A. Psychiatric aspects of Parkinson's disease—an update. J Neurol 2004;251: 795–804.

[15] Slaughter JR, Slaughter KA, Nichols D, et al. Prevalence, clinical manifestations, etiology, and treatment of depression in Parkinson's disease. J Neuropsychiatry Clin Neurosci 2001; 13:187–96.

[16] Starkstein SE, Mayberg HS, Preziosi TJ, et al. Reliability, validity, and clinical correlates of apathy in Parkinson's disease. J Neuropsychiatry Clin Neurosci 1992;4:134–9.

[17] Leentjens AF, Van den Akker M, Metsemakers JF, et al. Higher incidence of depression preceding the onset of Parkinson's disease: a register study. Mov Disord 2003;18:414–8.

[18] Shiba M, Bower JH, Maraganore DM, et al. Anxiety disorders and depressive disorders preceding Parkinson's disease: a case-control study. Mov Disord 2000;15:669–77.

[19] Nilsson FM, Kessing LV, Sorensen TM, et al. Major depressive disorder in Parkinson's disease: a register-based study. Acta Psychiatr Scand 2002;106:202–11.

[20] Gotham AM, Brown RG, Marsden CD. Depression in Parkinson's disease: a quantitative and qualitative analysis. J Neurol Neurosurg Psychiatry 1986;49:381–9.

[21] Fenelon G, Mahieux F, Huon R, et al. Hallucinations in Parkinson's disease: prevalence, phenomenology and risk factors. Brain 2000;123(Pt 4):733–45.

[22] Marsh L, Williams JR, Rocco M, et al. Psychiatric comorbidities in patients with Parkinson disease and psychosis. Neurology 2004;63:293–300.

[23] Kashihara K, Ohno M, Katsu Y. [Psychoses in patients with Parkinson's disease: their frequency, phenomenology, and clinical correlates]. Rinsho Shinkeigaku 2005;45:1–5.

[24] Merims D, Shabtai H, Korczyn AD, et al. Antiparkinsonian medication is not a risk factor for the development of hallucinations in Parkinson's disease. J Neural Transm 2004;111: 1447–53.

[25] Lieberman A. Managing the neuropsychiatric symptoms of Parkinson's disease. Neurology 1998;50:S33–8 [discussion: S44–8].

[26] Alexander GE, DeLong MR, Strick PL. Parallel organization of functionally segregated circuits linking basal ganglia and cortex. Annu Rev Neurosci 1986;9:357–81.

[27] Lindner MD, Cain CK, Plone MA, et al. Incomplete nigrostriatal dopaminergic cell loss and partial reductions in striatal dopamine produce akinesia, rigidity, tremor and cognitive deficits in middle-aged rats. Behav Brain Res 1999;102:1–16.

[28] Schneider JS, Kovelowski CJ 2nd. Chronic exposure to low doses of MPTP: I. cognitive deficits in motor asymptomatic monkeys. Brain Res 1990;519:122–8.

[29] Morissette M, Goulet M, Grondin R, et al. Associative and limbic regions of monkey striatum express high levels of dopamine D3 receptors: effects of MPTP and dopamine agonist replacement therapies. Eur J Neurosci 1998;10:2565–73.

[30] Steele TD, Hodges DB Jr, Levesque TR, et al. The D1 agonist dihydrexidine releases acetylcholine and improves cognition in rats. Ann N Y Acad Sci 1996;777:427–30.

[31] Kaasinen V, Rinne JO. Functional imaging studies of dopamine system and cognition in normal aging and Parkinson's disease. Neurosci Biobehav Rev 2002;26:785–93.

[32] Rinne JO, Myllykyla T, Lonnberg P, et al. A postmortem study of brain nicotinic receptors in Parkinson's and Alzheimer's disease. Brain Res 1991;547:167–70.

[33] Volkow ND, Wang GJ, Fowler JS, et al. Dopamine transporter occupancies in the human brain induced by therapeutic doses of oral methylphenidate. Am J Psychiatry 1998;155:1325–31.

[34] Kaasinen V, Nagren K, Hietala J, et al. Extrastriatal dopamine D2 and D3 receptors in early and advanced Parkinson's disease. Neurology 2000;54:1482–7.

[35] Antonini A, Schwarz J, Oertel WH, et al. Long-term changes of striatal dopamine D2 receptors in patients with Parkinson's disease: a study with positron emission tomography and [11C]raclopride. Mov Disord 1997;12:33–8.

[36] Kaasinen V, Aalto S, Någren K, et al. Extrastriatal dopamine D(2) receptors in Parkinson's disease: a longitudinal study. J Neural Transm 2003;110:591–601.

[37] Cools R, Barker RA, Sahakian BJ, et al. Enhanced or impaired cognitive function in Parkinson's disease as a function of dopaminergic medication and task demands. Cereb Cortex 2001;11:1136–43.

[38] Gotham AM, Brown RG, Marsden CD. 'Frontal' cognitive function in patients with Parkinson's disease 'on' and 'off' levodopa. Brain 1988;111(Pt 2):299–321.

[39] Lewis SJ, Cools R, Robbins TW, et al. Using executive heterogeneity to explore the nature of working memory deficits in Parkinson's disease. Neuropsychologia 2003;41:645–54.

[40] Swainson R, Rogers RD, Sahakian BJ, et al. Probabilistic learning and reversal deficits in patients with Parkinson's disease or frontal or temporal lobe lesions: possible adverse effects of dopaminergic medication. Neuropsychologia 2000;38:596–612.

[41] Mayberg HS, Starkstein SE, Sadzot B, et al. Selective hypometabolism in the inferior frontal lobe in depressed patients with Parkinson's disease. Ann Neurol 1990;28:57–64.

[42] Ring HA, Bench CJ, Trimble MR, et al. Depression in Parkinson's disease: a positron emission study. Br J Psychiatry 1994;165:333–9.

[43] Moskovitz C, Moses H 3rd, Klawans HL. Levodopa-induced psychosis: a kindling phenomenon. Am J Psychiatry 1978;135:669–75.

[44] Goetz CG, Tanner CM, Klawans HL. Pharmacology of hallucinations induced by long-term drug therapy. Am J Psychiatry 1982;139:494–7.

[45] Robinson TE, Kolb B. Persistent structural modifications in nucleus accumbens and prefrontal cortex neurons produced by previous experience with amphetamine. J Neurosci 1997;17:8491–7.

[46] Birkmayer W, Riederer P. Responsibility of extrastriatal areas for the appearance of psychotic symptoms (clinical and biochemical human post-mortem findings). J Neural Transm 1975;37:175–82.

[47] Wolters EC. Intrinsic and extrinsic psychosis in Parkinson's disease. J Neurol 2001;248(Suppl 3):III22–7.

[48] Perry EK, Marshall E, Kerwin J, et al. Evidence of a monoaminergic-cholinergic imbalance related to visual hallucinations in Lewy body dementia. J Neurochem 1990;55:1454–6.

[49] Jellinger K. The pathology of parkinsonism. In: Marsden CD, Fahn S, editors. Movement disorders. 2nd edition. London: Butterworth's; 1987. p. 124–65.

[50] Cash R, Dennis T, L'Heureux R, et al. Parkinson's disease and dementia: norepinephrine and dopamine in locus ceruleus. Neurology 1987;37:42–6.

[51] Zarow C, Lyness SA, Mortimer JA, et al. Neuronal loss is greater in the locus coeruleus than nucleus basalis and substantia nigra in Alzheimer and Parkinson diseases. Arch Neurol 2003;60:337–41.

[52] Scatton B, Javoy-Agid F, Rouquier L, et al. Reduction of cortical dopamine, noradrena-
line, serotonin and their metabolites in Parkinson's disease. Brain Res 1983;275:321–8.

[53] Stern Y, Mayeux R, Cote L. Reaction time and vigilance in Parkinson's disease: possible
role of altered norepinephrine metabolism. Arch Neurol 1984;41:1086–9.

[54] Chinaglia G, Landwehrmeyer B, Probst A, et al. Serotoninergic terminal transporters are
differentially affected in Parkinson's disease and progressive supranuclear palsy: an autora-
diographic study with [3H]citalopram. Neuroscience 1993;54:691–9.

[55] Paulus W, Jellinger K. The neuropathologic basis of different clinical subgroups of Parkinson's disease. J Neuropathol Exp Neurol 1991;50:743–55.

[56] Mayeux R. The "serotonin hypothesis" for depression in Parkinson's disease. Adv Neurol
1990;53:163–6.

[57] Riedel WJ, Klaassen T, Deutz NE, et al. Tryptophan depletion in normal volunteers produces selective impairment in memory consolidation. Psychopharmacology (Berl) 1999;
141:362–9.

[58] Mayberg HS, Solomon DH. Depression in Parkinson's disease: a biochemical and organic
viewpoint. Adv Neurol 1995;65:49–60.

[59] Torack RM, Morris JC. The association of ventral tegmental area histopathology with
adult dementia. Arch Neurol 1988;45:497–501.

[60] Candy JM, Perry RH, Perry EK, et al. Pathological changes in the nucleus of Meynert in
Alzheimer's and Parkinson's diseases. J Neurol Sci 1983;59:277–89.

[61] Dubois B, Ruberg M, Javoy-Agid F, et al. A subcortico-cortical cholinergic system is affected in Parkinson's disease. Brain Res 1983;288:213–8.

[62] Nakano I, Hirano A. Parkinson's disease: neuron loss in the nucleus basalis without concomitant Alzheimer's disease. Ann Neurol 1984;15:415–8.

[63] Perry EK, Curtis M, Dick DJ, et al. Cholinergic correlates of cognitive impairment in Parkinson's disease: comparisons with Alzheimer's disease. J Neurol Neurosurg Psychiatry
1985;48:413–21.

[64] Rinne JO, Laihinen A, Lonnberg P, et al. A post-mortem study on striatal dopamine receptors in Parkinson's disease. Brain Res 1991;556:117–22.

[65] Whitehouse PJ, Hedreen JC, White CL 3rd, et al. Basal forebrain neurons in the dementia
of Parkinson disease. Ann Neurol 1983;13:243–8.

[66] Pillon B, Boller F, Levy R, et al. Cognitive deficits and dementia in Parkinson's disease. In: Boller F, Cappa S, editors. Handbook of neuropsychology. Amsterdam: Elsevier; 2001. p. 311–71.

[67] Gibb WR, Scott T, Lees AJ. Neuronal inclusions of Parkinson's disease. Mov Disord 1991;
6:2–11.

[68] Duda JE, Giasson BI, Chen Q, et al. Widespread nitration of pathological inclusions in neurodegenerative synucleinopathies. Am J Pathol 2000;157:1439–45.

[69] Lennox G, Lowe J, Landon M, et al. Diffuse Lewy body disease: correlative neuropathology using anti-ubiquitin immunocytochemistry. J Neurol Neurosurg Psychiatry 1989;52:
1236–47.

[70] Spillantini MG, Crowther RA, Jakes R, et al. Alpha-Synuclein in filamentous inclusions of
Lewy bodies from Parkinson's disease and dementia with lewy bodies. Proc Natl Acad Sci
U S A 1998;95:6469–73.

[71] Hurtig HI, Trojanowski JQ, Galvin J, et al. Alpha-synuclein cortical Lewy bodies correlate
with dementia in Parkinson's disease. Neurology 2000;54:1916–21.

[72] Harding AJ, Halliday GM. Cortical Lewy body pathology in the diagnosis of dementia.
Acta Neuropathol (Berl) 2001;102:355–63.

[73] Jellinger KA. Morphological substrates of dementia in parkinsonism: a critical update.
J Neural Transm Suppl 1997;51:57–82.

[74] Hughes AJ, Daniel SE, Blankson S, et al. A clinicopathologic study of 100 cases of Parkinson's disease. Arch Neurol 1993;50:140–8.

[75] Yoshimura M. Cortical changes in the parkinsonian brain: a contribution to the delineation
of "diffuse Lewy body disease." J Neurol 1983;229:17–32.

[76] Apaydin H, Ahlskog JE, Parisi JE, et al. Parkinson disease neuropathology: later-developing dementia and loss of the levodopa response. Arch Neurol 2002;59:102–12.
[77] Colosimo C, Hughes AJ, Kilford L, et al. Lewy body cortical involvement may not always predict dementia in Parkinson's disease. J Neurol Neurosurg Psychiatry 2003;74:852–6.
[78] Richard IH, Papka M, Rubio A, et al. Parkinson's disease and dementia with Lewy bodies: one disease or two? Mov Disord 2002;17:1161–5.
[79] Mastaglia FL, Johnsen RD, Byrnes ML, et al. Prevalence of amyloid-beta deposition in the cerebral cortex in Parkinson's disease. Mov Disord 2003;18:81–6.
[80] Jellinger KA, Seppi K, Wenning GK, et al. Impact of coexistent Alzheimer pathology on the natural history of Parkinson's disease. J Neural Transm 2002;109:329–39.
[81] Kovari E, Gold G, Herrmann FR, et al. Lewy body densities in the entorhinal and anterior cingulate cortex predict cognitive deficits in Parkinson's disease. Acta Neuropathol (Berl) 2003;106:83–8.
[82] Samuel W, Galasko D, Masliah E, et al. Neocortical Lewy body counts correlate with dementia in the Lewy body variant of Alzheimer's disease. J Neuropathol Exp Neurol 1996; 55:44–52.
[83] Aarsland D, Ballard CG, Halliday G. Are Parkinson's disease with dementia and dementia with Lewy bodies the same entity? J Geriatr Psychiatry Neurol 2004;17:137–45.
[84] Geser F, Wenning GK, Poewe W, et al. How to diagnose dementia with Lewy bodies: state of the art. Mov Disord 2005;20(Suppl 12):S11–20.
[85] Londos E, Passant U, Gustafson L, et al. Neuropathological correlates to clinically defined dementia with Lewy bodies. Int J Geriatr Psychiatry 2001;16:667–79.
[86] Trembath Y, Rosenberg C, Ervin JF, et al. Lewy body pathology is a frequent co-pathology in familial Alzheimer's disease. Acta Neuropathol (Berl) 2003;105:484–8.
[87] McKeith IG, Dickson DW, Lowe J, et al. Diagnosis and management of dementia with Lewy bodies: third report of the DLB Consortium. Neurology 2005;65:1863–72.
[88] Aarsland D, Andersen K, Larsen JP, et al. Risk of dementia in Parkinson's disease: a community-based, prospective study. Neurology 2001;56:730–6.
[89] Levy G, Tang MX, Cote LJ, et al. Do risk factors for Alzheimer's disease predict dementia in Parkinson's disease? An exploratory study. Mov Disord 2002;17:250–7.
[90] Stern Y, Marder K, Tang MX, et al. Antecedent clinical features associated with dementia in Parkinson's disease. Neurology 1993;43:1690–2.
[91] Hughes TA, Ross HF, Musa S, et al. A 10-year study of the incidence of and factors predicting dementia in Parkinson's disease. Neurology 2000;54:1596–602.
[92] Aarsland D, Andersen K, Larsen JP, et al. Prevalence and characteristics of dementia in Parkinson disease: an 8-year prospective study. Arch Neurol 2003;60:387–92.
[93] Breteler MM, de Groot RR, van Romunde LK, et al. Risk of dementia in patients with Parkinson's disease, epilepsy, and severe head trauma: a register-based follow-up study. Am J Epidemiol 1995;142:1300–5.
[94] Giladi N, Treves TA, Paleacu D, et al. Risk factors for dementia, depression and psychosis in long-standing Parkinson's disease. J Neural Transm 2000;107:59–71.
[95] Levy G, Schupf N, Tang MX, et al. Combined effect of age and severity on the risk of dementia in Parkinson's disease. Ann Neurol 2002;51:722–9.
[96] Huckvale C, Richardson AM, Mann DM, et al. Debrisoquine hydroxylase gene polymorphism (CYP2D6*4) in dementia with Lewy bodies. J Neurol Neurosurg Psychiatry 2003;74:135–6.
[97] Huang X, Chen P, Kaufer DI, et al. Apolipoprotein E and dementia in Parkinson disease: a meta-analysis. Arch Neurol 2006;63:189–93.
[98] Mayeux R, Stern Y. Intellectual dysfunction and dementia in Parkinson disease. Adv Neurol 1983;38:211–27.
[99] Mortimer JA, Pirozzolo FJ, Hansch EC, et al. Relationship of motor symptoms to intellectual deficits in Parkinson disease. Neurology 1982;32:133–7.
[100] Stacy M, Jankovic J. Differential diagnosis of Parkinson's disease and the parkinsonism plus syndromes. Neurol Clin 1992;10:341–59.

[101] Starkstein SE, Preziosi TJ, Bolduc PL, et al. Depression in Parkinson's disease. J Nerv Ment Dis 1990;178:27–31.
[102] Cummings JL. Depression and Parkinson's disease: a review. Am J Psychiatry 1992;149: 443–54.
[103] Mayeux R, Stern Y, Williams JB, et al. Clinical and biochemical features of depression in Parkinson's disease. Am J Psychiatry 1986;143:756–9.
[104] Henderson R, Kurlan R, Kersun JM, et al. Preliminary examination of the comorbidity of anxiety and depression in Parkinson's disease. J Neuropsychiatry Clin Neurosci 1992;4: 257–64.
[105] Cummings JL. Behavioral complications of drug treatment of Parkinson's disease. J Am Geriatr Soc 1991;39:708–16.
[106] Barnes J, David AS. Visual hallucinations in Parkinson's disease: a review and phenomenological survey. J Neurol Neurosurg Psychiatry 2001;70:727–33.
[107] Goetz CG. Poor Beard! Charcot's internationalization of neurasthenia, the "American disease." Neurology 2001;57:510–4.
[108] Goetz CG, Aminoff MJ. The Brown-Sequard and S. Weir Mitchell letters. Neurology 2001; 57:2100–4.
[109] Goetz CG, Leurgans S, Pappert EJ, et al. Prospective longitudinal assessment of hallucinations in Parkinson's disease. Neurology 2001;57:2078–82.
[110] Holroyd S, Currie L, Wooten GF. Prospective study of hallucinations and delusions in Parkinson's disease. J Neurol Neurosurg Psychiatry 2001;70:734–8.
[111] Litvan I, MacIntyre A, Goetz CG, et al. Accuracy of the clinical diagnoses of Lewy body disease, Parkinson disease, and dementia with Lewy bodies: a clinicopathologic study. Arch Neurol 1998;55:969–78.
[112] Aarsland D, Ballard C, Larsen JP, et al. A comparative study of psychiatric symptoms in dementia with Lewy bodies and Parkinson's disease with and without dementia. Int J Geriatr Psychiatry 2001;16:528–36.
[113] Starkstein SE, Bolduc PL, Mayberg HS, et al. Cognitive impairments and depression in Parkinson's disease: a follow up study. J Neurol Neurosurg Psychiatry 1990;53:597–602.
[114] Troster AI, Paolo AM, Lyons KE, et al. The influence of depression on cognition in Parkinson's disease: a pattern of impairment distinguishable from Alzheimer's disease. Neurology 1995;45:672–6.
[115] Elizan TS, Sroka H, Maker H, et al. Dementia in idiopathic Parkinson's disease: variables associated with its occurrence in 203 patients. J Neural Transm 1986;65:285–302.
[116] Aarsland D, Larsen JP, Tandberg E, et al. Predictors of nursing home placement in Parkinson's disease: a population-based, prospective study. J Am Geriatr Soc 2000;48:938–42.
[117] Levy G, Tang MX, Louis ED, et al. The association of incident dementia with mortality in PD. Neurology 2002;59:1708–13.
[118] Louis ED, Marder K, Cote L, et al. Mortality from Parkinson disease. Arch Neurol 1997; 54:260–4.
[119] Hughes TA, Ross HF, Mindham RH, et al. Mortality in Parkinson's disease and its association with dementia and depression. Acta Neurol Scand 2004;110:118–23.
[120] Slawek J, Derejko M, Lass P. Factors affecting the quality of life of patients with idiopathic Parkinson's disease—a cross-sectional study in an outpatient clinic attendees. Parkinsonism Relat Disord 2005;11:465–8.
[121] Goetz CG, Stebbins GT. Risk factors for nursing home placement in advanced Parkinson's disease. Neurology 1993;43:2227–9.
[122] Wolters EC, Berendse HW. Management of psychosis in Parkinson's disease. Curr Opin Neurol 2001;14:499–504.
[123] Kuzuhara S. Drug-induced psychotic symptoms in Parkinson's disease: problems, management and dilemma. J Neurol 2001;248(Suppl 3):III28–31.
[124] Caap-Ahlgren M, Dehlin O. Factors of importance to the caregiver burden experienced by family caregivers of Parkinson's disease patients. Aging Clin Exp Res 2002;14:371–7.

[125] Happe S, Berger K. The association between caregiver burden and sleep disturbances in partners of patients with Parkinson's disease. Age Ageing 2002;31:349–54.

[126] Obeso JA, Olanow CW, Nutt JG. Levodopa motor complications in Parkinson's disease. Trends Neurosci 2000;23:S2–7.

[127] Dubois B, Pillon B. Cognitive deficits in Parkinson's disease. J Neurol 1997;244:2–8.

[128] Emre M. Dementia associated with Parkinson's disease. Lancet Neurol 2003;2:229–37.

[129] Emre M. Dementia in Parkinson's disease: cause and treatment. Curr Opin Neurol 2004;17: 399–404.

[130] Smith EE, Jonides J. Storage and executive processes in the frontal lobes. Science 1999;283: 1657–61.

[131] Boller F, Passafiume D, Keefe NC, et al. Visuospatial impairment in Parkinson's disease: role of perceptual and motor factors. Arch Neurol 1984;41:485–90.

[132] Bowen FP, Hoehn MM, Yahr MD. Parkinsonism: alterations in spatial orientation as determined by a route-walking test. Neuropsychologia 1972;10:355–61.

[133] Hovestadt A, de Jong GJ, Meerwaldt JD. Spatial disorientation as an early symptom of Parkinson's disease. Neurology 1987;37:485–7.

[134] Aarsland D, Litvan I, Salmon D, et al. Performance on the dementia rating scale in Parkinson's disease with dementia and dementia with Lewy bodies: comparison with progressive supranuclear palsy and Alzheimer's disease. J Neurol Neurosurg Psychiatry 2003;74:1215–20.

[135] Serrano C, Garcia-Borreguero D. Fluctuations in cognition and alertness in Parkinson's disease and dementia. Neurology 2004;63:S31–4.

[136] Mayeux R, Stern Y, Sano M, et al. Clinical and biochemical correlates of bradyphrenia in Parkinson's disease. Neurology 1987;37:1130–4.

[137] Stenager EN, Wermuth L, Stenager E, et al. Suicide in patients with Parkinson's disease: an epidemiological study. Acta Psychiatr Scand 1994;90:70–2.

[138] Walsh K, Bennett G. Parkinson's disease and anxiety. Postgrad Med J 2001;77:89–93.

[139] Poewe W. Psychosis in Parkinson's disease. Mov Disord 2003;18(Suppl 6):S80–7.

[140] Bosboom JL, Wolters E. Psychotic symptoms in Parkinson's disease: pathophysiology and management. Expert Opin Drug Saf 2004;3:209–20.

[141] Burns A, Lawlor B, Craig S. Rating scales in old age psychiatry. Br J Psychiatry 2002;180: 161–7.

[142] Feher EP, Mahurin RK, Doody RS, et al. Establishing the limits of the Mini-Mental State. Examination of 'subtests.' Arch Neurol 1992;49:87–92.

[143] Marinus J, Visser M, Verwey NA, et al. Assessment of cognition in Parkinson's disease. Neurology 2003;61:1222–8.

[144] Knopman DS, DeKosky ST, Cummings JL, et al. Practice parameter: diagnosis of dementia (an evidence-based review). Report of the Quality Standards Subcommittee of the American Academy of Neurology. Neurology 2001;56:1143–53.

[145] Roman GC, Tatemichi TK, Erkinjuntti T, et al. Vascular dementia: diagnostic criteria for research studies. Report of the NINDS-AIREN International Workshop. Neurology 1993; 43:250–60.

[146] McKhann GM, Albert MS, Grossman M, et al. Clinical and pathological diagnosis of frontotemporal dementia: report of the Work Group on Frontotemporal Dementia and Pick's Disease. Arch Neurol 2001;58:1803–9.

[147] Burn DJ, McKeith IG. Current treatment of dementia with Lewy bodies and dementia associated with Parkinson's disease. Mov Disord 2003;18(Suppl 6):S72–9.

[148] Aarsland D, Laake K, Larsen JP, et al. Donepezil for cognitive impairment in Parkinson's disease: a randomised controlled study. J Neurol Neurosurg Psychiatry 2002;72:708–12.

[149] Emre M, Aarsland D, Albanese A, et al. Rivastigmine for dementia associated with Parkinson's disease. N Engl J Med 2004;351:2509–18.

[150] McKeith IG, Grace JB, Walker Z, et al. Rivastigmine in the treatment of dementia with Lewy bodies: preliminary findings from an open trial. Int J Geriatr Psychiatry 2000;15: 387–92.

[151] Poewe W. Treatment of dementia with Lewy bodies and Parkinson's disease dementia. Mov Disord 2005;20(Suppl 12):S77–82.

[152] Singleton AB, Gibson AM, Edwardson JA, et al. Butyrylcholinesterase K: an association with dementia with Lewy bodies. Lancet 1998;351:1818.

[153] Andersen J, Aabro E, Gulmann N, et al. Anti-depressive treatment in Parkinson's disease: a controlled trial of the effect of nortriptyline in patients with Parkinson's disease treated with L-DOPA. Acta Neurol Scand 1980;62:210–9.

[154] Treatment of depression in idiopathic Parkinson's disease. Mov Disord 2002;17(Suppl 4): S112–9.

[155] Ceravolo R, Nuti A, Piccinni A, et al. Paroxetine in Parkinson's disease: effects on motor and depressive symptoms. Neurology 2000;55:1216–8.

[156] Dell'Agnello G, Ceravolo R, Nuti A, et al. SSRIs do not worsen Parkinson's disease: evidence from an open-label, prospective study. Clin Neuropharmacol 2001;24:221–7.

[157] Rampello L, Chiechio S, Raffaele R, et al. The SSRI, citalopram, improves bradykinesia in patients with Parkinson's disease treated with L-dopa. Clin Neuropharmacol 2002;25:21–4.

[158] Tesei S, Antonini A, Canesi M, et al. Tolerability of paroxetine in Parkinson's disease: a prospective study. Mov Disord 2000;15:986–9.

[159] Richard IH, Kurlan R, Tanner C, et al. Serotonin syndrome and the combined use of deprenyl and an antidepressant in Parkinson's disease. Parkinson Study Group. Neurology 1997;48:1070–7.

[160] de Smet Y, Ruberg M, Serdaru M, et al. Confusion, dementia and anticholinergics in Parkinson's disease. J Neurol Neurosurg Psychiatry 1982;45:1161–4.

[161] Drugs to treat dementia and psychosis: management of Parkinson's disease. Mov Disord 2002;17(Suppl 4):S120–7.

[162] Friedman JH, Factor SA. Atypical antipsychotics in the treatment of drug-induced psychosis in Parkinson's disease. Mov Disord 2000;15:201–11.

[163] Ballard C, Grace J, McKeith I, et al. Neuroleptic sensitivity in dementia with Lewy bodies and Alzheimer's disease. Lancet 1998;351:1032–3.

[164] McKeith I, Fairbairn A, Perry R, et al. Neuroleptic sensitivity in patients with senile dementia of Lewy body type. BMJ 1992;305:673–8.

[165] Low-dose clozapine for the treatment of drug-induced psychosis in Parkinson's disease. The Parkinson Study Group. N Engl J Med 1999;340:757–63.

[166] Clozapine in drug-induced psychosis in Parkinson's disease. The French Clozapine Parkinson Study Group. Lancet 1999;353:2041–2.

[167] Goetz CG, Blasucci LM, Leurgans S, et al. Olanzapine and clozapine: comparative effects on motor function in hallucinating PD patients. Neurology 2000;55:789–94.

[168] Fernandez HH, Trieschmann ME, Burke MA, et al. Quetiapine for psychosis in Parkinson's disease versus dementia with Lewy bodies. J Clin Psychiatry 2002;63:513–5.

[169] Morgante L, Epifanio A, Spina E, et al. Quetiapine and clozapine in parkinsonian patients with dopaminergic psychosis. Clin Neuropharmacol 2004;27:153–6.

[170] Bullock R, Cameron A. Rivastigmine for the treatment of dementia and visual hallucinations associated with Parkinson's disease: a case series. Curr Med Res Opin 2002;18:258–64.

[171] Hausdorff JM, Balash J, Giladi N. Effects of cognitive challenge on gait variability in patients with Parkinson's disease. J Geriatr Psychiatry Neurol 2003;16:53–8.

[172] Rubinstein TC, Giladi N, Hausdorff JM. The power of cueing to circumvent dopamine deficits: a review of physical therapy treatment of gait disturbances in Parkinson's disease. Mov Disord 2002;17:1148–60.

[173] Weiner WJ, Singer C. Parkinson's disease and nonpharmacologic treatment programs. J Am Geriatr Soc 1989;37:359–63.

ELSEVIER
SAUNDERS

Clin Geriatr Med 22 (2006) 797–812

CLINICS IN
GERIATRIC
MEDICINE

Postural Control, Gait, and Dopamine Functions in Parkinsonian Movement Disorders

Nicolaas I. Bohnen, MD, PhD[a],*, Rakié Cham, PhD[b]

[a]Departments of Radiology and Neurology, Functional Neuroimaging,
Cognitive and Mobility Laboratory, University of Michigan, 24 Frank Lloyd Wright Drive,
Box 362, Ann Arbor, MI 48106, USA
[b]Department of Bioengineering, Human Movement and Balance Laboratory,
University of Pittsburgh, 740 Benedum Hall, 3700 O'Hara Street, Pittsburgh, PA 15261, USA

Falling is a trademark of Parkinson's disease (PD). Almost 7 in 10 patients who have PD fall at least once each year [1]. The risk for falls in PD is a bell-shaped function of disease severity [2], reaching a maximum near Hoehn and Yahr stage 3 and decreasing in later stages because of immobilization [3,4]. Unlike falls in the general population that often result from slipping or tripping incidents, most falls in PD occur during walking, stopping, turning, standing up, and bending down maneuvers [5,6]. Clinical characteristics of parkinsonian locomotor patterns include a slow gait and a reduced angular excursion of the joints, such as those of the shoulder, knee, and trunk [7,8]. As the disease progresses, stooped posture, short steps, shuffling often resulting in reduced ground clearance, and festination become characteristic features of the parkinsonian gait [8–10].

Falls and balance impairment are largely unresponsive to L-dopa therapy. However, some gait abnormalities, such as stride length and gait velocity, can be improved with dopaminergic treatments [7,11–13]. Unfortunately, most postural control impairments associated with falls are resistance to treatment [12,14,15]. Balance impairments may even be worsened by the adverse effects of dopaminergic medication, such as orthostatic hypotension, violent dyskinesias, and confusion [16].

* Corresponding author.
E-mail address: nbohnen@umich.edu (N.I. Bohnen).

Normal postural control and locomotor functions

Walking necessitates complex neurobiomechanical processes involved in maintaining upright posture, initiating and terminating gait, and moving the body toward the desired location. When faced with balance perturbations, such as environmental changes or new task initiation, fast and appropriate postural corrective responses are required to prevent a fall. Various sensory, central neural, and motor systems work together to generate these responses [17]. This article reviews only the systems that are believed to be most affected by dopamine depletions and PD.

Postural control

Effective integration of sensory information about the visuospatial environment and body and limb position is essential for postural control. For example, standing posture is affected by perturbations to the visual, vestibular, and proprioceptive sensory systems [18–20]. Another correlate of these findings is that sensory information is used in a feedback control scheme to provide information about the body state. Evidence exists that the central nervous system (CNS) uses a "sensory re-weighting" strategy when integrating sensory channels, which may provide similar but also conflicting or inaccurate sensory information [20–22]. For example, if an individual is standing on a platform that rotates in the sagittal plane such that the ankle angle is always maintained at 90° (ie, ankle proprioceptive information related to body tilt is not reliable), and the eyes are closed (ie, no visual information), then the CNS must rely on vestibular inputs and ignore the destabilizing ankle proprioceptive channel to maintain balance [22]. In this example, the CNS must increase the "weight" of the vestibular channel and reduce the weight of the proprioceptive and visual channels [22].

The basal ganglia's specific role in postural control is complex and only beginning to be unraveled. Visser and Bloem [23] recently compiled evidence on how the postural control and locomotor systems are affected in people and animals that have basal ganglia lesions. In summary, the basal ganglia are believed to be involved in various aspects of postural control, including

1. Sensory channel integration
2. Selection of automatic postural reactions generated in response to motor and sensory perturbations (eg, moving visual environments)
3. Motor control flexibility and adaptability (ie, appropriate corrective postural reactions generated in an attempt to prevent a fall are dependent on the characteristics of the perturbation and environmental changes)
4. Regulation of muscle tone
5. Modulation of the impact of cognitive factors on balance and gait (eg, attention, multitasking, knowledge or expectation of a potential perturbation, fear of falling) [23]

In addition to these functional models of motor and postural control, several information processing theories have been proposed. One theory is that the function of the basal ganglia is to filter cortical input and feed back relevant output to the frontal cortex [24]. Another theory is that the basal ganglia act as a controller involving a desired model output and an error distribution system [25]. The clinical insights that these novel hypotheses provide have not been thoroughly examined.

Locomotor system

The stereotypic propulsive locomotor system is composed of a supraspinal part that initiates locomotion and maintains a certain degree of drive to the spinal networks generating the motor pattern [26]. Spinal networks are composed of excitatory and inhibitory interneurons that activate different groups of motor neurons in the appropriate sequence [26]. Stimulation of this network results in rhythmic alteration between flexor and extensor muscles. This basic reflex system is present even in anencephalic infants. Spinal cats that have been deafferented can be made to walk on the treadmill by the intravenous administration of L-dopa, which stimulates monoaminergic descending pathways from the brainstem [27]. Although the spinal pattern generators can produce basic locomotor rhythm, brainstem structures are necessary to activate and regulate the rhythm. The brain stem–spinal cord organization simplifies the control task for the brain, which only must decide when to locomote and the general level of activity [28].

The pedunculopontine nucleus (PPN) is a brainstem nucleus that probably plays a central role in generating movement [29]. The PPN is located in the dorsolateral part of the pontomesencephalic tegmentum [30] and is composed of two groups of neurons: one containing acetylcholine and the other containing noncholinergic neurotransmitters (eg, γ-aminobutyric acid, glutamate). The PPN is connected reciprocally with the limbic system, basal ganglia nuclei (eg, globus pallidus, substantia nigra, subthalamic nucleus), thalamus, and brainstem reticular formation [29]. The caudally directed corticolimbic–ventral striatal–ventral pallidal–PPN–pontomedullary reticular nuclei–spinal cord pathway seems to be involved in the initiation, acceleration, deceleration, and termination of locomotion [30]. During locomotion the cerebellum contributes to the timing adjustment of limb movements. The basal ganglia and thalamic circuits have reciprocal connections with the cortex [31]. In the natural, constantly varying environment, the discharge of motor cortical neurons is the result of interplay between the central and peripheral feedback signals ascending from the spinal cord and a feed-forward signal that provides information about the environment. The motor cortex control may range from subtle modifications to complete control of gait when walking over uneven ground [32].

Nigrostriatal dopaminergic denervation in Parkinson's disease

PD is a predominant nigrostriatal denervation syndrome resulting in a variable combination of clinical symptoms of tremor, rigidity, bradykinesia, and postural imbalance [33]. The greater the neuronal loss is in the substantia nigra, the lower the concentration of dopamine in the striatum and the more severe the parkinsonian symptoms [34]. Dopaminergic denervation is not evenly distributed in the striatum in PD. A posterior-to-anterior gradient exists, with the posterior putamen being more affected than the caudate [35]. Neurochemical imaging studies have also shown asymmetric nigrostriatal degeneration with more severe striatal dopaminergic losses contralateral to the clinically most affected body side [36]. In addition to presynaptic changes in the nigrostriatal neurons, postsynaptic striatal dopamine receptors alter in PD (Table 1). For instance, in early idiopathic PD, uptake of the D_2 receptor ligand ^{11}C-raclopride increases in the striatum contralateral to the predominant symptoms of PD, compared with uptake in the opposite striatum [37]. The relative increase in ^{11}C-raclopride binding may persist for 3 to 5 years after initial diagnosis, but may then decrease in patients who have more chronic idiopathic PD [37].

Although nigrostriatal dopaminergic denervation is a key pathobiologic mechanism in PD, evidence also exists of degeneration of other monoaminergic (serotonin and norepinephrine) and cholinergic systems [38]. For example, denervation of the cholinergic pedunculopontine nucleus in the brainstem has been implicated in the cause of the dopamine-resistant akinesia, such as gait ignition failure and freezing, in PD [39].

Pathophysiology of postural control and locomotor deficits in Parkinson's disease

Numerous standing and gait studies, motivated by the high incidence of falls in PD, have investigated the impact of PD on postural control and gait. Table 2 provides a summary of the major abnormalities in PD and the impact of L-dopa therapy on these abnormalities.

Table 1

Pre-and postsynaptic dopaminergic activity in idiopathic Parkinson's disease and atypical parkinsonism

	Presynaptic dopaminergic nigrostriatal innervation	Postsynaptic striatal dopamine receptor activity
Early idiopathic PD	↓	↑
Advanced PD	↓	↓
Atypical parkinsonism (eg, PSP or MSA)	↓	↓

Abbreviations: MSA, multiple systems atrophy; PSP, progressive supranuclear palsy; ↓, decreased activity; ↑, increased activity.

Standing balance

Spatial, velocity, and frequency characteristics of body sway during quiet (unperturbed) standing is abnormal in PD [40–43]. L-Dopa treatments improve some quiet standing sway abnormalities, but worsen others [40–42,44] (see Table 2). Postural reactions generated in response to external sensory and motor perturbations during standing are also impaired in PD. Visual destabilizing environments, such as moving scenes, yielded more pronounced body movements in patients who had PD than in controls [40,45]. Rotating the supporting floor in such a way that the ankle angle is kept nearly constant at 90° (ie, distorting proprioceptive inputs from the ankle) increased body sway in patients who had untreated PD compared with controls, particularly when vision is blocked, and these effects intensified with L-dopa treatment [42]. Other investigators exploited Achilles tendon–vibration protocols, which provide erroneous somatosensory inputs, but no significant sway differences were reported between patients medicated with L-dopa and age-matched controls under eyes-open and -closed conditions [44]. Motor perturbations such as "toes up" base-of-support tilts induced greater destabilizing body displacements, increased the gastrocnemius' medium latency, and delayed and reduced overall corrective responses in patients who had PD when they were not receiving dopaminergic treatment [46]. In general, these deficits either worsened or were not affected by dopaminergic therapies [40,46].

PD impairs (at least partially) the postural central set, which refers to the capacity of the nervous system to modulate postural adjustments that are adaptive or anticipatory in nature. Automatic postural adjustments generated in response to repeated exposures to erroneous ankle vibratory inputs were deemed normal in PD [44]. However, Bronstein and colleagues [45] suggested that the adaptive postural behavior is impaired in treated patients who have PD when they are repeatedly subjected to moving scenes. These findings are supported by other researchers using motor perturbations [43,47]. Thus, patients who have PD appear to be able to disregard some but not all types of balance-threatening inputs, even with repeated exposure. Dopaminergic therapies have limited impact on these adaptive postural reactions.

Gait

In addition to the clinical features of the parkinsonian gait mentioned earlier, other gait abnormalities exist in PD [48]. For example, gait variability often considered reflective of the ability to regulate gait deteriorates in PD [14,49,50]. One example of temporal gait variability relates to swing-phase duration in the gait cycle. Swing phase is the gait period when the left or right foot is not in contact with the floor (ie, starting at toe off and ends at heel contact). Yogev and colleagues [51] reported on the increased swing-phase duration variability in patients who have PD compared with controls. Gait kinetics are also abnormal in parkinsonian gait (see Table 2) [52].

Table 2
Summary of major postural and gait abnormalities in Parkinson's disease and the effects of L-dopa therapy on these abnormalities

Stance/Gait	General findings in Parkinson's disease compared with controls	Effects of L-dopa therapy
Quiet standing	Some disagreement in literature: Maurer and colleagues [40], reported increased sway whereas others suggested otherwise [42,43]. Increased sway velocity and frequency [40], with significant left/right asymmetries [41]	Reduces abnormalities in sway velocity/frequency [40,41]. Increases sway magnitude, especially in medial–lateral direction [40–42,44]. Worsens left/right asymmetry [41]
Standing/sensory perturbations (visual and/or proprioceptive perturbations)	Some disagreement in literature related to sway in the absence of vision: Sway normal [40,42,44,45]. Reduced sway [43]. Moving visual environments: Increased sway [40,45]. Floor sway-referenced (ie, ankles kept ~90°): Increased sway [42]. Achilles tendon vibration: Sway normal [44]	Increases sway [42]
Standing/motor perturbations (floor translations and/or rotations)	Floor rotations "toes up" [46]: Greater destabilizing body displacements, Increased gastrocnemius' medium latency, Delayed/reduced overall corrective responses. In contrast, floor translations [43]: Normal EMG latencies	Worsens or does not affect impairments [40,46]
Postural central set (adaptability/flexibility)	Repeated exposures to erroneous ankle vibratory inputs normal [44]. Repeated exposures to moving scenes impaired [45]. Repeated exposure to motor perturbations impaired [43,47]	Treatment-resistant

Gait	Steady state gait	Improves (closer to normal) stride length, gait velocity, rigidity and joint angular amplitudes [7,11–13,62]
	Reduced walking speed and short steps [7]	Temporal parameters, kinetic abnormalities and gait variability are treatment resistant [12,14,52]
	Reduced joint angular excursions [7]	Findings debated in literature [7,49,63]
	Stooped posture and gait shuffling resulting in reduced ground clearance and festination [8–10]	
	Increased gait variability [49,94]	
	Kinetic abnormalities [52]	
	Gait facilitated by simple sensory cueing (eg, visual or auditory) [53–57]	
	Complex tasks (eg, gait initiation, stops, turns):	
	Gait initiation: longer times to turn off postural muscles, reduced propulsion forces, reduced lateral body displacement over the supporting limb, reduced safety margin between the body's center of mass and the supporting area around the feet [58,60,61]	
	Turning: increased number of steps required to turn [48]	

Comparison of findings across studies may be limited. Although some studies used medicated patients, others did not. Also, the use of medication was not always reported in studies.

Gait in PD is facilitated (improved spatiotemporal characteristics) by simple sensory cues (eg, visual [guiding stripes on the floor], auditory) [53–57]. One interpretation of the beneficial impact of appropriate sensory cueing is that the dopamine-depleted basal ganglia is unable to integrate internal/external cues critical to gait and balance (sensory integration deficits) and that simple sensory cueing enhances this ability. An alternative explanation is that accurate external cues facilitate the focus of attentional resources on balance/gait during complex or simultaneous tasks and enable accurate visuospatial orientation.

PD also affects complex gait activities, such as gait initiation, breaking, and turning, which are gait tasks requiring coordinated sequential/simultaneous motor programs essential to maintain equilibrium and generate new movements. Healthy controls are able to harmoniously perform such complex motor tasks, whereas this ability is often impaired in patients who have PD, resulting in freezing, instability, and falls [9,10,58,59]. Examples of PD abnormalities observed during gait initiation include longer times needed to turn off postural muscles delaying movements, reduced propulsion forces, reduced lateral loading over the supporting limb, and reduced safety margin between the body's center of mass and the supporting area around the feet even in early stages of the disease [58,60,61].

Postural control strategies adopted by patients who have PD during stop-and-turn maneuvers have rarely been investigated. However, it is clinically known that patients who have PD have difficulty stopping and turning, especially in confined spaces [8]. The number of steps these patients take to turn is also greater compared with control subjects [48].

The modulating role of L-dopa therapy is of limited effectiveness when gait is a concern. Although some gait parameters, such as stride length, gait velocity, and movement amplitudes, improve with dopaminergic treatment [7,11–13,62], other characteristics, including temporal parameters (eg, cadence, swing and stance duration), kinetic abnormalities, and gait variability, are resistant to treatment [12,14,15]. Some of these findings are debated in the literature [7,49,63]. However, current concepts acknowledge that the effect of L-dopa treatment on balance and gait is limited by a ceiling effect as the disease progresses [62], suggesting postsynaptic dopaminergic denervation or partial implication of nondopaminergic lesions in postural control.

Nonmotor cognitive and visual deficits relevant to postural control and gait in Parkinson's disease

Cognitive impairment in Parkinson's disease and interference effects of dual-tasking on gait and balance

Selective cognitive impairments, especially executive and attentional deficits, are commonly present in patients who have PD [64,65]. These abnormalities might result from fundamental deficits involving the allocation of attentional resources, or the maintenance of representations in working memory [65,66]. Because of the primary basal ganglia involvement in PD, some experts have asserted that impairments in frontal executive functions and visuospatial deficits found in PD are mainly attributable to a dopaminergic loss [67]. However, cognitive slowing in patients who had PD and no dementia performing a complex visual discrimination task did not respond to L-dopa [68], suggesting that cognitive impairment in PD is multifactorial in nature and that alterations in other neurotransmitter systems may be responsible for some of the cognitive deficits in PD [69]. In addition to the well-known reductions in dopamine, norepinephrine, and serotonin, convergent evidence exists for alterations in cholinergic neurotransmission in PD, which has been associated with executive cognitive impairment [70].

Dual-tasking represents an executive type of cognitive function that is heavily dependent on basic operations of working memory and attention [71]. Gait and balance are challenged in patients who have PD when they must perform secondary tasks, which may lead to increased gait variability [51,72,73]. Significant differences in dual-task interference effects of cognitive or complex sensorimotor tasks (eg, carrying a tray) on gait parameters have been reported in PD [74–76]. Camicioli and colleagues [74] examined the effects of a simultaneous verbal fluency task on walking in patients who had PD who experienced gait freezing and found that these patients exhibited a greater increase in the number of steps to complete the walk with verbal fluency, even when the effect of medication was taken into account. However, Bloem and colleagues [77] suggested that the task of walking when talking is a poor predictor of falls in patients who have PD who are cognitively normal. Thus, the comorbid presence of cognitive impairment, especially the limited ability of dual-tasking, may negatively affect gait and postural control functions in PD [4,78].

Visual, visuospatial, and oculomotor functions in Parkinson's disease

Balance and gait deficits in patients who have PD may also be partially caused by various types of visual dysfunction found in PD, such as impaired ability to perceive colors, reduced dynamic visual contrast sensitivity, and edge-detection disability, which some experts have suggested result from dopamine deficiencies in the retina and are sometimes reversed by L-dopa treatments [79,80]. Functional neuroimaging studies have also shown reduced activity in the occipital lobe in PD, which may be related to visuoperceptual difficulties [79,81].

Dopamine impacts visuospatial orientation abilities. Studies have shown that left/right asymmetries in striatal dopamine availability is associated with preferred turning/veering toward the side with less dopamine, or in other words, with preferential spatial orientation away from the cerebral hemisphere side with more dopamine [82,83]. As a result, the basal ganglia's impaired ability to integrate sensorimotor information has been suggested to be at the source of the parkinsonian deficits related to spatial orientation [84]. Some experts suspect that dopaminergic lesions in the left hemisphere will cause less neglect than lesions in the right hemisphere. Left hemi-neglect is predominant in PD with right brain–predominant dopamine depletion. Thus, patients may veer more when they turn to the left visuospatial field than to the right [83]. A relationship exists between visuospatial disturbances and oculomotor abnormalities, such as hypometric saccades and slowing of maximum saccadic velocity [85–88].

Potential causes of dopaminergic treatment resistance on parkinsonian imbalance

PD provides a hypodopaminergic model for further experimental research into the functional role of the dopaminergic system of the basal ganglia in postural control. The impact of dopamine loss on postural instability is often debated in the literature because of several balance-related deficits resistant to L-dopa treatments. Thus, based on those findings and the fact that falls occur most often in mobile patients who have moderately advanced PD and during the medicated "on" state [5], nondopaminergic lesions and extrastriatal dopaminergic deficits have been hypothesized to be the major cause of balance and gait abnormalities in PD. However, this hypothesis can be challenged by several factors.

First, dopaminergic therapy is dependent on the availability of postsynaptic dopamine receptors. In early PD, dopamine receptors are up-regulated to compensate for presynaptic deficits [89]. However, as the disease progresses, these patients also lose postsynaptic dopamine receptors, thus decreasing dopamine binding and resulting in less effective dopaminergic therapies [89]. Second, dopaminergic treatments improve some aspects of postural control in PD, especially during the performance of centrally initiated tasks or generation of voluntary movements [90]. Third, patients who do not have PD who have dopaminergic lesions have postural abnormalities similar to those observed in patients who have PD [90]. Thus, the role of dopamine in postural control appears important; however, the specifics of this role are unclear. Additionally, dopaminergic drugs have been associated with increasing risk for falls. However, the impact of L-dopa on postural control may be confounded by secondary factors. For example, falls in PD often occur while patients consider their symptoms under control [1] (ie, improved mobility while in a medicated "on" state). Patients often tend to become overactive in an "on" state before fluctuating to a less mobile "off" state. The medicated "on" state can also be complicated by involuntary truncal movements (dyskinesias), which may limit effective center-of-mass or center-of-gravity control. Furthermore, the impact of L-dopa on balance and gait is dependent on several aspects of its pharmacology, including its short half-time (<2–3 hours), which results in highly fluctuating dopamine brain levels even in patients who are fully medicated, and its delayed kick-in and early wearing off effects (motor fluctuations). The highly variable brain dopamine levels throughout the day in patients who have PD may somewhat explain the apparent lack of effect of dopaminergic therapy on balance and gait functions. Finally, some mobility deficits might only be seemingly L-dopa–resistant, because dose-limiting side-effects in advanced disease stages prevent clinicians from prescribing adequate dosages to overcome the increasing underlying dopaminergic deficit.

Atypical parkinsonian disorders

Although idiopathic PD accounts for most patients who have parkinsonian symptoms, parkinsonism can also be seen with other neurodegenerative disorders, such as progressive supranuclear palsy (PSP) and multiple systems atrophy (MSA). Idiopathic PD distinguishes itself from other parkinsonian syndromes by marked left–right asymmetry in symptom severity and good symptomatic response to L-dopa therapy [33]. The additional presence of certain clinical findings may raise the clinical suspicion for an atypical parkinsonian syndrome [33]. For example, PSP is an atypical parkinsonian syndrome characterized by falls predominantly in the backward direction, severe gait and balance impairments occurring in early stages of the disease, and supranuclear gaze palsy. MSA presents as a clinical spectrum of parkinsonism in variable combination with symptoms of cerebellar ataxia and dysautonomia. Presynaptic dopaminergic denervation seen in patients who have PD has also been shown in those who have MSA or PSP [91–93]. However, unlike up-regulation of postsynaptic dopamine receptors in early idiopathic PD, expression of dopamine receptors is generally decreased in patients who have atypical parkinsonism (see Table 1) [93], which also explains the limited clinical effectiveness of dopaminergic pharmacotherapy in atypical parkinsonian disorders. In addition to more prominent postsynaptic dopamine receptor losses, degeneration of other neural systems, such as cerebellar ataxia in MSA and the supranuclear gaze palsy and axial dystonia (limited ability to visually explore the environment) in PSP, further contribute to the balance impairments in these disorders.

Summary

Postural instability is an important contributor to incapacitation in patients who have parkinsonian disorders. The precise underlying mechanisms of postural instability in these disorders are not fully understood. Several hypothesized integrative functions of the basal ganglia and its dopaminergic system have been proposed; however, those theories have not been fully validated using balance-related experimental data. Because the effectiveness of traditional dopaminergic therapies in reducing falls is limited and often debated in the literature, little agreement exists on how to intervene to address postural deficits. One explanation for the limited effectiveness of dopaminergic pharmacotherapy is loss of postsynaptic dopaminergic receptors with advancing PD and in atypical parkinsonian disorders. Nonmotor cognitive and visual disturbances are now being recognized as new risk factors for falls in PD. Recent evidence also suggests degeneration of the cholinergic pedunculopontine nucleus in PD, which has been associated with akinesia, including gait ignition failure and gait freezing, in this disorder. Degeneration of other neural systems, such as cerebellar ataxia in MSA and the supranuclear gaze palsy in PSP, further contribute to the balance impairments in these atypical parkinsonian disorders.

References

[1] Bloem BR, Steijns JA, Smits-Engelsman BC. An update on falls. Curr Opin Neurol 2003;16: 15–26.
[2] Pickering RM, Mazibrada G, Wood BH, et al. A meta-analysis of six prospective studies of falls in Parkinson's disease. Mov Disord 2004;19:S262.
[3] Bloem BR, van Vugt JP, Beckley DJ. Postural instability and falls in Parkinson's disease. Adv Neurol 2001;87:209–23.
[4] Wood BH, Bilclough JA, Bowron A, et al. Incidence and prediction of falls in Parkinson's disease: a prospective multidisciplinary study. J Neurol Neurosurg Psychiatry 2002;72: 721–5.
[5] Bloem BR, Grimbergen YA, Cramer M, et al. Prospective assessment of falls in Parkinson's disease. J Neurol 2001;248:950–8.
[6] Morris ME. Movement disorders in people with Parkinson disease: a model for physical therapy. Phys Ther 2000;80:578–97.
[7] Azulay JP, Van Den Brand C, Mestre D, et al. Automatic motion analysis of gait in patients with Parkinson disease: effects of levodopa and visual stimulations. Rev Neurol (Paris) 1996; 152:128–34 [in French].
[8] Kemoun G, Defebvre L. Clinical description, analysis of posture, initiation of stabilized gait. Presse Med 2001;30:452–9 [in French].
[9] Murray MP, Sepic SB, Gardner GM, et al. Walking patterns of men with parkinsonism. Am J Phys Med 1978;57:278–94.
[10] Nieuwboer A, Dom R, De Weerdt W, et al. Abnormalities of the spatiotemporal characteristics of gait at the onset of freezing in Parkinson's disease. Mov Disord 2001;16:1066–75.
[11] Bowes SG, Clark PK, Leeman AL, et al. Determinants of gait in the elderly parkinsonian on maintenance levodopa/carbidopa therapy. Br J Clin Pharmacol 1990;30:13–24.
[12] O'Sullivan JD, Said CM, Dillon LC, et al. Gait analysis in patients with Parkinson's disease and motor fluctuations: influence of levodopa and comparison with other measures of motor function. Mov Disord 1998;13:900–6.
[13] Shan DE, Lee SJ, Chao LY, et al. Gait analysis in advanced Parkinson's disease—effect of levodopa and tolcapone. Can J Neurol Sci 2001;28:70–5.
[14] Blin O, Ferrandez AM, Pailhous J, et al. Dopa-sensitive and dopa-resistant gait parameters in Parkinson's disease. J Neurol Sci 1991;103:51–4.
[15] Ebersbach G, Heijmenberg M, Kindermann L, et al. Interference of rhythmic constraint on gait in healthy subjects and patients with early Parkinson's disease: evidence for impaired locomotor pattern generation in early Parkinson's disease. Mov Disord 1999;14:619–25.
[16] Bloem BR, Bhatia KP. Gait and balance in basal ganglia disorders. In: Bronstein AM, Brandt T, Nutt JG, et al, editors. Clinical disorders of balance, posture, and gait. 2nd edition. London: Arnold; 2004. p. 173–206.

[17] Bronstein AM, Brandt J, Woollacott MH. Clinical disorders of balance, postural control and gait. 1st edition. London: Arnold; 1996.

[18] Latt LD, Sparto PJ, Furman JM, et al. The steady-state postural response to continuous sinusoidal galvanic vestibular stimulation. Gait Posture 2003;18:64–72.

[19] Horak FB, Shupert CL, Dietz V, et al. Vestibular and somatosensory contributions to responses to head and body displacements in stance. Exp Brain Res 1994;100:93–106.

[20] Mahboobin A, Loughlin PJ, Redfern MS, et al. Sensory re-weighting in human postural control during moving-scene perturbations. Exp Brain Res 2005;167:260–7.

[21] Peterka RJ, Loughlin PJ. Dynamic regulation of sensorimotor integration in human postural control. J Neurophysiol 2004;91:410–23.

[22] Peterka RJ. Sensorimotor integration in human postural control. J Neurophysiol 2002;88: 1097–118.

[23] Visser JE, Bloem BR. Role of the basal ganglia in balance control. Neural Plast 2005;12: 161–74.

[24] Bar-Gad I, Havazelet-Heimer G, Goldberg JA, et al. Reinforcement-driven dimensionality reduction–a model for information processing in the basal ganglia. J Basic Clin Physiol Pharmacol 2000;11:305–20.

[25] Baev KV, Greene KA, Marciano FF, et al. Physiology and pathophysiology of cortico-basal ganglia-thalamocortical loops: theoretical and practical aspects. Prog Neuropsychopharmacol Biol Psychiatry 2002;26:771–80.

[26] Grillner S, Parker D, el Manira A. Vertebrate locomotion—a lamprey perspective. Ann N Y Acad Sci 1998;16(860):1–18.

[27] Zangger P. The effect of 4-aminopyridine on the spinal locomotor rhythm induced by l-DOPA. Brain Res 1981;215:211–23.

[28] Grillner S. Control of locomotion in bipeds, tetrapods, and fish. Baltimore (MD): Waverly Press; 1981.

[29] Lee MS, Rinne JO, Marsden CD. The pedunculopontine nucleus: its role in the genesis of movement disorders. Yonsei Med J 2000;41:167–84.

[30] Pahapill PA, Lozano AM. The pedunculopontine nucleus and Parkinson's disease. Brain 2000;123:1767–83.

[31] Alexander GE, DeLong MR, Strick PL. Parallel organization of functionally segregated circuits linking basal ganglia and cortex. Annu Rev Neurosci 1986;9:357–81.

[32] Grillner S, Wallen P. Cellular bases of a vertebrate locomotor system-steering, intersegmental and segmental co-ordination and sensory control. Brain Res Brain Res Rev 2002;40:92–106.

[33] Quinn N. Parkinsonism-recognition and differential diagnosis. BMJ 1995;310:447–52.

[34] Bernheimer H, Birkmayer W, Hornykiewicz O, et al. Brain dopamine and the syndromes of Parkinson and Huntington. Clinical, morphological and neurochemical correlations. J Neurol Sci 1973;20:415–55.

[35] Kish SJ, Shannak K, Hornykiewicz O. Uneven pattern of dopamine loss in the striatum of patients with idiopathic Parkinson's disease. N Engl J Med 1988;318:876–80.

[36] Frey KA, Koeppe RA, Kilbourn MR, et al. Presynaptic monoaminergic vesicles in Parkinson's disease and normal aging. Ann Neurol 1996;40:873–84.

[37] Antonini A, Schwarz J, Oertel WH, et al. Long-term changes of striatal dopamine D2 receptors in patients with Parkinson's disease: a study with positron emission tomography and [^{11}C]raclopride. Mov Disord 1997;12:33–8.

[38] Jellinger K. The pedunculopontine nucleus in Parkinson's disease, progressive supranuclear palsy and Alzheimer's disease. J Neurol Neurosurg Psychiatry 1988;51:540–3.

[39] Jenkinson N, Nandi D, Miall RC, et al. Pedunculopontine nucleus stimulation improves akinesia in a Parkinsonian monkey. Neuroreport 2004;15:2621–4.

[40] Maurer C, Mergner T, Xie J, et al. Effect of chronic bilateral subthalamic nucleus (STN) stimulation on postural control in Parkinson's disease. Brain 2003;126:1146–63.

[41] Rocchi L, Chiari L, Horak FB. Effects of deep brain stimulation and levodopa on postural sway in Parkinson's disease. J Neurol Neurosurg Psychiatry 2002;73:267–74.

[42] Bronte-Stewart HM, Minn AY, Rodrigues K, et al. Postural instability in idiopathic Parkinson's disease: the role of medication and unilateral pallidotomy. Brain 2002;125: 2100–14.

[43] Horak FB, Nutt JG, Nashner LM. Postural inflexibility in parkinsonian subjects. J Neurol Sci 1992;111:46–58.

[44] Smiley-Oyen AL, Cheng HY, Latt LD, et al. Adaptation of vibration-induced postural sway in individuals with Parkinson's disease. Gait Posture 2002;16:188–97.

[45] Bronstein AM, Hood JD, Gresty MA, et al. Visual control of balance in cerebellar and parkinsonian syndromes. Brain 1990;113:767–79.

[46] Bloem BR, Beckley DJ, van Dijk JG, et al. Influence of dopaminergic medication on automatic postural responses and balance impairment in Parkinson's disease. Mov Disord 1996;11:509–21.

[47] Chong RK, Horak FB, Woollacott MH. Parkinson's disease impairs the ability to change set quickly. J Neurol Sci 2000;175:57–70.

[48] Morris ME, Huxham F, McGinley J, et al. The biomechanics and motor control of gait in Parkinson disease. Clin Biomech (Bristol, Avon) 2001;16:459–70.

[49] Hausdorff JM, Schaafsma JD, Balash Y, et al. Impaired regulation of stride variability in Parkinson's disease subjects with freezing of gait. Exp Brain Res 2003;149:187–94.

[50] Hausdorff JM, Cudkowicz ME, Firtion R, et al. Gait variability and basal ganglia disorders: stride-to-stride variations of gait cycle timing in Parkinson's disease and Huntington's disease. Mov Disord 1998;13:428–37.

[51] Yogev G, Giladi N, Peretz C, et al. Dual tasking, gait rhythmicity, and Parkinson's disease: which aspects of gait are attention demanding? Eur J Neurosci 2005;22:1248–56.

[52] Nieuwboer A, De Weerdt W, Dom R, et al. Plantar force distribution in Parkinsonian gait: a comparison between patients and age-matched control subjects. Scan J Rehab Med 1999; 31:185–92.

[53] Azulay JP, Mesure S, Amblard B, et al. Visual control of locomotion in Parkinson's disease. Brain 1999;122:111–20.

[54] Lewis GN, Byblow WD, Walt SE. Stride length regulation in Parkinson's disease: the use of extrinsic, visual cues. Brain 2000;123:2077–90.

[55] McIntosh GC, Brown SH, Rice RR, et al. Rhythmic auditory-motor facilitation of gait patterns in patients with Parkinson's disease. J Neurol Neurosurg Psychiatry 1997;62:22–6.

[56] Thaut MH, McIntosh GC, Rice RR, et al. Rhythmic auditory stimulation in gait training for Parkinson's disease patients. Mov Dis 1996;11:193–200.

[57] Howe TE, Lovgreen B, Cody FW, et al. Auditory cues can modify the gait of persons with early-stage Parkinson's disease: a method for enhancing parkinsonian walking performance? Clin Rehabil 2003;17:363–7.

[58] Burleigh-Jacobs A, Horak FB, Nutt JG, et al. Step initiation in Parkinson's disease: influence of levodopa and external sensory triggers. Mov Disord 1997;12:206–15.

[59] Giladi N, Treves TA, Simon ES, et al. Freezing of gait in patients with advanced Parkinson's disease. J Neural Transm 2001;108:53–61.

[60] Ueno E, Yanagisawa N, Takami M. Gait disorders in parkinsonism. A study with floor reaction forces and EMG. Adv Neurol 1993;60:414–8.

[61] Martin M, Shinberg M, Kuchibhatla M, et al. Gait initiation in community-dwelling adults with Parkinson disease: comparison with older and younger adults without the disease. Phys Ther 2002;82:566–77.

[62] Ferrandez AM, Blin O. A comparison between the effect of intentional modulations and the action of L-dopa on gait in Parkinson's disease. Behav Brain Res 1991;45:177–83.

[63] Knutsson E, Martensson A. Quantitative effects of L-dopa on different types of movements and muscle tone in Parkinsonian patients. Scand J Rehabil Med 1971;3:121–30.

[64] Lees AJ, Smith E. Cognitive deficits in the early stages of Parkinson's disease. Brain 1983; 106:257–70.

[65] Dubois B, Pillon B. Cognitive deficits in Parkinson's disease. J Neurol 1997;244:2–8.

[66] Stern Y, Mayeux R, Rosen J, et al. Perceptual motor dysfunction in Parkinson's disease: a deficit in sequential and predictive voluntary movement. J Neurol Neurosurg Psychiatry 1983;46:145–51.

[67] Cools R, Barker RA, Sahakian BJ, et al. Enhanced or impaired cognitive function in Parkinson's disease as a function of dopaminergic medication and task demands. Cereb Cortex 2001;11:1136–43.

[68] Boller F, Mizutani T, Roessmann U, et al. Parkinson's disease, dementia and Alzheimer's disease: clinicopathologic correlations. Ann Neurol 1980;7:329–35.

[69] Cooper JA, Sagar HJ, Doherty SM, et al. Different effects of dopaminergic and anticholinergic therapies on cognitive and motor function in Parkinson's disease. A follow-up study of untreated patients. Brain 1992;115:1701–25.

[70] Dubois B, Pillon B, Lhermitte F, et al. Cholinergic deficiency and frontal dysfunction in Parkinson's disease. Ann Neurol 1990;28:117–21.

[71] Stuss DT, Alexander MP. Executive functions and the frontal lobes: a conceptual view. Psychol Res 2000;63:289–98.

[72] Bloem BR, Valkenburg VV, Slabbekoorn M, et al. The multiple tasks test. Strategies in Parkinson's disease. Exp Brain Res 2001;137:478–86.

[73] Marchese R, Bove M, Abbruzzese G. Effect of cognitive and motor tasks on postural stability in Parkinson's disease: a posturographic study. Mov Disord 2003;18:652–8.

[74] Camicioli R, Oken BS, Sexton G, et al. Verbal fluency task affects gait in Parkinson's disease with motor freezing. J Geriatr Psychiatry Neurol 1998;11:181–5.

[75] Bond JM, Morris M. Goal-directed secondary motor tasks: their effects on gait in subjects with Parkinson disease. Arch Phys Med Rehabil 2000;81:110–6.

[76] O'Shea S, Morris ME, Iansek R. Dual task interference during gait in people with Parkinson disease: effects of motor versus cognitive secondary tasks. Phys Ther 2002;82(9):888–97.

[77] Bloem BR, Grimbergen YA, Cramer M, et al. "Stops walking when talking" does not predict falls in Parkinson's disease. Ann Neurol 2000;48:268.

[78] Hausdorff JM, Balash J, Giladi N. Effects of cognitive challenge on gait variability in patients with Parkinson's disease. J Geriatr Psychiatry Neurol 2003;16:53–8.

[79] Rodnitzky RL. Visual dysfunction in Parkinson's disease. Clin Neurosci 1998;5:102–6.

[80] Bodis-Wollner I, Tagliati M. The visual system in Parkinson's disease. Adv Neurol 1993;60:390–4.

[81] Peppard RF, Martin WR, Carr GD, et al. Cerebral glucose metabolism in Parkinson's disease with and without dementia. Arch Neurol 1992;49:1262–8.

[82] Bracha HS, Shults C, Glick SD, et al. Spontaneous asymmetric circling behavior in hemiparkinsonism; a human equivalent of the lesioned-circling rodent behavior. Life Sci 1987;40:1127–30.

[83] Ebersbach G, Trottenberg T, Hättig H, et al. Directional bias of initial visual exploration. A symptom of neglect in Parkinson's disease. Brain 1996;119:79–87.

[84] Leiguarda R, Merello M, Balej J, et al. Disruption of spatial organization and interjoint coordination in Parkinson's disease, progressive supranuclear palsy, and multiple system atrophy. Mov Disord 2000;15:627–40.

[85] White OB, Saint-Cyr JA, Tomlinson RD, et al. Ocular motor deficits in Parkinson's disease. III. Coordination of eye and head movements. Brain 1988;111:115–29.

[86] Shibasaki H, Tsuji S, Kuroiwa Y. Oculomotor abnormalities in Parkinson's disease. Arch Neurol 1979;36:360–4.

[87] Geldmacher DS. Visuospatial dysfunction in the neurodegenerative diseases. Front Biosci 2003;8:e428–36.

[88] Briand KA, Strallow D, Hening W, et al. Control of voluntary and reflexive saccades in Parkinson's disease. Exp Brain Res 1999;129:38–48.

[89] Antonini A, Schwarz J, Oertel WH, et al. [^{11}C]raclopride and positron emission tomography in previously untreated patients with Parkinson's disease: Influence of L-dopa and lisuride therapy on striatal dopamine D2-receptors. Neurology 1994;44:1325–9.

[90] Bloem BR, Hausdorff JM, Visser JE, et al. Falls and freezing in Parkinson's disease: a review of two interconnected, episodic phenomena. Mov Disord 2004;19:871–84.

[91] Brooks DJ, Ibanez V, Sawle GV, et al. Striatal D2 receptor status in patients with Parkinson's disease, striatonigral degeneration, and progressive supranuclear palsy, measured with ^{11}C-raclopride and positron emission tomography. Ann Neurol 1992;31:184–92.

[92] Pirker W, Asenbaum S, Bencsits G, et al. [^{123}I]beta-CIT SPECT in multiple system atrophy, progressive supranuclear palsy, and corticobasal degeneration. Mov Disord 2000;15: 1158–67.

[93] Schulz JB, Klockgether T, Petersen D, et al. Multiple system atrophy: natural history, MRI morphology, and dopamine receptor imaging with ^{123}IBZM-SPECT. J Neurol Neurosurg Psychiatry 1994;57:1047–56.

[94] Blin O, Ferrandez AM, Serratrice G. Quantitative analysis of gait in Parkinson patients: increased variability of stride length. J Neurol Sci 1990;98:91–7.

ELSEVIER
SAUNDERS

Clin Geriatr Med 22 (2006) 813–825

CLINICS IN
GERIATRIC
MEDICINE

Surgical Treatment of Movement Disorders

Alberto J. Espay, MD, MSc[a],
George T. Mandybur, MD[b], Fredy J. Revilla, MD[a],*

[a]Department of Neurology, Movement Disorders Center, The Neuroscience Institute,
University of Cincinnati College of Medicine, 231 Albert Sabin Way,
ML 0525, Cincinnati, OH 45267-0525, USA
[b]Department of Neurosurgery, Movement Disorders Center,
The Neuroscience Institute and Mayfield Clinic, University of Cincinnati College
of Medicine, 231 Albert Sabin Way, Cincinnati, OH 45267-0525, USA

Since the serendipitous discovery that lesions within specific areas of the motor system can improve parkinsonian deficits (especially tremor) without the expense of motor paresis, interest in exploring and expanding surgical techniques has existed. An often-quoted turning point was the accidental interruption and forced ligation of the anterior choroidal artery during an aborted pedunculotomy performed in 1952 by Cooper [1]. The unexpected postoperative resolution of this patient's tremor and rigidity prompted Cooper to ligate this artery deliberately in subsequent patients with Parkinson's disease (PD) to reduce their tremor. After levodopa was introduced in the late 1960s, a hiatus in surgical interventions for PD ensued. When the limitations of levodopa were noted and as newer therapies for movement disorders became recognized, renewed interest emerged for the surgical treatment of PD and subsequently of essential tremor (ET) and dystonia. In recent years, the number of surgical indications has increased largely on anecdotal evidence. Controlled clinical trials have justified adequately, however, widespread use of stereotactic neurosurgery in PD, ET, and idiopathic dystonia (Table 1). The alternative to ablative surgery in the form of high-frequency deep brain stimulation (DBS) became an accepted and effective therapy in the early 1990s with the pioneering work of Benabid and colleagues [2].

* Corresponding author.
E-mail address: fredy.revilla@uc.edu (F.J. Revilla).

0749-0690/06/$ - see front matter © 2006 Elsevier Inc. All rights reserved.
doi:10.1016/j.cger.2006.06.002

Table 1
Established and emerging indications and targets for deep brain stimulation

Established indications	Targets of surgery		
	GPi	STN	Thalamus
Parkinson's disease	Bilateral	Bilateral	Vim unilateral
Essential tremor			Vim unilateral
Dystonia	Unilateral or bilateral		
Emerging indications	Proposed targets		
Tourette's syndrome (motor tics and OCS)			CM and SPV nuclei [55] CM-PF complex [56]
Huntington's disease [21]	Bilateral		
Myoclonus dystonia [57]	Bilateral		
Proposed indications	Proposed targets		
Posthypoxic myoclonus [58]			VL nucleus
Refractory Meige syndrome [59]	Bilateral		

Abbreviations: CM, centromedian (part of the intralaminar thalamic nuclei); CM-PF, centro-median-parafascicular; GPi, internal segment of the globus pallidus; OCS, obsessive-compulsive symptoms; SPV, substantia periventricularis (part of the intralaminar thalamic nuclei); STN, subthalamic nucleus; Vim, ventral intermediate thalamic nucleus; VL, ventral lateral. (Courtesy of the Mayfield Clinic, Cincinnatti, OH.)

Rationale for neurosurgery in movement disorders

The efficacy and tolerability shortcomings of medical treatment have been the crucial encouragement for surgical treatments in movement disorders. Oral medications for dystonia and ET, none of which are disease-specific, have variable efficacy and elicit intolerable side effects in a significant proportion of patients. In PD, levodopa is highly efficacious, but among other limitations, motor complications in the form of motor fluctuations (wearing-off phenomenon, delayed or no "on" response, unpredictable "off" episodes, and freezing) and dyskinesias eventually appear, regardless of age at onset [3]. These treatment-related complications often exhibit suboptimal response to a variety of drug manipulations and become the source of substantial disability. These motor complications have been managed successfully first with ablative procedures and later with subthalamic nucleus (STN) and globus pallidus pars interna (GPi) DBS directly or through the postoperative reduction in medication requirements [4–7].

Methodologic factors that provide a solid basis on which surgery can be justified include (1) advances in the safety of stereotactic neurosurgical procedures; (2) improvements in techniques for accurate target localization, including neuroimaging and microelectrode recording techniques of single cell and multiple neuronal discharges; and (3) greater understanding of the organization of the basal ganglia (see later) [8]. Ultimately, the striking responses reported with DBS placement in PD, ET, and dystonia have cemented widespread interest in its use for these and other movement disorders.

Candidates for surgery

Traditionally, when medical treatment fails to provide benefit or is associated with intolerable side effects, surgical options are considered. Factors to be considered when selecting individual patients for neurosurgical treatment include the potential surgical morbidity and mortality; short-term and long-term costs of DBS; the considerable time and effort required by the patient, caregivers, and medical staff in the postoperative period for programming and drug adjustments; and the need for ongoing assessment of device-related complications [9]. These factors are sufficiently comprehensive in addressing suitability for surgery in patients with disabling ET and dystonia.

The selection of PD patients for surgery is more complicated than the relatively simple assessment of the various elements previously mentioned. In contrast to ET and dystonia, one important exclusion criterion for any neurosurgical therapy is the failure of levodopa and other dopaminergic agents to elicit a good response in PD patients. Poor response to levodopa often indicates the presence of an atypical parkinsonism (eg, multiple system atrophy, progressive supranuclear palsy, and dementia with Lewy bodies); these patients typically do not respond well to surgery. Response to surgery at best matches but never exceeds the maximal benefit obtained from levodopa [10]. Adequate response to levodopa has been defined as at least a 33% improvement in motor function as measured by the motor subscale of the Unified Parkinson's Disease Rating Scale (UPDRS) [11].

Eligibility criteria for DBS in PD used by most centers rely on the recommendations made by the Core Assessment Program for Surgical Interventional Therapies in Parkinson's disease (CAPSIT-PD) [12]. This protocol proposes that the disease should be present for at least 5 years before the patient is considered to undergo DBS implantation. This time frame is sufficient not only to allow exclusion of atypical forms of parkinsonism whose early course may be indistinguishable from PD, but also to achieve optimization of levodopa therapy. In addition, dementia and poorly controlled psychiatric disorders are important exclusion criteria. Candidates with significant cognitive impairment are less likely to have long-lasting improvement and may be unable to tolerate and cooperate with all aspects of surgery and postoperative care [9]. This aspect has received substantial attention and has made the neuropsychologist a crucial participant in the screening and outcome evaluation of patients with PD and other movement disorders.

An 18-item questionnaire based on CAPSIT-PD has been created to standardize the ascertainment of surgical eligibility (Box 1) [13]. Strict application of this questionnaire showed that less than 2% of all PD patients evaluated in a movement disorders clinic (those whose response is "yes"

Box 1. Questionnaire to determine eligibility for DBS in PD patients (from the CAPSIT-PD)

Items
Clinically definite PD
Disease duration >5 years
Age <70 years
Refractory motor complications (eg, wearing off or
   levodopa-induced dyskinesia)
Hoehn-Yahr scale ≥3 (bilateral disease with postural impairment)
UPDRS "off" ≥40 (motor subscale range 0–108)
Severe motor disability
Good clinical levodopa response
Absence of (or adequately treated) major depression
   or psychosis
Absence of current (or adequately treated previous)
   drug-induced psychosis
Good compliance of patient and family
Strong personal motivation
Poor quality of life
Absence of (or minimal) cognitive impairment
Absence of alcohol or drug abuse
Absence of systemic diseases or illnesses
Absence of major cerebrovascular risk factors
Absence of anticoagulant therapy

All items need to be checked "Yes" for candidates to become
   eligible for STN DBS.

Adapted from Morgante L, Morgante F, Moro E, et al. How many parkinsonian patients are suitable candidates for deep brain stimulation of subthalamic nucleus? Results of a screening questionnaire. Mov Disord 2006, in press; with permission.

---

to all items listed) could be considered suitable candidates for STN DBS implantation [13]. Less stringent adherence to these criteria may be applied in select cases.

Organization of basal ganglia

Modern surgical approaches to surgery for movement disorders were developed from fortuitous strokes and neurophysiologic observations made during neurosurgery and on the basis of physiologic and neuroanatomic studies in primate models of disease. Albin and colleagues [8] and DeLong

[14] generated a model of basal ganglia function whereby basal ganglia and thalamocortical circuits were segregated to serve specific functions. This model facilitated the understanding of the underlying pathophysiology of PD, dystonia, and other conditions (Fig. 1A). The basal ganglia are a group of interconnected nuclei believed to regulate or control movements. The striatum (caudate nucleus and putamen) receives and projects from and to several brain regions. The topographically organized output pathways are

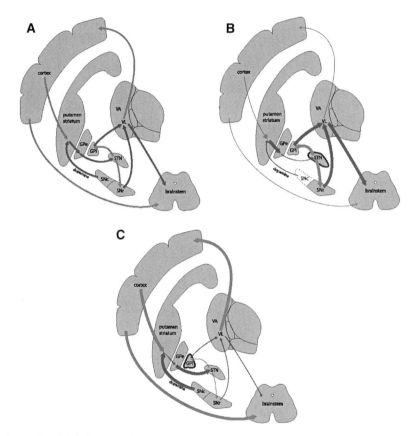

Fig. 1. Simplified diagram of abnormalities in the basal ganglia circuitry in a normal health state (*A*), PD (*B*), and dystonia (*C*). *Green arrows* indicate excitatory pathways, and *red arrows* show inhibitory pathways. The SNr and GPi represent the common basal ganglia output to the cortex via motor thalamus and to the brainstem. The cortex ultimately drives the production of movement from the spinal cord via the corticospinal system. Most internal connections within the basal ganglia are GABAergic (inhibitory) with the exception of the glutamatergic output from the STN. The so-called direct pathway, which contains an excitatory D1 dopaminergic pathway between SNpc and the putamen, has been suppressed from this figure to facilitate clarity. (*Adapted from* Obeso JA, Rodriguez-Oroz MC, Rodriguez M, et al. The basal ganglia and disorders of movement: pathophysiological mechanisms. News Physiol Sci 2002;17:51–5 and Vitek JL. Pathophysiology of dystonia: a neuronal model. Mov Disord 2002;17(Suppl 3): S49–62.)

directed to either the external (GPe) or internal segment of the globus pallidus (GPi) and substantia nigra pars reticulata (SNr), also known as the indirect and direct pathways. GPi and SNr share a similar embryologic origin and represent the final common basal ganglia output to the cortex through an inhibitory (GABAergic) pathway to the motor thalamus [15]. In PD, degeneration of the nigrostriatal dopaminergic neurons with subsequent dopamine deficiency leads to increased inhibitory activity from the putamen onto the GPe and disinhibition of the STN. Excessive glutamatergic action of the STN produces overexcitation of the GPi/SNr output neurons, which overinhibit the thalamocortical and ultimately the cortical projections to the brainstem and spinal cord (Fig. 1B) [16]. Conversely, dystonia often develops after striatal lesions or dysfunction, particularly of the putamen, which reduces the inhibitory activity of the putamen-GPe connection and enhances the inhibition of the STN. The resulting understimulation of GPi (and SNr) leads to disinhibition of the thalamocortical projections and, finally, increased cortical excitatory influence to the brainstem and spinal cord (Fig. 1C) [17]. This simplified circuitry forms the pathophysiologic basis for the hypokinetic and hyperkinetic disorders that PD and dystonia represent.

The aforementioned schema explains the dramatic improvement in motor control in patients with PD after inducing a reduction of the excessive neuronal activity in the GPi and STN [18,19]. Similar disruption of the GPi output leads to functional improvement in hyperkinetic disorders (eg, primary generalized dystonia [20] and chorea caused by Huntington's disease [21] or levodopa-induced dyskinesias [5]). The reduction in chorea through pallidotomy or GPi DBS contradicts the prediction of the model and is held as one of the shortcomings in the functional predictions of the basal ganglia diagram discussed previously [17]. To conciliate this discrepancy, several lines of research have suggested that the benefits of GPi DBS do not result from a reduction in the increased *rate* of firing from chronic high-frequency stimulation, long argued to be the crucial mechanism of action. Rather, the benefit may result from disruption of the GPi output *pattern* and degree of synchronization of neuronal activity [22,23]. A new basal ganglia model has been proposed [24] that also accounts for selective facilitation and surround inhibition of competing motor patterns; however, complexities suggested therein require further testing before general acceptance.

Targets and outcomes in deep brain stimulation surgery

In part stemming from the functional organization of the basal ganglia, DBS treatment is aimed at three targets (Table 1): the ventral intermediate nucleus of the thalamus (Vim), the GPi, and the STN. Long-term stimulation of the thalamic Vim, which receives tremor-generating neurons from the cerebellum, is used primarily to treat essential tremor safely and efficaciously [25]. In PD patients, Vim DBS improves contralateral tremor almost exclusively, largely to the neglect of rigidity and bradykinesia. As a result, Vim DBS has been replaced by DBS of the two other targets, even when tremor is the most disabling symptom [26].

Although it has been suggested that stimulation of the STN may be superior to stimulation of the GPi in the surgical treatment of PD, comparative trials are limited. This notion was generated partly by the reports of three patients who were successfully improved by STN DBS after pallidotomy or GPi DBS failed to provide adequate motor relief [27,28]. GPi DBS exerts the largest effect by reducing the total "on" state (during maximum effect of medication) dyskinesia score [29]. STN DBS induces a large degree of motor improvement in the "off" state (when medication effect has worn off). In many cases, this effect permits a dramatic decrease in levodopa dose requirement after surgery [7]. The levodopa dose remains relatively unchanged after GPi DBS placement [30]. In a retrospective study comparing the 1-year postoperative outcome of these two targets, there was no difference in motor symptoms during the "off" state, dyskinesias during the "on" state, and motor fluctuations [19]. Significantly less electrical power in STN DBS was required, however; this reduction provides a benefit-to-cost ratio advantage versus GPi DBS that may be counterbalanced by the need for more intensive postoperative monitoring and, possibly, a higher incidence of adverse events associated with levodopa withdrawal [19].

A nonrandomized multicenter study describing the response of 96 PD patients to STN DBS and 38 PD patients to GPi DBS found that median improvement in the motor score (compared with no stimulation) was 49% in the STN and 37% in the GPi group at 3 months after surgery, a significant improvement within each group [31]. Between the preoperative and 6-month visits, the percentage of time during the day that patients had good mobility increased from 27% to 74% with STN DBS and from 28% to 64% with GPi DBS. Only levodopa-induced dyskinesias were equal in both groups. In a randomized and blinded study aimed at comparing the safety and efficacy of DBS between STN and GPi in 10 patients, "on" state motor scores (measured by UPDRS) were more improved by GPi than by STN stimulation, and axial symptoms were clinically improved in the GPi group but not the STN group [32]. Levodopa-induced dyskinesia and "off" state motor scores were reduced by DBS of either site. Medication requirement was reduced only in the STN group, however [32]. A more recent and larger randomized clinical trial comparing GPi and STN DBS showed a motor improvement (based on UPDRS blinded rating of "off-drug" PD patients) of 39% and 48% after 12 months [33]. Although levodopa dose was reduced by 38% in STN stimulation patients compared with only 3% in patients with GPi stimulation (confirmed in a 4-year follow-up study in which no GPi-related levodopa reduction occurred [34]), levodopa-induced dyskinesia was reduced to a greater extent by stimulation of GPi than that of STN (89% versus 62%) [33]. The greater antidyskinetic effect from the procedure that affords little or no levodopa dose reduction suggests that the reduction of levodopa-induced dyskinesias is the consequence of independent mechanisms in these two targets: target-specific in GPi and dependent on postoperative levodopa reduction in STN. Patients with primary generalized dystonia improve significantly in motor function and disability after GPi DBS placement, whose efficacy and safety have been well shown in a prospective controlled manner [20].

Intraoperative evaluations

Anatomic targets for STN, GPi, and Vim are obtained initially by applying pre-established coordinates to special sequences of brain MRI with the aid of stereotactic planning software. These targets are confirmed intraoperatively using microelectrode recording (MER) and, in some centers, microstimulation to evoke motor, oculomotor, or sensory responses that alert the surgical team as to the appropriate neural "neighborhood" [35]. Intraoperative stimulation also may be used to define optimal stimulation parameters when the electrodes are implanted with the aid of a stereotactic guidance system. Several clinical and electrophysiologic variables are evaluated in awake patients undergoing DBS implantation. In the case of STN DBS for PD, the improvement of segmental bradykinesia and the elicitation of dyskinesias by stimulation during the operation are the best predictors of postoperative benefit [36]. A permanent quadripolar electrode is implanted at the site where stimulation adequately improves motor symptoms without obvious side effects at therapeutic current levels. The electrode is connected to an implantable pulse generator (which generates high-frequency current) that is positioned under the skin in the subclavicular area. Some centers confirm electrode placement after surgery with a brain imaging study, MRI or CT. These images are fused with preoperative imaging studies using stereotactic software. Some controversy exists, however, as to whether intraoperative MER reliably enhances the accuracy of electrode placement, minimizes lesion size, and reduces the risks and side effects associated with surgery. A large review comparing MER-guided and non–MER-guided procedures suggested that MER techniques may increase the risks of surgery without enhancing its accuracy compared with MRI-based macrostimulation techniques [37]. The value of MER will remain undetermined in the absence of controlled clinical studies that compare outcomes with and without this instrument.

Mechanism of action of deep brain stimulation surgery

DBS produces clinical benefits approximately similar in magnitude to lesioning the same structures through ablative procedures. It has been hypothesized that long-term stimulation of these targets produces a lesion-like inactivation (depolarization block and "jamming" of abnormal neuronal output are among the mechanisms proposed) [38]. Although there is no consensus on the exact mechanism of action, more recent microscopic, neurophysiologic, and neuroimaging evidence favors excitation of the target neural structures, perhaps leading to normalization in the pattern of neuronal activity [22,39–41].

Stimulator programming

Programming of DBS settings is a time-consuming and labor-intensive task of the neurology team in charge of the postoperative care of patients. Several programming sessions are needed to set up optimally the active electrode contact combination and stimulation parameters (amplitude, pulse width, and frequency) on the implantable pulse generator. This pacemaker-like device is placed under the chest skin and connected to the DBS electrode, which is implanted in the brain and fixed to the skull [42]. Adequate programming of the implantable pulse generator is required not only to maximize the motor benefits, but also to avoid or restrict cognitive adverse effects [43]. For PD, an appropriate estimation of the clinical effect of stimulation may require at least 3 hours off STN DBS [44]. Tremor improves within minutes, followed by a slower improvement of bradykinesia and rigidity over $\frac{1}{2}$ hour to 1 hour, and finally a slow and steady improvement of axial signs (speech, neck rigidity, rising from a chair, posture, gait, and postural stability) occurs over 3 to 4 hours, after turning stimulation "on" [44]. On turning off the DBS current, 90% of the baseline UPDRS motor score is reached after 2 hours. Motor deficits deteriorate with a similar sequence and timing, but slower than their rate of "on" DBS improvement, when switching the stimulator "off" [44].

Potential complications from surgery

In a large series of 300 PD patients with STN, GPi, or Vim DBS (212 with bilateral implantation), 2 deaths were indirectly related to surgery (pulmonary embolism and frontal hematoma during surgery and death 3 years later) [26]. In stereotactic neurosurgery, the most severe inherent complication is intracranial hematoma. This complication was estimated to occur in 2% to 8% of patients in the older literature [45] when ablative and stimulation procedures were practiced approximately equally. Estimates with DBS, mostly of the STN, place this risk at about 1% [46]. The incidence of permanent severe morbidity may range from none [46] to about 6% [47]. Sources of temporary morbidity, besides intracranial hematoma, include seizures, postoperative confusion, device infections, wound hematomas, skin erosions over implanted hardware, and need for electrode revisions and battery failures. These sources of morbidity require minor interventions and generally resolve with little or no sequelae. The most dreaded form of morbidity is dementia possibly caused by surgery-related acceleration of subclinical cognitive dysfunction. Other adverse events are speech difficulty, instability, gait disorders, and depression, which seem to be more common in patients treated with DBS of the STN [33,34]. Besides these and other behavioral problems (see later), the 5-year complications include eyelid opening apraxia, weight gain, addiction to levodopa treatment, hypomania and disinhibition, depression, dysarthria, and apathy [48].

Behavior and cognition after deep brain stimulation

The relationship between neuropsychologic measures and response to DBS surgery is not only related to the target (STN versus GPi versus Vim), but, importantly, also to premorbid function. In PD, early studies reported negligible or no changes in cognition owing to DBS implantation. Studies have reported improvement in psychomotor speed and working memory for patients with STN or GPi DBS and no measurable cognitive deficit 12 months after STN DBS surgery except for reduced lexical fluency [49]. Thorough examination after bilateral STN DBS may document, however, declines in set alternation, lexical fluency and switching, and verbal/nonverbal memory [50,51]. Elderly patients (>69 years old) may have improved mood but significant declines in cognitive processes involving executive functioning (eg, working memory, phonemic fluency, associative learning, speed of processing, set switching, bimanual coordination under divided attention) [50]. More recent studies have shown that after 60 months, cognitive performance (as measured by the Mattis Dementia Rating Scale and the frontal score) can decline significantly [48]. This decline emphasizes the importance of selecting candidates with little or no cognitive impairment.

Patients with tremor treated with unilateral Vim DBS may experience improvements in fine visuomotor and visuoperceptual functions, verbal memory, and mood [52]; decrement in word recall occurs related to left-sided thalamic stimulation (which disappears when the stimulator is turned off) [53]. Although data on neuropsychologic outcomes in dystonia patients undergoing bilateral GPi DBS are scarce, no measurable deterioration using large cognitive and neuropsychiatric batteries at 1 year after the procedure has been reported [20,54].

Summary

DBS procedures for movement disorders, particularly PD, ET, and primary dystonia, have become established therapeutic options because of their safety and efficacy. Patient selection is of utmost concern, however, because of the inherent risks of stereotactic procedures and the relationship between response and presurgical motor and cognitive status. For PD, the most reliable indicator of response to surgery is the extent of improvement in response to levodopa, which is matched but not outperformed by any surgical treatment. Eligibility criteria in current use limit the surgical treatment to about 2% of all patients. These criteria intend to maximize the motor benefits and restrict the potential procedure-related and disease-specific complications. Only a few randomized controlled clinical trials are available comparing the benefits of the two major surgical targets for PD (STN and GPi), but each affords significant improvement compared with the baseline function. STN DBS also allows for dopaminergic dose reduction. The need for time-intensive postoperative DBS programming must be considered when deciding in favor of this therapeutic modality given the active involvement required of patients.

Acknowledgments

The authors thank Tonya Hines, Art Director, and Mary Kemper, medical editor of The Neuroscience Institute, for providing the figures and editorial review of this manuscript, respectively.

References

[1] Cooper IS. Anterior choroidal artery ligation for involuntary movements. Science 1953;118: 193.
[2] Benabid AL, Pollak P, Gervason C, et al. Long-term suppression of tremor by chronic stimulation of the ventral intermediate thalamic nucleus. Lancet 1991;337:403–6.
[3] Wagner ML, Fedak MN, Sage JI, et al. Complications of disease and therapy: a comparison of younger and older patients with Parkinson's disease. Ann Clin Lab Sci 1996;26:389–95.
[4] Vitek JL, Bakay RA, Freeman A, et al. Randomized trial of pallidotomy versus medical therapy for Parkinson's disease. Ann Neurol 2003;53:558–69.
[5] Lang AE, Lozano AM, Montgomery E, et al. Posteroventral medial pallidotomy in advanced Parkinson's disease. N Engl J Med 1997;337:1036–42.
[6] Kleiner-Fisman G, Fisman DN, Sime E, et al. Long-term follow up of bilateral deep brain stimulation of the subthalamic nucleus in patients with advanced Parkinson disease. J Neurosurg 2003;99:489–95.
[7] Moro E, Scerrati M, Romito LM, et al. Chronic subthalamic nucleus stimulation reduces medication requirements in Parkinson's disease. Neurology 1999;53:85–90.
[8] Albin RL, Young AB, Penney JB. The functional anatomy of basal ganglia disorders. Trends Neurosci 1989;12:366–75.
[9] Lang AE, Widner H. Deep brain stimulation for Parkinson's disease: patient selection and evaluation. Mov Disord 2002;17(Suppl 3):S94–101.
[10] Welter ML, Houeto JL, Tezenas du MS, et al. Clinical predictive factors of subthalamic stimulation in Parkinson's disease. Brain 2002;125:575–83.
[11] Fahn S, Elton RL. Unified Parkinson's Disease Rating Scale. In: Fahn S, Goldstein M, Marsden D, et al, editors. Recent developments in Parkinson's disease. Florham Park, NJ: MacMillan; 1987. p. 153–63.
[12] Defer GL, Widner H, Marie RM, et al. Core assessment program for surgical interventional therapies in Parkinson's disease (CAPSIT-PD). Mov Disord 1999;14:572–84.
[13] Morgante L, Morgante F, Moro E, et al. How many parkinsonian patients are suitable candidates for deep brain stimulation of subthalamic nucleus? Results of a screening questionnaire. Mov Disord 2006, in press.

[14] DeLong MR. Primate models of movement disorders of basal ganglia origin. Trends Neurosci 1990;13:281–5.

[15] Wichmann T, DeLong MR. Functional and pathophysiological models of the basal ganglia. Curr Opin Neurobiol 1996;6:751–8.

[16] Obeso JA, Rodriguez-Oroz MC, Rodriguez M, et al. The basal ganglia and disorders of movement: pathophysiological mechanisms. News Physiol Sci 2002;17:51–5.

[17] Vitek JL. Pathophysiology of dystonia: a neuronal model. Mov Disord 2002;17(Suppl 3): S49–62.

[18] Lozano AM, Lang AE, Galvez-Jimenez N, et al. Effect of GPi pallidotomy on motor function in Parkinson's disease. Lancet 1995;346:1383–7.

[19] Volkmann J, Allert N, Voges J, et al V. Safety and efficacy of pallidal or subthalamic nucleus stimulation in advanced PD. Neurology 2001;56:548–51.

[20] Vidailhet M, Vercueil L, Houeto JL, et al. Bilateral deep-brain stimulation of the globus pallidus in primary generalized dystonia. N Engl J Med 2005;352:459–67.

[21] Moro E, Lang AE, Strafella AP, et al. Bilateral globus pallidus stimulation for Huntington's disease. Ann Neurol 2004;56:290–4.

[22] Hashimoto T, Elder CM, Okun MS, et al. Stimulation of the subthalamic nucleus changes the firing pattern of pallidal neurons. J Neurosci 2003;23:1916–23.

[23] Wichmann T, DeLong MR. Pathophysiology of Parkinson's disease: the MPTP primate model of the human disorder. Ann N Y Acad Sci 2003;991:199–213.

[24] Mink JW. The basal ganglia and involuntary movements: impaired inhibition of competing motor patterns. Arch Neurol 2003;60:1365–8.

[25] Koller WC, Lyons KE, Wilkinson SB, et al. Long-term safety and efficacy of unilateral deep brain stimulation of the thalamus in essential tremor. Mov Disord 2001;16:464–8.

[26] Pollak P, Fraix V, Krack P, et al. Treatment results: Parkinson's disease. Mov Disord 2002; 17(Suppl 3):S75–83.

[27] Houeto JL, Bejjani PB, Damier P, et al. Failure of long-term pallidal stimulation corrected by subthalamic stimulation in PD. Neurology 2000;55:728–30.

[28] Moro E, Esselink RA, Van Blercom N, et al. Bilateral subthalamic nucleus stimulation in a parkinsonian patient with previous unilateral pallidotomy and thalamotomy. Mov Disord 2000;15:753–5.

[29] Kumar R, Lang AE, Rodriguez-Oroz MC, et al. Deep brain stimulation of the globus pallidus pars interna in advanced Parkinson's disease. Neurology 2000;55:S34–9.

[30] Volkmann J, Sturm V, Weiss P, et al. Bilateral high-frequency stimulation of the internal globus pallidus in advanced Parkinson's disease. Ann Neurol 1998;44:953–61.

[31] The Deep-Brain Stimulation for Parkinson's Disease Study Group. Deep-brain stimulation of the subthalamic nucleus or the pars interna of the globus pallidus in Parkinson's disease. N Engl J Med 2001;345:956–63.

[32] Burchiel KJ, Anderson VC, Favre J, et al. Comparison of pallidal and subthalamic nucleus deep brain stimulation for advanced Parkinson's disease: results of a randomized, blinded pilot study. Neurosurgery 1999;45:1375–82.

[33] Anderson VC, Burchiel KJ, Hogarth P, et al. Pallidal vs subthalamic nucleus deep brain stimulation in Parkinson disease. Arch Neurol 2005;62:554–60.

[34] Rodriguez-Oroz MC, Obeso JA, Lang AE, et al. Bilateral deep brain stimulation in Parkinson's disease: a multicentre study with 4 years follow-up. Brain 2005;128:2240–9.

[35] Kaplitt MG, Hutchinson WD, Lozano AM. Target localization in movement disorders surgery. In: Tarsy D, Vitek JL, Lozano AM, editors. Surgical treatment of Parkinson's disease and other movement disorders. Totowa (NJ): Humana Press; 2003. p. 87–98.

[36] Houeto JL, Welter ML, Bejjani PB, et al. Subthalamic stimulation in Parkinson disease: intraoperative predictive factors. Arch Neurol 2003;60:690–4.

[37] Hariz MI, Fodstad H. Do microelectrode techniques increase accuracy or decrease risks in pallidotomy and deep brain stimulation? A critical review of the literature. Stereotact Funct Neurosurg 1999;72:157–69.

[38] Benazzouz A, Piallat B, Pollak P, et al. Responses of substantia nigra pars reticulata and globus pallidus complex to high frequency stimulation of the subthalamic nucleus in rats: electrophysiological data. Neurosci Lett 1995;189:77–80.

[39] Hershey T, Revilla FJ, Wernle AR, et al. Cortical and subcortical blood flow effects of subthalamic nucleus stimulation in PD. Neurology 2003;61:816–21.

[40] Windels F, Bruet N, Poupard A, et al. Effects of high frequency stimulation of subthalamic nucleus on extracellular glutamate and GABA in substantia nigra and globus pallidus in the normal rat. Eur J Neurosci 2000;12:4141–6.

[41] Molnar GF, Sailer A, Gunraj CA, et al. Changes in cortical excitability with thalamic deep brain stimulation. Neurology 2005;64:1913–9.

[42] Kumar R. Methods of programming and patient management with deep brain stimulation. In: Tarsy D, Vitek JL, Lozano AM, editors. Surgical treatment of Parkinson's disease and other movement disorders. Totowa (NJ): Humana Press; 2003. p. 189–212.

[43] Francel P, Ryder K, Wetmore J, et al. Deep brain stimulation for Parkinson's disease: association between stimulation parameters and cognitive performance. Stereotact Funct Neurosurg 2004;82:191–3.

[44] Temperli P, Ghika J, Villemure JG, et al. How do parkinsonian signs return after discontinuation of subthalamic DBS? Neurology 2003;60:78–81.

[45] Obeso JA, Rodriguez MC, Gorospe A, et al. Surgical treatment of Parkinson's disease. Baillieres Clin Neurol 1997;6:125–45.

[46] Goodman RR, Kim B, McClelland S III, et al. Operative techniques and morbidity with subthalamic nucleus deep brain stimulation in 100 consecutive patients with advanced Parkinson's disease. J Neurol Neurosurg Psychiatry 2006;77:12–7.

[47] Beric A, Kelly PJ, Rezai A, et al. Complications of deep brain stimulation surgery. Stereotact Funct Neurosurg 2001;77:73–8.

[48] Schupbach WM, Chastan N, Welter ML, et al. Stimulation of the subthalamic nucleus in Parkinson's disease: a 5 year follow up. J Neurol Neurosurg Psychiatry 2005;76:1640–4.

[49] Pillon B, Ardouin C, Damier P, et al. Neuropsychological changes between "off" and "on" STN or GPi stimulation in Parkinson's disease. Neurology 2000;55:411–8.

[50] Saint-Cyr JA, Trepanier LL. Neuropsychologic assessment of patients for movement disorder surgery. Mov Disord 2000;15:771–83.

[51] Hershey T, Revilla FJ, Wernle A, et al. Stimulation of STN impairs aspects of cognitive control in PD. Neurology 2004;62:1110–4.

[52] Fields JA, Troster AI, Woods SP, et al. Neuropsychological and quality of life outcomes 12 months after unilateral thalamic stimulation for essential tremor. J Neurol Neurosurg Psychiatry 2003;74:305–11.

[53] Loher TJ, Gutbrod K, Fravi NL, et al. Thalamic stimulation for tremor: subtle changes in episodic memory are related to stimulation per se and not to a microthalamotomy effect. J Neurol 2003;250:707–13.

[54] Halbig TD, Gruber D, Kopp UA, et al. Pallidal stimulation in dystonia: effects on cognition, mood, and quality of life. J Neurol Neurosurg Psychiatry 2005;76:1713–6.

[55] Vandewalle V, Van der LC, Groenewegen HJ, et al. Stereotactic treatment of Gilles de la Tourette syndrome by high frequency stimulation of thalamus. Lancet 1999;353:724.

[56] Houeto JL, Karachi C, Mallet L, et al. Tourette's syndrome and deep brain stimulation. J Neurol Neurosurg Psychiatry 2005;76:992–5.

[57] Magarinos-Ascone CM, Regidor I, Martinez-Castrillo JC, et al. Pallidal stimulation relieves myoclonus-dystonia syndrome. J Neurol Neurosurg Psychiatry 2005;76:989–91.

[58] Frucht SJ, Trost M, Ma Y, et al. The metabolic topography of posthypoxic myoclonus. Neurology 2004;62:1879–81.

[59] Houser M, Waltz T. Meige syndrome and pallidal deep brain stimulation. Mov Disord 2005; 20:1203–5.

ELSEVIER
SAUNDERS

Clin Geriatr Med 22 (2006) 827–842

CLINICS IN
GERIATRIC
MEDICINE

Parkinsonian Syndromes

Sid Gilman, MD, FRCP[a,b,*]

[a]*Department of Neurology, University of Michigan, 300 North Ingalls,
3D15, Ann Arbor, MI 48109-0489, USA*
[b]*Michigan Alzheimer's Disease Research Center, 300 North Ingalls Street,
3D15, Ann Arbor, MI 48109-0489, USA*

Several neurodegenerative disorders share with idiopathic Parkinson's disease (IPD) the features of bradykinesia, rigidity, hypokinetic speech, and unsteady gait, which are crucial aspects of parkinsonism. A clear beneficial response to dopaminergic medications characterizes IPD, and although some of these disorders can show a good response initially, usually the response diminishes and disappears with time. Albin discusses the initial evaluation of parkinsonism elsewhere in this issue. At autopsy examination, IPD shows degenerative changes in the substantia nigra, but the neuropathologic changes are more widespread in the other disorders [1]. As these disorders bear clinical similarity to IPD, they have been termed *Parkinson-plus syndromes* [2]. However, this term is misleading, because these disorders have clinical and neuropathologic features that are different from those of IPD. This article uses the term *parkinsonian syndromes* to discuss the most common types encountered clinically: multiple system atrophy (MSA), progressive supranuclear palsy (PSP), corticobasal degeneration (CBD), and vascular parkinsonism (VP). In one major autopsy series of patients who had parkinsonism, MSA, PSP, and CBD accounted for virtually all cases not attributable to IPD, with VP comprising a very small fraction of the ascertained cases [3].

Multiple system atrophy

A sporadic neurodegenerative disorder of undetermined cause, MSA can begin with parkinsonian features, cerebellar ataxia, or, less commonly,

This work was supported in part by Grants No. AG08671 and NS15655 from the National Institutes of Health.

* Department of Neurology, University of Michigan, 300 North Ingalls, 3D15, Ann Arbor, MI 48109-0489.

E-mail address: sgilman@umich.edu

autonomic failure. MSA was first described as several different diseases, including sporadic olivopontocerebellar atrophy [4], parkinsonism with autonomic failure [5], and striatonigral degeneration [6]. Graham and Oppenheimer [7] later introduced the term *multiple system atrophy* to delineate a neurodegenerative disease characterized clinically by combinations of parkinsonian, cerebellar, autonomic, and corticospinal ("pyramidal") symptoms and signs, with cell loss and gliosis extensively in the basal ganglia, inferior olives, pons, and cerebellum. Papp and colleagues [8] then showed that all forms of MSA possess a distinctive neuropathologic feature, glial cytoplasmic inclusions [8], consisting principally of alpha-synuclein [9–11]. MSA is an alpha-synucleinopathy, along with IPD and dementia with Lewy bodies. The incidence of MSA is 0.6 cases per 100,000 population [12], but is 3.0 cases per 100,000 in people older than age 50 [13,14]. Estimates of the prevalence of MSA vary from 1.9 to 4.9 per 100,000 [14,15].

Clinical presentation

MSA begins with parkinsonian features in most cases, and with cerebellar ataxia in a minority [16–18]. Autonomic failure consisting of urinary insufficiency, orthostatic hypotension, or both accompanies the motor disorder in approximately 50% of patients at disease onset. The parkinsonian features consist of bradykinesia, rigidity, gait unsteadiness, and hypokinetic (soft) speech. Patients complain of difficulty turning over in bed and rising from soft seats, usually needing to push off with their hands. Falls occur, but not as often as in PSP. Some patients show a postural tremor, but typical parkinsonian resting tremor is unusual. Patients usually show a poor response to levodopa, although some show a good, and occasionally an excellent, response, although it is usually short-lived [19].

MSA beginning with parkinsonism, designated *MSA-P* [20], is the most common motor subtype, ranging from 40% to 66% in various series [19]. Most individuals (85%–100%) develop parkinsonism some time along the disease course, even if the disorder begins with cerebellar ataxia [19]. MSA beginning with cerebellar ataxia, designated *MSA-C*, occurs in 10% to 15% of cases [19,20]. The cerebellar disorder includes ataxia of gait, limb movements, and speech, and oculomotor disorders, including gaze-evoked nystagmus, overshoot dysmetria, and saccadic intrusions into smooth pursuit movements. Most people who have MSA-C initially complain of imbalance, unsteadiness of gait, bumping into walls when walking in narrow passageways, and deterioration of handwriting and other fine motor skills. When patients who have MSA-C first seek medical attention, brain imaging often shows atrophy of the superior cerebellar vermis and pons. People who have MSA-C who survive sufficiently long develop progressively increasing parkinsonian features of bradykinesia, rigidity, and hypokinetic speech.

Autonomic dysfunction can appear as presenting symptoms of MSA or develop early in the course, usually in the form of urinary retention with incomplete bladder emptying and, later, urinary incontinence [21]. Fecal incontinence occurs less frequently (2%–12%) despite frequent denervation of the external anal sphincter [19]. Impotence in men occurs nearly uniformly in MSA, appearing sometimes 5 to 10 years before other symptoms. Patients who have MSA complain commonly of constipation and occasionally of impaired sweating. Symptomatic orthostatic hypotension usually appears later in the course, but measurable postural hypotension can be found early and should be sought in patients presenting with parkinsonian or cerebellar features. Blood pressure and pulse should be measured after patients have been recumbent for 2 to 3 minutes, and then measured again 2 to 3 minutes after standing. Measurements while seated are not helpful. The consensus conference diagnosis for autonomic failure requires an orthostatic fall in blood pressure by 30 mm Hg systolic or 15 mm Hg diastolic; urinary incontinence consisting of persistent, involuntary partial or total bladder emptying accompanied by erectile dysfunction in men; or blood pressure changes and urinary difficulties [20]. Patients who have MSA remain asymptomatic often despite large systolic and diastolic decreases in blood pressure. With advanced disease, orthostatic syncope is common and associated with sudden death. Dopaminergic drugs can provoke or worsen orthostatic hypotension and must be administered in low doses initially with cautious escalation. Recumbent arterial hypertension has been reported in a few patients who had severe cardiovascular autonomic failure [16].

Rapid eye movement sleep behavioral disorder (RBD) is found through history in a large fraction of patients who have MSA, and in almost all through polysomnography [22–24]. It can appear in advance of other features of MSA. RBD consists of dream enactment with motor outbursts that can be violent and injure the patient or bed partner. Most people who have MSA also have obstructive sleep apnea, which is an ominous feature of this disease because it is associated with sudden death [23,25,26].

Additional clinical findings reported in MSA include extensor plantar reflexes and hyperreflexia, but limb weakness and spasticity are uncommon. Less frequent features include upgaze palsy, emotional lability, truncal dystonia with a tendency to lean laterally while seated, antecollis, myoclonus, stridor, polyneuropathy, distal limb cyanosis, postprandial hypotension, poor lacrimation and salivation, and Raynaud phenomenon [19].

Pathophysiology

The neuropathologic findings consist of widespread loss of neurons and gliosis, accompanied by glial cytoplasmic inclusions, occurring most prominently in the substantia nigra, striatum, cerebellar cortex, pyramidal tract, Edinger-Westphal nucleus, locus ceruleus, inferior olives, dorsal motor nucleus of the vagus, intermediolateral cell column of the spinal cord, and Onuf's nucleus [8,27]. The pathogenesis of the cell loss is not known. Oligodendroglial inclusions stain heavily for alpha-synuclein [9], and their distribution relative to that of the neuronal pathology suggests that the glial defect may be the primary event [27]. MSA is currently defined as a sporadic disease, and familial cases are rare [28].

Diagnostic evaluation

Diagnosis is based on consensus criteria [20]. Purely based on clinical examination, the criteria include four domains: autonomic/urinary dysfunction, parkinsonism, cerebellar ataxia, and corticospinal dysfunction. The criteria were developed to define the relative importance of these features. The diagnosis of possible MSA requires one criterion plus two features from separate domains. The diagnosis of probable MSA requires the criterion of autonomic failure/urinary dysfunction plus poorly levodopa-responsive parkinsonism or cerebellar ataxia. The diagnosis of definite MSA requires pathologic confirmation. The exclusion criteria include onset before the age of 30 years, family history, hallucinations unrelated to medication, dementia, vertical supranuclear gaze dysfunction, focal cortical dysfunction, and clinical or radiographic evidence for alternate diagnoses. In more than half of those who have MSA-C, MRI scans show cerebellar and brainstem atrophy, iron deposition appearing as a low T2 signal in the putamen, and gliosis appearing as a high-T2 "slit" at the posterolateral border of the putamen [29]. In MSA-P, an even greater percentage of patients show the putaminal changes [30]. These findings have high sensitivity and specificity in patients clinically diagnosed with MSA [31,32]. Newer MRI techniques have the potential for additional objective criteria for diagnosis [33]. Positron emission tomography (PET) and single-photon emission computed tomography (SPECT) imaging with striatal dopamine terminal ligands show a marked decrease of striatal dopaminergic terminals, but do not differentiate MSA from IPD [34–36]. Nerve conduction and electromyogram studies may show subclinical polyneuropathy, but this is seldom helpful diagnostically. External urethral sphincter electromyogram shows denervation in almost all patients who have MSA [18,37], but denervation can also be found in advanced IPD and PSP [38,39]. If denervation is found in the first 5 years of the disorder, however, the test can differentiate MSA from IPD [40].

Management and prognosis

MSA shortens life expectancy. In one series, patients who had autopsy-proven MSA survived a mean of 8 years [41], and a meta-analysis of 433 patients showed a mean survival of 6.2 years [42], with no difference between the MSA-P and MSA-C types. People who have this disease must be aware that MSA limits life span, although the duration from onset in any single individual cannot be determined. Patients should be aware of the availability of treatment for certain features to assist with some of the disabling symptoms. In MSA-P, levodopa may improve rigidity, bradykinesia, and postural instability, but it is effective in only about half of the patients [41,43]. Treatment should be initiated slowly and cautiously because of the danger of worsening autonomic symptoms. Orthostatic hypotension should be treated with pressure stockings to increase central venous volume, and liberal use of sodium and water in the diet to expand the blood volume, unless a danger exists of renal insufficiency or congestive heart failure. Affected individuals should sleep with the head of the bed elevated 6 in, rise slowly from the recumbent position, and have multiple small meals rather than three large meals to reduce postprandial splanchnic blood flow. Dietary fiber supplementation and stool softening agents treat constipation and avoid straining at stool, reducing risk for syncope. Extreme heat should be avoided because of impaired sweating.

When orthostatic hypotension is symptomatic, fludrocortisone, a mineralocorticoid, should be added at a dose of 0.1 mg daily and increased as needed to a maximum of 0.4 mg per day in two divided doses. Midodrine, an α-adrenergic agonist, can also be effective [44] when initiated at a dose of 2.5 mg three times a day and increased as needed to 10 mg three times a day. Supine hypertension is rarely a problem, but can be treated with the α-adrenergic agonist clonidine at a dose of 0.1 mg twice a day, increasing to 0.3 mg twice a day as needed. Propranolol can also be used, beginning with a dose of 20 mg twice a day and increasing gradually as needed.

Urinary function should be evaluated through urodynamic studies. If bladder emptying is incomplete, treatment is mandatory to prevent recurrent infection. If detrusor hyperreflexia is found, urinary frequency or incontinence can be treated with a peripherally acting anticholinergic medication, such as oxybutynin, 5 mg to 10 mg, or propantheline, 15 mg to 30 mg. Sildenafil can be hazardous as a treatment for male impotence because of the risk for exacerbating orthostatic hypotension [45].

Depression is an almost universal reaction to the physical, occupational, and social losses associated with MSA, and referral to psychiatry or direct treatment with a selective serotonin reuptake inhibitor can be helpful. Although RBD rarely needs treatment other than separate beds for the patient and spouse, it does respond to clonazepam, 0.5 mg, at bedtime.

Progressive supranuclear palsy

PSP is a sporadic neurodegenerative disorder of undetermined cause usually presenting with parkinsonian features and frequent falls, and then progressing to include supranuclear gaze palsy. One of the neurofibrillary degenerations, PSP is characterized by neuronal loss, gliosis, and neurofibrillary tangles consisting of paired helical filaments and straight filaments of tau protein [46,47]. The average annual incidence rate for PSP in individuals older than age 50 is 5.3 per 100,000 population [13] and the prevalence is approximately 5 per 100,000 population [48].

Clinical presentation

PSP usually begins with bradykinesia, rigidity, postural instability, dysarthria, and dysphagia. The dysarthria includes hypokinetic, ataxic, and spastic elements [49]. Patients persistently overfill their mouths when eating, and dysphagia is a prominent early feature. PSP does not usually cause tremor, and postural instability with frequent falls, often backward, begins early in the course. In unusual cases, PSP begins with a cerebellar ataxia, with the diagnosis becoming clear after a few years as parkinsonian features intervene and then supranuclear palsy appears. Falls are the most disabling initial feature of PSP. PSP is also associated with personality change, frequently apathy and depression, and mild dementia characterized principally by executive dysfunction [50]. Impaired abstract thought, decreased verbal fluency, motor perseveration, apathy, and disinhibition are observed at an early stage. Sleep disturbances, notably insomnia, shorter sleep latency, and increased number of awakenings, which all become more severe with increased motor impairment, worsen quality of life [51].

Supranuclear gaze palsy is the most definitive diagnostic feature of PSP, but often develops 3 to 4 years after the initial symptoms. Slowing of vertical saccades precedes the development of vertical gaze palsy, and staircase movements with vertical gaze suggest the diagnosis. Impairment of downward opticokinetic nystagmus can help distinguish PSP from IPD [52]. The supranuclear gaze palsy initially involves only upgaze or downgaze, but ocular movements in both vertical and horizontal planes gradually become affected. Dissociation between impaired voluntary and pursuit gaze and preservation of oculocephalic reflexes shows the supranuclear origin of the oculomotor disorder. Associated oculomotor abnormalities include square-wave jerks, convergence insufficiency, reduced blink rate, eyelid apraxia (difficulty opening the closed eyelids) accompanied by compensatory eyebrow elevation with frontalis overactivity, and blepharospasm. Many patients have difficulty reading because of problems with visual tracking and trouble understanding the material. Approximately one third of patients present with relative asymmetry, mild tremor, and a moderate but transient response to levodopa [53].

Pathophysiology

The neuropathologic changes include brainstem atrophy with neuronal loss, neurofibrillary tangles, and glial inclusions in the brainstem, basal ganglia, and diencephalon [47]. The neurofibrillary tangles of PSP have a different distribution and ultrastructure from those of Alzheimer's disease [54]. The primary constituent of neurofibrillary tangles is the microtubule-associated protein tau (MAPT). The gene for MAPT is located on chromosome 17, and the region containing MAPT consists of two haplotypes, H1 and H2, which are defined by linkage disequilibrium among several polymorphisms over the entire MAPT gene [55]. PSP is associated with the full H1 tau haplotype [56], and single nucleotide polymorphisms from this region are associated with a higher risk for the disease [57].

Diagnostic evaluation

The National Institute of Neurological Disorders and Stroke and the Society for PSP established clinical diagnostic criteria that were validated in a large autopsy series [58]. The criteria specify three degrees of diagnostic certainty: possible, probable, and definite. Possible PSP requires the presence of a gradually progressive disorder with onset at the age of 40 years or later; either vertical supranuclear gaze palsy or slowing of vertical saccades and prominent postural instability with falls in the first year of onset; and no evidence of other diseases that could explain these features. Probable PSP requires vertical supranuclear gaze palsy, prominent postural instability, and falls in the first year of onset, in addition to the features of possible PSP. Definite PSP requires a history of probable or possible PSP and histopathologic confirmation. Diagnosis is clinical, but MRI frequently shows midbrain atrophy, which is a specific but not highly sensitive sign of the disorder [59]. Atrophy of the superior cerebellar peduncle can help differentiate between PSP and MSA [60]. A few individuals show an "eye-of-the-tiger" sign in MRI, consisting of a high T2 signal in a V formed by the lateral and medial putamen with a normal signal between them [59].

Management and prognosis

Early management should focus on preventing falls by encouraging patients to use a four-wheel walker with a heavy base and handbrakes. Apart from antidepressants, medications are largely ineffective in PSP. Levodopa therapy can be attempted, but is effective in only approximately one third of cases and the beneficial response rarely persists more than 1 or 2 years [61]. Care is otherwise assistive, focusing on adapting to the deficits. The disorder progresses inexorably, with death occurring at a median interval of 9.7 years from onset [62].

Corticobasal degeneration

Initially described by Rebeiz and colleagues [63], CBD is a sporadic neurodegenerative disorder characterized by the parkinsonian features of bradykinesia and rigidity, usually markedly asymmetrical, with limb apraxias leading to severe motor dysfunction and a progressive cognitive disorder. Along with PSP, CBD is a tauopathy, with neuropathologic changes consisting of an intracellular filament accumulation composed of MAPT [64]. Epidemiologic data are limited, with a single study reporting a prevalence of 1.93 per 100,000 [65]. Incidence data are conflicting; one study reported a CBD:PSP ratio of 1:6.7 [3], but another reported a ratio of 1:2.5 [65].

Clinical presentation

CBD begins usually with asymmetric parkinsonian symptoms or cognitive decline. When motor dysfunction appears initially, the symptoms include rigidity, akinesia, and gait disorder, coupled with marked difficulty using the involved side of the body because of limb apraxia [66]. Subjects complain that the affected limbs are clumsy, and that they have difficulty with fine motions of the fingers, along with abnormal reaching movements owing to incorrect orientation and trajectory during movements projected into space. Some patients exhibit the "alien limb" phenomenon in which the affected limb, usually an arm, moves involuntarily, appearing to float in space without the individual's awareness [67]. The limb can also develop abnormal (dystonic) postures with spasms, myoclonic movements, or both [68]. In many cases, cognitive dysfunction is the presenting feature, and is characterized by a progressive general cognitive decline, with prominent executive dysfunction and learning deficits [69]. Hemispatial neglect can be a feature, along with disinhibition and dysphasia [70]. Irrespective of the mode of onset, once the disorder has become established, rigidity, bradykinesia, gait disorder, or tremor affect all subjects; myoclonus or dystonia appear in 89%; and cognitive dysfunction can be found in 93% [71]. Multiple oculomotor abnormalities have been described, including oculomotor apraxia, optic ataxia, supranuclear gaze palsy, and simultanagnosia [72].

Pathophysiology

The neuropathologic features of CBD consist of ballooned neurons, cortical and striatal tau-containing neuronal and glial inclusions, astrocytic plaques and threadlike lesions, and loss of neurons in the substantia nigra, cerebral cortex, and cervical spinal cord [73–75]. As in PSP, patients who have CBD have a tau H1 haplotype with overrepresentation of the H1/H1 genotype, suggesting a similar genomic cause [76]. The tau aggregates in corticobasal degeneration are different from those of Alzheimer's disease and similar to those of PSP [76,77].

Diagnostic evaluation

The diagnosis of CBD is based principally on clinical findings, but the disorder can be difficult to distinguish from other neurologic diseases, particularly PSP, frontotemporal dementia, Creutzfeldt-Jakob disease, and Alzheimer's disease [78]. Anatomic imaging with CT or MR shows generalized cerebral or focal atrophy, but the findings are nonspecific unless quantified [79,80]. Functional imaging with SPECT scans show asymmetrical blood flow to the cerebral cortex and basal ganglia in CBD, and symmetrical flow in PSP [81,82]. SPECT with [123I]beta-CIT, a ligand for dopamine terminals, shows asymmetric striatal binding in CBD, but also in IPD [83]. PET with [18F]fluorodeoxyglucose shows asymmetric hypometabolism in the parietal lobe and thalamus or in the frontal lobe and striatum, more severe on the side contralateral to the most affected limbs [84]. Neuropsychologic tests show asymmetric apraxias, executive dysfunctioning, and learning deficits, but rigorous studies have not shown these tests to differentiate CBD from other dementias [85–87].

Management and prognosis

Medication does not ameliorate the cognitive dysfunction or apraxia. Dopaminergic agents can be provided to improve the parkinsonian features, but have been effective in fewer than 25% of cases [71]. Clonazepam can be helpful for dystonia, and selective injection of botulinum toxin into muscles of dystonic limbs can help avoid the strong fist clenching that occurs later in the disorder [71,88]. Depression occurs almost universally in this disorder and can be ameliorated with appropriate treatment [89]. The disease progresses relentlessly to death within 6 to 9 years without influence by medications [90].

Vascular parkinsonism

VP, also termed *arteriosclerotic parkinsonism* or *lacunar parkinsonism*, is a neurologic disorder that affects people in the seventh to eighth decade of life and is characterized by the parkinsonian signs of bradykinesia, rigidity, and gait disorder resulting from multiple lacunar infarctions bilaterally in the basal ganglia and subcortical white matter. VP differs clinically from IPD in showing plastic (lead-pipe) rigidity rather than cogwheel rigidity, symmetric rather than asymmetric symptoms, absence of tremor, and poor or no response to dopaminergic medications. VP frequently affects the lower body more than the upper and is often associated with pseudobulbar palsy, pyramidal tract signs, and dementia. Critchley [91] originally described the disorder, and many subsequent case reports and autopsy series confirmed the finding that multiple infarctions can cause a parkinsonian syndrome [92–95]. VP accounts for a small fraction of cases of parkinsonism [1,3,92–96].

Clinical presentation

Patients who have VP frequently have a history of hypertension-related stroke, usually lacunar syndromes, and develop parkinsonian symptoms of akinesia rigidity, masked face, and gait disorder. The symptoms often exhibit stepwise progression; however, gradual slow progression and sudden onset, followed by improvement are described [93,97–99]. The variable course relates to variations in the development of lacunar infarcts. These lacunar infarcts begin stepwise within 3 hours in one third of cases; develop gradually over 2 to 6 days in another third; and are preceded by a transient ischemic attack within 24 hours in another third [100–103]. Many lacunar infarcts are silent. Although VP characteristically responds poorly to dopaminergic medications, some patients experience an initial response to levodopa with a gradual decline in responsiveness [104]. Patients who have VP are unsteady while standing, their balance is poor, and their gait consists of small, short steps, often with a "glued to the floor" quality [105]. Associated neurologic signs include impaired cognition; frontal release signs; pseudobulbar palsy with dysarthria, dysphagia, and emotional lability; and extensor plantar reflexes [1,95,96,99].

Pathophysiology

VP usually results from lacunar infarctions. Arterial hypertension and intracranial atherosclerosis are the key factors in the pathogenesis of lacunes, which are small infarcts (<1 cm) accompanying occlusion of perforating vessels [100,101]. Hypertension is the most important risk factor for lacunar infarcts. Other risk factors include older age, diabetes mellitus, ischemic heart disease, transient ischemic attacks, and cigarette smoking. Multiple small infarctions deep in the white matter of the cerebral hemispheres and basal ganglia bilaterally affect the long descending pathways to the brainstem and spinal cord in addition to the basal ganglia circuits, thereby evoking bilaterally symmetric parkinsonian symptomatology with the associated abnormalities of impaired cognition, frontal release signs, pseudobulbar palsy, and extensor plantar reflexes.

Cerebral autosomal-dominant arteriopathy, a rare disorder associated with lacunes, results from a dominant mutation in the notch 3 gene [106,107]. Diffuse white-matter changes and lacunar infarcts often lead to progressive dementia, occasionally with parkinsonian features. Other vascular disorders, including dissection, vasculitis, drug abuse, and neurosyphilis, have also been associated with lacunar infarctions.

Diagnostic evaluation

The diagnosis should be considered in people who have a symmetric parkinsonian syndrome, particularly when accompanied by cognitive impairment, pseudobulbar palsy, extensor plantar responses, and a poor or absent response to levodopa. The disorder can be differentiated from MSA by the absence of autonomic impairment, from PSP by the absence of oculomotor disorders, and from CBD by the symmetric presentation and absence of focal dystonias. CT is less sensitive than MRI for detecting small subcortical lacunes. MR scans show multiple lacunes or larger infarctions in the deep white matter bilaterally and within the basal ganglia. Patients who are suspected of having VP should undergo CT or MR angiography of the large intracranial arteries to detect nonlacunar pathology, and this should be performed as an emergency if the patient presents with an acute stroke, particularly if clinical progression or fluctuation occurs. The carotid arteries should be evaluated with ultrasonography and MR angiography after a lacunar stroke. The finding of moderate to severe stenosis of an extracranial internal carotid artery should lead to consideration of carotid endarterectomy. Echocardiography should be considered if there is reason to suspect cardiogenic or paradoxical embolism.

Management and prognosis

People who have VP usually do not experience a response to dopaminergic medications, but a clinical trial is worth the effort, even if the benefits are short-lived. Physical therapy and speech therapy can be helpful, and a four-wheel walker with a heavy base and hand brakes can prevent falls. Management of hypertension is the most important medical strategy in VP to prevent additional lacunar infarctions. Diuretics, angiotensin-converting–enzyme inhibitors, β-blockers, or calcium channel blockers can be used. Other risk factors should also be addressed. Individuals who smoke should stop, and if unable, should be treated with progressively decreasing doses of nicotine through patches, chewing gum, nasal spray, or inhalant spray. Diabetes mellitus should be treated vigorously with intensive glucose monitoring to maintain strict glycemic control, thereby reducing microvascular complications. Moderate- to high-grade asymptomatic carotid stenosis shown on catheter angiogram should be considered for carotid endarterectomy. The usefulness of endarterectomy is unclear, however, because no data specifically address prevention of lacunar stroke in asymptomatic carotid disease. Antithrombotic therapy (warfarin or aspirin) should be considered for nonvalvular atrial fibrillation. Elevated cholesterol levels should be treated with statins, which have not only lipid-lowering benefits but also improved endothelial function, plaque stabilization, antithrombotic, and neuroprotective properties. Additional risk factors for stroke include obesity, physical inactivity, alcohol abuse, hyperhomocysteinemia, and drug abuse [108], and each must be evaluated and treated. For secondary prevention, aspirin (160 mg or 325 mg) reduces the risk for early recurrent ischemic stroke [109], but for secondary prevention of lacunar infarcts, aspirin in a dose as low as 30 mg daily, dipyridamole, and the combination of extended release dipyridamole with aspirin are recommended [110]. Lacunar strokes are associated with low mortality and recurrence rates, and with good recovery and functional outcomes [111]. By the time people develop VP, however, they have a large burden of vascular disease.

Summary

The most common non-IPD neurodegenerative disorders presenting with parkinsonian features are MSA, PSP, and CBD. VP constitutes a small fraction of parkinsonian syndromes. In the early stages, the parkinsonian syndromes can be difficult to distinguish, but distinctive clinical features often gradually emerge, underscoring the importance of careful documentation of findings and prolonged follow-up. Treatment is primarily supportive care, but accurate diagnoses are necessary to provide patients with crucial information to plan their lives.

References

[1] Hughes AJ, Daniel SE, Kilford L, et al. Accuracy of clinical diagnosis of idiopathic Parkinson's disease: a clinico-pathologic study of 100 cases. J Neurol Neurosurg Psychiatry 1992; 55(3):181–4.

[2] Mark MH. Lumping and splitting the Parkinson plus syndromes: dementia with Lewy bodies, multiple system atrophy, progressive supranuclear palsy, and cortical-basal ganglionic degeneration. Neurol Clin 2001;19(3):607–27.

[3] Hughes AJ, Daniel SE, Ben-Shlomo Y, et al. The accuracy of diagnosis of parkinsonian syndromes in a specialist movement disorder service. Brain 2002;125(Pt 4):861–70.

[4] Dejerine J, Thomas A. L'atrophie olivopontocerebelleuse. Nouv Iconogr Salpet 1900;13: 330–70.

[5] Shy GM, Drager GA. A neurological syndrome associated with orthostatic hypotension: a clinical-pathologic study. Arch Neurol 1960;2:511–27.

[6] van der Eecken H, Adams RD, van Bogaert L. Striopallidal-nigral degeneration. A hitherto undescribed lesion in paralysis agitans. J Neuropathol Exp Neurol 1960;19:159–61.

[7] Graham JG, Oppenheimer DR. Orthostatic hypotension and nicotine sensitivity in a case of multiple system atrophy. J Neurol Neurosurg Psychiatry 1969;32(1):28–34.

[8] Papp MI, Kahn JE, Lantos PL. Glial cytoplasmic inclusions in the CNS of patients with multiple system atrophy (striatonigral degeneration, olivopontocerebellar atrophy and Shy-Drager syndrome). J Neurol Sci 1989;94(1–3):79–100.

[9] Gai WP, Power JH, Blumbergs PC, et al. Multiple-system atrophy: a new alpha-synuclein disease? Lancet 1998;352(9127):547–8.

[10] Spillantini MG, Crowther RA, Jakes R, et al. Filamentous alpha-synuclein inclusions link multiple system atrophy with Parkinson's disease and dementia with Lewy bodies. Neurosci Lett 1998;251(3):205–8.

[11] Dickson DW, Liu W, Hardy J, et al. Widespread alterations in alpha-synuclein in multiple system atrophy. Am J Pathol 1999;155(4):1241–51.

[12] Vanacore N, Bonifati V, Fabbrini G, et al. Epidemiology of multiple system atrophy. ESGAP Consortium. European Study Group on Atypical Parkinsonisms. Neurol Sci 2001;22(1):97–9.

[13] Bower JH, Maraganore DM, McDonnell SK, et al. Incidence of progressive supranuclear palsy and multiple system atrophy in Olmsted County, Minnesota, 1976 to 1990. Neurology 1997;49(5):1284–8.

[14] Vanacore N. Epidemiological evidence on multiple system atrophy. J Neural Transm 2005; 112(12):1605–12.

[15] Schrag A, Ben-Shlomo Y, Quinn NP. Prevalence of progressive supranuclear palsy and multiple system atrophy: a cross-sectional study. Lancet 1999;354(9192):1771–5.

[16] Wenning GK, Colosimo C, Geser F, et al. Multiple system atrophy. Lancet Neurol 2004; 3(2):93–103.

[17] Wenning GK, Ben Shlomo Y, Magalhaes M, et al. Clinical features and natural history of multiple system atrophy: an analysis of 100 cases. Brain 1994;117(Pt 4):835–45.

[18] Wenning GK, Kraft E, Beck R, et al. Cerebellar presentation of multiple system atrophy. Mov Disord 1997;12(1):115–7.

[19] Colosimo C, Geser F, Benarroch EE, et al. Multiple system atrophy. In: Gilman S, editor. Neurobiology of disease. San Diego (CA): Academic Press; 2007, in press.

[20] Gilman S, Low PA, Quinn N, et al. Consensus statement on the diagnosis of multiple system atrophy. J Neurol Sci 1999;163(1):94–8.

[21] Beck RO, Betts CD, Fowler CJ. Genitourinary dysfunction in multiple system atrophy: clinical features and treatment in 62 cases. J Urol 1994;151(5):1336–41.

[22] Plazzi G, Corsini R, Provini F, et al. REM sleep behavior disorders in multiple system atrophy. Neurology 1997;48(4):1094–7.

[23] Ghorayeb I, Bioulac B, Tison F. Sleep disorders in multiple system atrophy. J Neural Transm 2005;112(12):1669–75.

[24] Gilman S, Koeppe RA, Chervin RD, et al. REM sleep behavior disorder is related to striatal monoaminergic deficit in MSA. Neurology 2003;61(1):29–34.

[25] Munschauer FE, Loh L, Bannister R, et al. Abnormal respiration and sudden death during sleep in multiple system atrophy with autonomic failure. Neurology 1990;40(4):677–9.

[26] Gilman S, Chervin RD, Koeppe RA, et al. Obstructive sleep apnea is related to a thalamic cholinergic deficit in MSA. Neurology 2003;61(1):35–9.

[27] Papp MI, Lantos PL. The distribution of oligodendroglial inclusions in multiple system atrophy and its relevance to clinical symptomatology. Brain 1994;117(Pt 2):235–43.

[28] Soma H, Yabe I, Takei A, et al. Heredity in multiple system atrophy. J Neurol Sci 2006;240: 107–10.

[29] Konagaya M, Konagaya Y, Iida M. Clinical and magnetic resonance imaging study of extrapyramidal symptoms in multiple system atrophy. J Neurol Neurosurg Psychiatry 1994; 57(12):1528–31.

[30] Macia F, Yekhlef F, Ballan G, et al. T2-hyperintense lateral rim and hypointense putamen are typical but not exclusive of multiple system atrophy. Arch Neurol 2001;58(6): 1024–6.

[31] Schrag A, Kingsley D, Phatouros C, et al. Clinical usefulness of magnetic resonance imaging in multiple system atrophy. J Neurol Neurosurg Psychiatry 1998;65(1):65–71.

[32] Kraft E, Schwarz J, Trenkwalder C, et al. The combination of hypointense and hyperintense signal changes on T2-weighted magnetic resonance imaging sequences: a specific marker of multiple system atrophy? Arch Neurol 1999;56(2):225–8.

[33] Seppi K, Schocke MF, Wenning GK, et al. How to diagnose MSA early: the role of magnetic resonance imaging. J Neural Transm 2005;112(12):1625–34.

[34] Gilman S, Koeppe RA, Junck L, et al. Decreased striatal monoaminergic terminals in multiple system atrophy detected with PET. Ann Neurol 1999;45(6):769–77.

[35] Brucke T, Asenbaum S, Pirker W, et al. Measurement of the dopaminergic degeneration in Parkinson's disease with [123I] beta-CIT and SPECT. Correlation with clinical findings and comparison with multiple system atrophy and progressive supranuclear palsy. J Neural Transm Suppl 1997;50:9–24.

[36] Cilia R, Marotta G, Benti R, et al. Brain SPECT imaging in multiple system atrophy. J Neural Transm 2005;112(12):1635–45.

[37] Kirby R, Fowler C, Gosling J, et al. Urethro-vesical dysfunction in progressive autonomic failure with multiple system atrophy. J Neurol Neurosurg Psychiatry 1986;49(5):554–62.

[38] Giladi N, Simon ES, Korczyn AD, et al. Anal sphincter EMG does not distinguish between multiple system atrophy and Parkinson's disease. Muscle Nerve 2000;23(5):731–4.

[39] Vodušek DB. How to diagnose MSA early: the role of sphincter EMG. J Neural Transm 2005;112(12):1657–68.

[40] Polinsky RJ. Shy-Drager syndrome. In: Jankovic J, Tolosa E, editors. Parkinson's disease and movement disorders. Baltimore (MD): Williams and Wilkins; 1993. p. 191–204.

[41] Hughes AJ, Colosimo C, Kleedorfer B, et al. The dopaminergic response in multiple system atrophy. J Neurol Neurosurg Psychiatry 1992;55(11):1009–13.

[42] Ben-Shlomo Y, Wenning GK, Tison F, et al. Survival of patients with pathologically proven multiple system atrophy: a meta-analysis. Neurology 1997;48(2):384–93.

[43] Parati EA, Fetoni V, Geminiani GC, et al. Response to L-DOPA in multiple system atrophy. Clin Neuropharmacol 1993;16(2):139–44.

[44] Jankovic J, Gilden JL, Hiner BC, et al. Neurogenic orthostatic hypotension: a double-blind placebo-controlled study with midodrine. Am J Med 1993;95(1):38–48.

[45] Hussain IF, Brady CM, Swinn MJ, et al. Treatment of erectile dysfunction with sildenafil citrate (Viagra) in parkinsonism due to Parkinson's disease or multiple system atrophy with observations on orthostatic hypotension. J Neurol Neurosurg Psychiatry 2001;71(3):371–4.

[46] Steele JC, Richardson JC, Olszewski J. Progressive supranuclear palsy: a heterogeneous degeneration involving the brain stem, basal ganglia and cerebellum with vertical gaze and pseudobulbar palsy, nuchal dystonia and dementia. Arch Neurol 1964; 10:333–59.

[47] Litvan I, Hauw JJ, Bartko JJ, et al. Validity and reliability of the preliminary NINDS neuropathological criteria for progressive supranuclear palsy and related disorders. J Neuropathol Exp Neurol 1996;55(1):97–105.

[48] Nath U, Ben-Shlomo Y, Thomson RG, et al. The prevalence of progressive supranuclear palsy (Steele-Richardson-Olszewski syndrome) in the UK. Brain 2001;124(Pt 7):1438–49.

[49] Kluin KJ, Foster NL, Berent S, et al. Perceptual analysis of speech disorders in progressive supranuclear palsy. Neurology 1993;43(3 Pt 1):563–6.

[50] Grafman J, Litvan I, Gomez C, et al. Frontal lobe function in progressive supranuclear palsy. Arch Neurol 1990;47(5):553–8.

[51] Aldrich MS, Foster NL, White RF, et al. Sleep abnormalities in progressive supranuclear palsy. Ann Neurol 1989;25(6):577–81.

[52] Garbutt S, Riley DE, Kumar AN, et al. Abnormalities of optokinetic nystagmus in progressive supranuclear palsy. J Neurol Neurosurg Psych 2004;75(10):1386–94.

[53] Williams DR, de Silva R, Paviour DC, et al. Characteristics of two distinct clinical phenotypes in pathologically proven progressive supranuclear palsy: Richardson's syndrome and PSP-parkinsonism. Brain 2005;128(Pt 6):1247–58.

[54] Avila J, Lucas JJ, Perez M, et al. Role of tau protein in both physiological and pathological conditions. Physiol Rev 2004;84(2):361–84.

[55] Pittman AM, Myers AJ, Duckworth J, et al. The structure of the tau haplotype in controls and in progressive supranuclear palsy. Hum Moler Genet 2004;13(12):1267–74.

[56] Pastor P, Ezquerra M, Perez JC, et al. Novel haplotypes in 17q21 are associated with progressive supranuclear palsy. Ann Neurol 2004;56(2):249–58.

[57] Odetti P, Garibaldi S, Norese R, et al. Lipoperoxidation is selectively involved in progressive supranuclear palsy. J Neuropathol Exp Neurol 2000;59(5):393–7.

[58] Litvan I, Agid Y, Calne D, et al. Clinical research criteria for the diagnosis of progressive supranuclear palsy (Steele-Richardson-Olszewski syndrome): report of the NINDS-SPSP international workshop. Neurology 1996;47(1):1–9.

[59] Savoiardo M, Strada L, Girotti F, et al. MR imaging in progressive supranuclear palsy and Shy-Drager syndrome. J Comput Assist Tomogr 1989;13(4):555–60.

[60] Paviour DC, Price SL, Stevens JM, et al. Quantitative MRI measurement of superior cerebellar peduncle in progressive supranuclear palsy. Neurology 2005;64(4):675–9.

[61] Nieforth KA, Golbe LI. Retrospective study of drug response in 87 patients with progressive supranuclear palsy. Clin Neuropharmacol 1993;16(4):338–46.

[62] Golbe LI, Davis PH, Schoenberg BS, et al. Prevalence and natural history of progressive supranuclear palsy. Neurology 1988;38(7):1031–4.

[63] Rebeiz JJ, Kolodny EH, Richardson EP Jr. Corticodentatonigral degeneration with neuronal achromasia. Arch Neurol 1968;18(1):20–33.

[64] Mahapatra RK, Edwards MJ, Schott JM, et al. Corticobasal degeneration. Lancet Neurol 2004;3(12):736–43.

[65] Morimatsu M. Diseases other than Parkinson's disease presenting with parkinsonism. Nippon Ronen Igakkai Zasshi 2004;41(6):589–93.

[66] Zadikoff C, Lang AE. Apraxia in movement disorders. Brain 2005;128(Pt 7):1480–97.

[67] Doody RS, Jankovic J. The alien hand and related signs. J Neurol Neurosurg Psychiatry 1992;55(9):806–10.

[68] Grosse P, Kuhn A, Cordivari C, et al. Coherence analysis in the myoclonus of corticobasal degeneration. Mov Disord 2003;18(11):1345–50.

[69] Graham NL, Bak TH, Hodges JR. Corticobasal degeneration as a cognitive disorder. Mov Disord 2003;18(11):1224–32.

[70] Graham NL, Bak T, Patterson K, et al. Language function and dysfunction in corticobasal degeneration. Neurology 2003;61(4):493–9.

[71] Kompoliti K, Goetz CG, Boeve BF, et al. Clinical presentation and pharmacological therapy in corticobasal degeneration. Arch Neurol 1998;55(7):957–61.

[72] Mendez MF. Corticobasal ganglionic degeneration with Balint's syndrome. J Neuropsych Clin Neurosci 2000;12(2):273–5.

[73] Dickson DW, Bergeron C, Chin SS, et al. Office of Rare Diseases neuropathologic criteria for corticobasal degeneration. J Neuropathol Exp Neurol 2002;61(11):935–46.

[74] Iwasaki Y, Yoshida M, Hattori M, et al. Widespread spinal cord involvement in corticobasal degeneration. Acta Neuropathol (Berl) 2005;109(6):632–8.

[75] Lowe J, Errington DR, Lennox G, et al. Ballooned neurons in several neurodegenerative diseases and stroke contain alpha B crystallin. Neuropathol Appl Neurobiol 1992;18(4):341–50.

[76] Houlden H, Baker M, Morris HR, et al. Corticobasal degeneration and progressive supranuclear palsy share a common tau haplotype. Neurology 2001;56(12):1702–6.

[77] Yang L, Ksiezak-Reding H. Ubiquitin immunoreactivity of paired helical filaments differs in Alzheimer's disease and corticobasal degeneration. Acta Neuropathol (Berl) 1998;96(5):520–6.

[78] Litvan I, Bhatia KP, Burn DJ, et al. Movement Disorders Society Scientific Issues Committee report: SIC Task Force appraisal of clinical diagnostic criteria for Parkinsonian disorders. Mov Disord 2003;18(5):467–86.

[79] Yekhlef F, Ballan G, Macia F, et al. Routine MRI for the differential diagnosis of Parkinson's disease, MSA, PSP, and CBD. J Neural Transm 2003;110(2):151–69.

[80] Boxer AL, Geschwind MD, Belfor N, et al. Patterns of brain atrophy that differentiate corticobasal degeneration syndrome from progressive supranuclear palsy. Arch Neurol 2006;63:81–6.

[81] Zhang L, Murata Y, Ishida R, et al. Differentiating between progressive supranuclear palsy and corticobasal degeneration by brain perfusion SPET. Nucl Med Commun 2001;22(7):767–72.

[82] Hossain AK, Murata Y, Zhang L, et al. Brain perfusion SPECT in patients with corticobasal degeneration: analysis using statistical parametric mapping. Mov Disord 2003;18(6):697–703.

[83] Pirker W, Asenbaum S, Bencsits G, et al. [123I]beta-CIT SPECT in multiple system atrophy, progressive supranuclear palsy, and corticobasal degeneration. Mov Disord 2000;15(6):1158–67.

[84] Coulier IM, de Vries JJ, Leenders KL. Is FDG-PET a useful tool in clinical practice for diagnosing corticobasal ganglionic degeneration? Mov Disord 2003;18(10):1175–8.

[85] Pillon B, Blin J, Vidailhet M, et al. The neuropsychological pattern of corticobasal degeneration: comparison with progressive supranuclear palsy and Alzheimer's disease. Neurology 1995;45(8):1477–83.

[86] Massman PJ, Kreiter KT, Jankovic J, et al. Neuropsychological functioning in corticobasal degeneration: differentiation from Alzheimer's disease. Neurology 1996;46(3):720–8.

[87] Denes G. Comparison of apraxia in corticobasal degeneration and progressive supranuclear palsy. Neurology 2002;58(8):1317.

[88] Cordivari C, Misra VP, Catania S, et al. Treatment of dystonic clenched fist with botulinum toxin. Mov Disord 2001;16(5):907–13.

[89] Hargrave R, Rafal R. Depression in corticobasal degeneration. Psychosomatics 1998;39(5):481–2.

[90] Gibb WR, Luthert PJ, Marsden CD. Corticobasal degeneration. Brain 1989;112(Pt 5):1171–92.

[91] Critchley M. Arteriosclerotic parkinsonism. Brain 1929;52:23–83.

[92] Parkes JD, Marsden CD, Rees JE, et al. Parkinson's disease, cerebral arteriosclerosis, and senile dementia: clinical features and response to levodopa. Q J Med 1974;43(169):49–61.

[93] Tolosa ES, Santamaria J. Parkinsonism and basal ganglia infarcts. Neurology 1984;34(11): 1516–8.

[94] Jellinger K. Overview of morphological changes in Parkinson's disease. Adv Neurol 1987; 45:1–18.

[95] Hughes AJ, Daniel SE, Blankson S, et al. A clinicopathologic study of 100 cases of Parkinson's disease. Arch Neurol 1993;50(2):140–8.

[96] Sibon I, Tison F. Vascular parkinsonism. Curr Opin Neurol 2004;17(1):49–54.

[97] Fitzgerald PM, Jankovic J. Lower body parkinsonism: evidence for a vascular etiology. Mov Disord 1989;4(3):249–60.

[98] Zijlmans JC, Thijssen HO, Vogels OJ, et al. MRI in patients with suspected vascular parkinsonism. Neurology 1995;45(12):2183–8.

[99] Yamanouchi H, Nagura H. Neurological signs and frontal white matter lesions in vascular parkinsonism. A clinicopathologic study. Stroke 1997;28(5):965–9.

[100] Fisher CM. Lacunes: small, deep cerebral infarcts. Neurology 1965;15:774–84.

[101] Fisher CM. The arterial lesions underlying lacunes. Acta Neuropathol (Berl) 1968;12(1): 1–15.

[102] Fisher CM. Lacunar strokes and infarcts: a review. Neurology 1982;32(8):871–6.

[103] Fisher CM. A career in cerebrovascular disease: a personal account. Stroke 2001;32(11): 2719–24.

[104] Mark MH, Sage JI, Walters AS, et al. Binswanger's disease presenting as levodopa-responsive parkinsonism: clinicopathologic study of three cases. Mov Disord 1995;10(4):450–4.

[105] Thompson PD, Marsden CD. Gait disorder of subcortical arteriosclerotic encephalopathy: Binswanger's disease. Mov Disord 1987;2(1):1–8.

[106] Amberla K, Waljas M, Tuominen S, et al. Insidious cognitive decline in CADASIL. Stroke 2004;35(7):1598–602.

[107] Peters N, Opherk C, Danek A, et al. The pattern of cognitive performance in CADASIL: a monogenic condition leading to subcortical ischemic vascular dementia. Am J Psychiatry 2005;162(11):2078–85.

[108] Goldstein LB, Adams R, Becker K, et al. Primary prevention of ischemic stroke: a statement for healthcare professionals from the Stroke Council of the American Heart Association. Circulation 2001;103(1):163–82.

[109] Coull BM, Williams LS, Goldstein LB, et al. Anticoagulants and antiplatelet agents in acute ischemic stroke: report of the Joint Stroke Guideline Development Committee of the American Academy of Neurology and the American Stroke Association (a division of the American Heart Association). Stroke 2002;33(7):1934–42.

[110] Albers GW, Easton JD, Sacco RL, et al. Antithrombotic and thrombolytic therapy for ischemic stroke. Chest 1998;114(5 Suppl):683S–98S.

[111] Petty GW, Brown RD, Whisnant JP, et al. Ischemic stroke subtypes: a population-based study of functional outcome, survival, and recurrence. Stroke 2000;31(5):1062–8.

ELSEVIER
SAUNDERS

Clin Geriatr Med 22 (2006) 843–857

CLINICS IN
GERIATRIC
MEDICINE

Essential Tremor

Elan D. Louis, MD, MS[a,b,*]

[a]*Department of Neurology, College of Physicians and Surgeons, Columbia University,
710 West 168th Street, New York, NY 10032, USA*
[b]*G.H. Sergievsky Center, College of Physicians and Surgeons, Columbia University,
630 West 168th Street, New York, NY 10032, USA*

Essential tremor (ET) is a common neurologic disorder that geriatricians and neurologists see frequently. The traditional paradigm has been that ET is a benign, monosymptomatic condition that is of little consequence. This view, however, is slowly being replaced. The emerging view of ET is that it is a progressive and often disabling neurologic disorder characterized by several motor and nonmotor features that accompany the readily recognizable tremor.

History of tremor

For thousands of years, human beings have provided written commentary on their tremors. The writings of ancient India, Egypt, Israel, and Greece contain references to tremor [1]. The hallmark feature of ET is the kinetic tremor (ie, tremor that occurs during voluntary movement) of the arms, in contrast to tremor at rest. Early physicians were seeing these types of tremors in their patients, as evident in the writings of Galen of Pergamon (130–200 AD) and much later in the writings of Sylvius de la Boe (1680), Van Swieten (1745), and Sauvages (1768) [1], who each distinguished kinetic tremor from rest tremor. In the nineteenth century, the word *essential* was applied to several medical entities that, like ET, seemed to have no clear medical cause and were viewed as an inherent or innate characteristic of the affected individual. The most complete early account of ET was that of Dr. Charles Dana, the New York neurologist who in 1887 documented

This article was supported by NIH grants R01 NS39422 and R01 NS42859.

* Department of Neurology, Columbia University Medical Center, The Neurological Institute of New York, Unit 198, 710 West 168th Street, New York, NY, 10032
E-mail address: EDL2@columbia.edu

doi:10.1016/j.cger.2006.06.012   *geriatric.theclinics.com*

the presence of this tremor in several large families [1,2]. The term *essential tremor* has been used with some degree of consistency by physicians since the mid-twentieth century to denote a form of kinetic tremor that is often familial and for which no cause has been established.

Epidemiology and genetics

A wide range of prevalence estimates exist in the now more than 20 prevalence studies from around the world [3], with much of this wide range explainable by the absence of a uniform methodology. In a recent population-based study that used improved methods, the prevalence of ET was 4% among individuals aged 40 years or older [4], making ET the most common tremor disorder. In this and other studies, the prevalence increased with advancing age, making ET highly prevalent in the sixth through eighth decades of life (with prevalence estimates often ranging from 6%–9%) [3,4]. One population-based study that estimated the rate at which new cases arise (incidence) found an adjusted annual incidence of 616 cases per 100,000 person-years [5].

Although experts often state that ET cases have no increased risk for mortality compared with similarly-aged controls, few data support this belief [6]. A prospective study of mortality in ET has not been conducted, nor has a study that assesses risk for mortality in patients who have ET compared with a contemporaneously enrolled control group. The association between ET and prevalent and incident dementia (discussed later) [7,8] suggests that some increased risk for mortality in ET is likely.

Epidemiologic studies have identified several risk factors for ET. First, age is clearly a risk factor; studies have shown an age-associated rise in the incidence [6] and prevalence [3,4] of ET. Second, ethnicity may be a risk factor for ET, with a higher prevalence in whites than in African-Americans [9,10]. Third, a family history of ET is a risk factor for ET, because the disease is in some cases familial [11,12]. Traditionally, genetic factors have been viewed as important in the etiology of ET because the disease can aggregate in families, many of which show an autosomal dominant pattern of inheritance [11–14]. Specific genes for ET have not yet been identified, although linkage has been reported on two different chromosomes, 3q13 and 2p22 [13,14]. Other investigators have shown the absence of linkage to either of these two loci in families that have a history of ET, indicating that genetic heterogeneity exists [15]. Twin studies have shown that the pairwise concordance was only 60% to 63% among monozygotic twins [11,16], suggesting that environmental factors are also important [12]. Recent epidemiologic studies [17,18] have implicated several specific environmental factors (toxicants), namely β-carboline alkaloids (eg, harmine and harmane, a group of highly tremorogenic chemicals) and lead, but further studies of putative environmental toxins are needed. In sum, the cause of ET is likely to be genetic in some instances and environmental in others.

Clinical presentation

The most recognizable and defining feature in patients who have ET is a kinetic tremor of the arms. This tremor may appear during various daily activities (eg, writing [Fig. 1], pouring, eating), and patients who have severe ET may also have a postural tremor (elicited by asking them to hold their arms outstretched in front of their body) [19]. This kinetic tremor may also have an intentional component (eg, during the finger–nose–finger maneuver, the tremor may worsen when patients approach their noses or the examiner's finger). The frequency of the tremor (4 and 12 Hz) is inversely related to age, with older patients generally exhibiting slower tremors [19]. In general, the tremor in ET is gradually progressive [20–22]. More than 90% of patients who seek medical attention report disability [23], and severely affected end-stage patients are physically unable to feed or dress themselves [20]. Between 15% and 25% of clinic patients are forced to retire prematurely, and 60% choose not to apply for a job or promotion because of uncontrollable shaking [21,22]. Far from being benign, most patients who have this disorder must adjust the way they perform their daily activities.

Although this tremor is most commonly seen in the arms, other body regions can be involved, especially the head or voice, but also occasionally the chin, tongue, and lower extremities [20]. Between 34% and 53% of patients have head involvement, with arm involvement also occurring in most (ie, isolated head tremor occurs in as few as 1% of patients) [21,24–27]. Another characteristic feature of ET is the gradual somatotopic spread of tremor. Head tremor typically evolves several years after the onset of arm tremor, with the converse (spread of tremor from the head to the arms) distinctly unusual [20,27–29].

Although ET is a progressive disorder [20,30], longitudinal studies are scant. In one study [31] that followed-up patients prospectively for 4 years, a 7% increase in tremor amplitude was seen each year, confirming the clinical anecdotal sense that the kinetic tremor in ET worsens gradually.

Although the most traditionally recognized feature of ET is the kinetic tremor, a more complex picture of a disorder with myriad clinical features is beginning to emerge. The presence of these clinical features is not uniform among patients, even at the same disease stage (ie, clinical heterogeneity exists). These features may be divided into motor versus nonmotor features.

Motor features include cerebellar signs (eg, ataxic gait, eye movement abnormalities) and tremor at rest. Several studies [32–34] have shown that patients who have ET experience postural instability and mild to moderate ataxic gait beyond that seen in normal aging. Furthermore, subtle eye-movement abnormalities have also been observed in patients who have ET [35]. It is well-known that some patients who have ET develop a tremor at rest [36,37]. At one tertiary referral center [38], 18.8% of the patients who had ET experienced rest tremor. These patients had disease of longer duration and greater severity than did those who did not experience rest tremor.

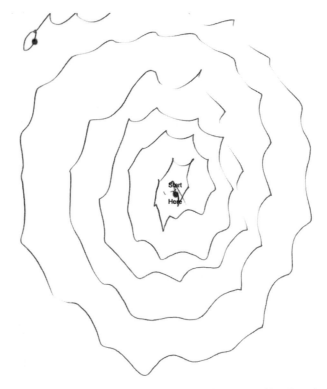

Fig. 1. An attempt by a patient who has ET to draw an Archimedes spiral.

Several recent studies have shown mild cognitive and neuropsychologic differences between patients who have ET and controls. Problems with verbal fluency, recent memory, working memory, and mental set-shifting have been described in these patients, suggesting that frontal cortical or frontal cortical–cerebellar pathways are involved [39–44]. In addition, changes in personality may occur. Patients who have ET have been shown to have higher harm-avoidance scores on a personality inventory [45], suggesting that, similar to several other progressive movement disorders (Parkinson's disease and Huntington's disease), cognitive–neuropsychologic features are part of the disorder in addition to involuntary movements. Even more than subtle cognitive changes, two recent studies have shown that the risk for dementia is elevated in patients who have ET compared with controls. In particular, patients who had older onset were 70% more likely to have dementia than were age-matched controls [7,8]. Finally, an olfactory deficit has been reported to occur in patients who have ET, and the deficit appears to be milder than that seen in patients who have Parkinson's disease [46–48]. This deficit seems to be unrelated to disease duration or severity, suggesting that, similar to Parkinson's disease, the deficit occurs early in the disease process.

In summary, the traditional view of ET as no more than a bland tremor is being replaced with a view of ET as a disease entity with a more varied set of clinical characteristics. Understanding of the pathophysiology of this disorder has also progressed.

Pathophysiology

Until recently, only 25 published postmortem studies of ET brains existed. Many were published 50 to 100 years ago, most did not use rigorous methodologies, and none used age-matched control brains [29,49–56]. No consistent pathologic abnormality had been identified. The Essential Tremor Centralized Brain Repository was recently established at Columbia University to collect postmortem tissue from patients who had ET. Initial studies on 11 ET brains and 12 control brains have shown that postmortem materials can be divided into two groups: those with cerebellar degenerative changes ("ET with cerebellar pathology") and those with brain stem Lewy bodies ("Lewy body variant of ET") [57–59]. The distribution of the Lewy bodies differs from that seen in Parkinson's disease; in ET the Lewy bodies occur primarily in the locus ceruleus (in the pons), whereas in Parkinson's disease, they occur in the substantia nigra pars compacta (in the midbrain) and other structures. The neurons of the locus ceruleus are the major source of norepinephrine in the brain; these neurons also synapse with cerebellar Purkinje cells. Alterations in the locus ceruleus could result in a diminution of stimulatory output from that locus to the Purkinje cells. Because the Purkinje cells are inhibitory output neurons, the net result would be a reduction in the normal inhibitory output from the cerebellum. Whether the pathologic lesion in ET is a primary cerebellar lesion ("ET with cerebellar pathology") or a lesion that results in secondary involvement of the cerebellum ("Lewy body variant of ET"), the net effect may the deregulation (through decreased cerebellar inhibitory output) of the neuronal pathway that involves the cerebellum, thalamus, and motor cortex (ie, the cerebellar–thalamic–cortical pathway). Stroke studies indicate that clinical lesioning of these structures ablates tremor [60], and the use of continuous deep-brain (thalamic) stimulation as an effective treatment for the tremor of ET (discussed later) also suggests that this loop is involved in ET.

Ultimately, ET might represent a family or complex of diseases rather than a single disease entity, and this disease complex may be more appropriately referred to as *the essential tremors*. Clinical, genetic, and pharmacologic heterogeneity suggest that this entity may be a composite of several entities unified by the presence of kinetic tremor [13,14,61–63]. Whether specific clinical manifestations can be linked with specific pathologic subtypes is unknown, but it is conceivable that patients who have ET with olfactory dysfunction, tremor at rest, and dementia may have the Lewy body variant of the disease. However, further clinical–pathologic correlations are needed.

Investigations and differential diagnosis

The diagnostic approach to patients who have ET includes obtaining a medical history, a physical examination and, in select instances, laboratory tests [64]. While taking the history, the clinician can collect information on localization of tremor ("Do you have head tremor?", "Do you have a shaky voice?", "Do your hands shake?"), progression of tremor over time ("When did your tremor start and how has it worsened over the years?"), and family history ("Does anyone else in your family shake?"). Caffeine, cigarettes, and numerous medications (eg, lithium, prednisone, sodium valproate, asthma inhalers) can exacerbate enhanced physiologic tremor (ie, normal tremor), which can resemble ET. A complete inventory of all current medications and caffeine and tobacco use is suggested for patients who experience tremor. Kinetic tremor may also be caused by hyperthyroidism, so the medical history should elicit symptoms of this condition (eg, diarrhea, weight loss, heat intolerance).

During the physical examination, the clinician should carefully assess the characteristics of the tremor. First, the clinician should determine that the movement is a tremor. Tremor is a rhythmic and oscillatory movement. *Rhythmic* means regularly recurrent (eg, normal sinus rhythm is a regularly recurrent heart pattern, whereas atrial fibrillation is arrhythmic) and *oscillatory* means that the movement alternates around a central plane. Patients who have ET must be distinguished from those who have Parkinson's disease (Table 1). Although patients who have Parkinson's disease often manifest a mild to moderate postural tremor (eg, tremor occurring during sustained arm extension) or kinetic tremor (eg, tremor occurring during voluntary movements such as writing or touching finger to nose) [61,65], rest tremor (eg, tremor occurring when the limb is fully relaxed) is also present in approximately 85% [66] of patients who have autopsy-proven Parkinson's disease. Although rest tremor can accompany ET, it usually occurs in the setting of severe kinetic tremor of long duration, and although mild cogwheeling can occur in ET, it does not occur in the setting of increased tone, as it does in Parkinson's disease. Other features of Parkinson's disease that generally do not occur in patients who have ET are hemibody

Table 1
Clinical differentiation of essential tremor and Parkinson's disease

	Essential tremor	Parkinson's disease
Kinetic tremor in arms, hands, or head	++	++
Hemi-body (arm and leg) tremor	0	++
Kinetic tremor > rest tremor	++	+
Rest tremor > kinetic tremor	0	++
Rigidity or bradykinesia (excluding cogwheeling without rigidity)	0	++

Abbreviations: ET, essential tremor; 0, does not occur; +, sometimes occurs; ++, often occurs.

involvement (eg, ipsilateral arm and leg tremor) and bradykinesia. The postural tremor of ET also tends to involve wrist flexion and extension, whereas in Parkinson's disease, wrist rotation often occurs.

Differentiation between patients who have ET and gait ataxia and patients who have spinocerebellar ataxia is based on the observation that patients who have ET do not exhibit nystagmus or scanning or dysarthric speech as they often do in these other types of ataxia.

Distinguishing ET from enhanced physiologic tremor is also important. Although the amplitude of kinetic tremor in ET is generally higher and the frequency lower than those of enhanced physiologic tremor, mild ET and severe enhanced physiologic tremor may have similar tremor amplitudes. In this setting, quantitative computerized tremor analysis with accelerometers attached to the arms, which is available at some tertiary care centers, may guide clinicians. Inertial loading of the limbs causes decreased tremor frequency in ET, but not in enhanced physiologic tremor.

Hence, examination of patients experiencing tremor should include maneuvers to elicit postural arm tremor (eg, having patients hold their arms extended in front of their bodies for 10 seconds), kinetic tremor (eg, having patients perform the finger-to-nose maneuver, draw spirals or write, or pour water between cups), rest tremor (eg, examining the arms while they are resting in the patients' laps or as patients walk to assess whether a rest tremor occurs). Clinicians can assess tone by passively moving the wrists and elbows while the patients relax their arms, and bradykinesia can be assessed by asking patients to perform rapid alternating movements (eg, finger taps, foot taps, pronation–supination of the arm).

The final step in evaluating patients suspected of having ET is the laboratory workup. If symptoms or signs of hyperthyroidism are present, then thyroid function tests should be performed. In younger patients who have kinetic tremor (younger than 40 years), the possibility of Wilson's disease should be explored with a serum ceruloplasmin. This disease is usually not an issue in older patients. Striatal dopamine transporter imaging may be useful in distinguishing ET from Parkinson's disease. Values in patients who have Parkinson's disease are lower than those of controls. Although some patients who have ET may have reduced values, their values are generally similar to those of controls [67,68], but this testing is rarely necessary because Parkinson's disease can generally be diagnosed based on a careful history and physical examination.

Treatment

The treatment of ET involves pharmacotherapy (Table 2) and surgery. Medications may be used to lessen functional disability and reduce embarrassment [69,70]. When these symptoms are not present, medications are generally not indicated. Surgery has a role in severe, disabling cases that are refractory to medications.

Current data suggest that two neurochemical systems may play a role in the pathophysiology and modulation of ET: the γ-aminobutyric acid (GABA)-ergic system in the central nervous system (CNS) and the adrenergic system (β_2 muscular adrenoreceptors) on the muscle spindles [71]. Because of the abundance of GABA terminals in the cerebellum (eg, on Purkinje cells), the tremor in ET could conceivably have its genesis in a disturbance of the GABA system, which is the major inhibitory neurotransmitter in the CNS. Medications that enhance CNS GABAergic activity, such as primidone, benzodiazepines, and barbiturates, have therapeutic value in patients who have ET, as does ethanol, which binds to the GABA type A (GABA$_A$) receptor and facilitates GABAergic neurotransmission [71]. The adrenoreceptors involved in the modulation ET are located deep in the striated muscle (outside of the nervous system). They probably play a role in the peripheral modulation of ET.

Several treatment issues require special emphasis. First, a large proportion of patients do not experience benefit from any medication, and factors that predict this lack of response have not been identified. Second, patients who respond to medications often only experience partial response, and tremor is rarely reduced to asymptomatic levels. The discussion that follows is largely limited to medications that have undergone scrutiny in double-blind trials.

Propranolol and primidone are the two front-line agents (see Table 2). Peripheral β-adrenergic receptors [72] probably mediate the effects of β-adrenergic blocking agents such as propranolol. When propranolol is given in doses of 120 mg/d or more, a significant reduction occurs in tremor severity [73]. In elderly patients, these doses may be difficult to achieve because of dose-dependent bradycardia. In addition, several relative contraindications exist [74] that do not preclude the use of propranolol, but make its use more difficult. These contraindications are asthma, congestive heart failure, diabetes mellitus, and atrioventricular block. Several β_1-selective β-blockers, including sotalol and atenolol, appear to be effective in managing ET, but

Table 2
Oral medications used in the treatment of essential tremor

Medication	Usual starting dose	Usual therapeutic dose	Side effects
Propranolol	10 mg/d	160–320 mg/d	Fatigue, bradycardia, hypotension, depression, exercise intolerance
Primidone	62.5 mg/d	62.5–1,000 mg/d	Sedation, nausea, vomiting, unsteadiness
Gabapentin	300 mg/d	1,200–3,600 mg/d	Drowsiness, nausea, dizziness, unsteadiness
Topiramate	25 mg/d	200–400 mg/d	Paresthesias, weight loss, taste perversion, fatigue, nausea, somnolence
Alprazolam	0.75 mg/d	0.75–2.75 mg/d	Sedation, fatigue

propranolol, a nonselective antagonist, has been the most consistently studied and is more effective than relatively selective β_1 antagonists [72]. In one recent crossover study, arotinolol was found to be as effective as propranolol [75]. One study showed that sustained-release propranolol is as effective as conventional propranolol [76].

Primidone, an anticonvulsant medication, is partially metabolized to phenylethylmalonamide and phenobarbital. The barbiturate metabolite and the parent compound are believed to mediate most of the therapeutic effect [77–79]. Primidone is superior to phenobarbital in reducing tremor [80]. In doses of up to 750 mg/d, primidone significantly reduces tremor compared with placebo [77–80]. Tolerability can be a common problem. Even at a low starting dose (62.5 mg/d), an acute toxic reaction consisting of nausea, vomiting, or ataxia has been reported in 22.7% [77] to 72.7% [78] of patients. One study found that the use of a very low initial dose (2.5 mg in suspension) and a graduated titration schedule did not appear to improve primidone tolerability [81]. Sedation is another side effect, which often limits the attainable dose in elderly patients.

Several studies have compared the two front-line agents, propranolol and primidone [79,82]; however, neither agent has been conclusively shown to be superior to the other. Although initial tolerability is a sizeable problem with primidone, one study provides tentative evidence that long-term tolerability of primidone is superior to that of propranolol. In a study of 25 patients who had ET, acute adverse reactions occurred in 8% treated with propranolol and 32% treated with primidone; however, 0% treated with primidone experienced "significant" side effects after 1 year compared with 17% treated with propranolol [83].

Several additional agents have been used with variable efficacy to treat patients who have ET. Gabapentin is an anticonvulsant medication that is structurally similar to the inhibitory neurotransmitter GABA. In two of three clinical trials, gabapentin (1200 to 3600 mg/d) resulted in a significant reduction in tremor compared with placebo, and in one of these two, its effect was similar to that of propranolol [84–86]. Gabapentin is generally well tolerated. In a single-center study, topiramate, an anticonvulsant agent with mixed effects (including effects of $GABA_A$ receptors), was administered to 24 patients and showed a significant antitremor effect [87]. A recent multicenter, randomized, double-blind trial in 208 patients found that topiramate (mean maintenance dose = 292 mg/d) was more effective than placebo in treating ET, although side effects (eg, paresthesia, fatigue, somnolence) were very common [88]. Benzodiazepines potentiate the effect of GABA by binding to the $GABA_A$ receptor. In one trial [89], alprazolam (dose ranging from 0.75 to 2.75 mg/d) resulted in significant reduction in tremor compared with placebo, and 75% of patients showed at least some improvement. However, another agent, clonazepam, has shown variable efficacy in clinical trials [90,91], with one of these trials showing no improvement compared with placebo [90]. One problem with the benzodiazepines is that their antitremor effect often requires a dose that is associated with sedation or cognitive slowing.

Calcium channel blockers have had variable success in treating ET. In one trial, flunarizine resulted in a significant reduction in tremor compared with placebo, with 13 of 15 patients experiencing improvement. However, none of the patients experienced improvement in a second trial [92]. In one trial [93], nimodipine (30 mg/d) resulted in a significant reduction in tremor compared with placebo, with 8 of 15 patients experiencing improvement. However, no further data exist regarding its efficacy. Clozapine, an atypical neuroleptic agent, effectively reduced tremor in one clinical trial [94], although no further data exist and the possibility of agranulocytosis has limited the use of this agent. More recently, zonisamide, an anticonvulsant with multiple mechanisms of action, was used in a crossover trial (zonisamide or arotinolol) and resulted in significant tremor reduction [95]. Levetiracetam is another anticonvulsant whose exact mechanism of action is unknown. In a recent double-blind, placebo-controlled trial, a single 1000-mg dose of levetiracetam significantly reduced hand tremor for at least 2 hours [96]. Follow-up studies are needed. In summary, propranolol and primidone remain the two front-line agents in treating ET. Several other agents have shown promise and further studies are needed to examine their efficacies and compare them with the two front-line agents.

Intramuscular botulinum toxin injections have the potential to reduce arm tremor by producing weakness. One trial randomized patients who had ET to receive 50 to 100 U of botulinum toxin per arm [97]. Although significant reduction in tremor amplitude occurred, studies have not always shown a significant improvement in function, and moderate hand and finger weakness is a common side effect. Intramuscular botulinum toxin injections may play more of a role in treating head tremor, particularly because oral medications tend to be less effective in treating the head tremor than that of the arm in ET.

Because ET may be mediated by neuronal loops that pass from the cerebellum to the cortex by way of the ventral intermediate nucleus of the thalamus, the main surgical approach currently used is continuous deep-brain stimulation through an electrode implanted in the ventral intermediate nucleus of the thalamus [98]. The procedure is effective in reducing tremor [98]. Patients who have moderate to severe tremor at baseline show complete resolution of tremor after treatment [98]. The clinician has the ability to adjust the stimulator settings during follow-up care [99]. Several studies also have evaluated the use of gamma knife thalamotomy, reporting favorable results [100,101], although deep-brain stimulation remains the preferred surgical treatment.

Nonprescription agents such as ethanol have also traditionally played a role in treating ET. Several studies have shown the effect of ethanol on tremor [102,103], although many patients are reluctant to use ethanol. Older patients take medications for which the concurrent use of ethanol is often contraindicated. Also, concerns about dependence and the social stigma of ethanol use exist. These factors all limit the use of ethanol.

1-Octanol is an alcohol that is currently used as a food-flavoring agent. In a recent randomized, placebo-controlled trial of 12 patients who had ET, a single 1 mg/kg oral dose of 1-octanol significantly decreased tremor amplitude for up to 90 minutes with no observed significant side effects or signs of intoxication [104]. Further studies are warranted.

Summary

ET is one of the most commonly encountered neurologic disorders in elderly individuals. The traditional view of ET as no more than a mono-symptomatic condition of little consequence is being replaced. As with other progressive neurologic disorders of later life, ET may represent a family of related diseases rather than a single disease. A better understanding of the causes and mechanism of the disease will lead to advances in treatment development.

References

[1] Louis ED. Essential tremor (Seminal Citations Section). Arch Neurol 2000;57:1522–4.
[2] Dana CL. Hereditary tremor, a hitherto undescribed form of motor neurosis. Am J Med Sci 1887;94:386–9.
[3] Louis ED, Ottman R, Hauser WA. How common is the most common adult movement disorder?: Estimates of the prevalence of essential tremor throughout the world. Mov Disord 1998;13:5–10.
[4] Dogu O, Sevim S, Camdeviren H, et al. Prevalence of essential tremor: door-to-door neurological exams in Mersin Province, Turkey. Neurology 2003;61:1804–7.
[5] Benito-Leon J, Bermejo-Pareja F, Louis ED. Incidence of essential tremor in three elderly populations of central Spain. Neurology 2005;64:1721–5.
[6] Rajput AH, Offord KP, Beard CM, et al. Essential tremor in Rochester, Minnesota: a 45-year study. J Neurol Neurosurg Psychiatry 1984;47:466–70.
[7] Benito-Leon J, Louis ED, Bermejo-Pareja F. Elderly onset essential tremor is associated with dementia. the NEDICES study. Neurology 2006; In press.
[8] Benito-Leon J, Bermejo-Pareja F, Louis ED. Essential tremor is associated with increased risk of incident dementia in a community-based longitudinal study. Neurology 2005; 64(Suppl 1):A253–4.
[9] Louis ED, Marder K, Cote L, et al. Differences in the prevalence of essential tremor among elderly African-Americans, Whites and Hispanics in Northern Manhattan, NY. Arch Neurol 1995;52:1201–5.
[10] Haerer AF, Anderson DW, Schoenberg BS. Prevalence of essential tremor. Results from the Copiah county study. Arch Neurol 1992;39:750–1.
[11] Tanner CM, Goldman SM, Lyons KE, et al. Essential tremor in twins: an assessment of genetic vs. environmental determinants of etiology. Neurology 2001;57:1389–91.
[12] Louis ED. Etiology of essential tremor: Should we be searching for environmental causes? Mov Disord 2001;16:822–9.
[13] Gulcher JR, Jonsson P, Kong A, et al. Mapping of a familial essential tremor gene, FET1, to chromosome 3q13. Nature Genetics 1997;17:84–7.

[14] Higgins JJ, Loveless JM, Jankovic J, Patel PI. Evidence that a gene for essential tremor maps to chromosome 2p in four families 1998;13:972–7.

[15] Kovach MJ, Ruiz J, Kimonis K. Genetic heterogeneity in autosomal dominant essential tremor. Genet Med 2001;3:197–9.

[16] Lorenz D, Frederiksen H, Moises H, et al. High concordance for essential tremor in monozygotic twins of old age. Neurology 2004;62:208–11.

[17] Louis ED, Zheng W, Jurewicz EC, et al. Elevation of blood β-carboline alkaloids in essential tremor. Neurology 2002;59:1940–4.

[18] Louis ED, Jurewicz EC, Applegate L, et al. Association between essential tremor and blood lead concentration. Environ Health Perspect 2003;111:1707–11.

[19] Brennan KC, Jurewicz E, Ford B, et al. Is essential tremor predominantly a kinetic or a postural tremor? A clinical and electrophysiological study. Mov Disord 2002;17:313–6.

[20] Critchley M. Observations on essential tremor (heredofamilial tremor). Brain 1949;72:113–39.

[21] Bain PG, Findley LJ, Thompson PD, et al. A study of heredity of essential tremor. Brain 1994;117:805–24.

[22] Rautakorpi I. Essential tremor. An epidemiological, clinical and genetic study. Research Reports from the Department of Neurology, University of Turku, Finland. Finland: University of Turkey; 1978.

[23] Louis ED, Barnes LF, Albert SM, et al. Correlates of functional disability in essential tremor. Mov Disord 2001;16:914–20.

[24] Lou JS, Jankovic J. Essential tremor: clinical correlates in 350 patients. Neurology 1991;41:234–8.

[25] Hubble JP, Busenbark KL, Pahwa R, et al. Clinical expression of essential tremor: effects of gender and age. Mov Disord 1997;12:969–72.

[26] Ashenhurst EM. The nature of essential tremor. Can Med Assoc J 1973;109:876–8.

[27] Louis ED, Ford B, Frucht S. Factors associated with increased risk of head tremor in essential tremor: a community-based study in northern Manhattan. Mov Disord 2003;18:432–6.

[28] Larsson T, Sjogren T. Essential tremor: a clinical and genetic population study. Acta Psychiatr Scand 1960;36(Suppl 144):1–176.

[29] Rajput A, Robinson C, Rajput AH. Essential tremor course and disability: a clinicopathologic study of 20 cases. Neurology 2004;62:932–6.

[30] Louis ED, Jurewicz EC, Watner D. Community-based data on associations of disease duration and age with severity of essential tremor: implications for disease pathophysiology. Mov Disord 2003;18:90–3.

[31] Elble RJ. Essential tremor frequency decreases with time. Neurology 2000;55:1547–51.

[32] Stolze H, Petersen G, Raethjen J, et al. Gait analysis in essential tremor- further evidence for a cerebellar dysfunction. Mov Disord 2000;15(Suppl 3):87.

[33] Deuschl G, Wenzelburger R, Loffler K, et al. Essential tremor and cerebellar dysfunction. Clinical and kinematic analysis of intention tremor. Brain 2000;123:1568–80.

[34] Singer C, Sanchez-Ramos J, Weiner WJ. Gait abnormality in essential tremor. Mov Dis 1994;9:193–6.

[35] Helmchen C, Hagenow A, Miesner J, et al. Eye movement abnormalities in essential tremor may indicate cerebellar dysfunction. Brain 2003;126:1319–32.

[36] Rajput AH, Rozdilsky B, Ang L, et al. Significance of Parkinsonian manifestations in essential tremor. Can J Neurol Sci 1993;20:114–7.

[37] Koller WC, Rubino FA. Combined resting postural tremors. Arch Neurol 1985;42:683–4.

[38] Cohen O, Pullman S, Jurewicz E, et al. Rest tremor in essential tremor patients: prevalence, clinical correlates, and electrophysiological characteristics. Arch Neurol 2003;60:405–10.

[39] Gasparini M, Bonifati V, Fabrizio E, et al. Frontal lobe dysfunction in essential tremor. A preliminary study. J Neurol 2001;248:399–402.

[40] Lombardi WJ, Woolston DJ, Roberts JW, et al. Cognitive deficits in patients with essential tremor. Neurology 2001;57:785–90.

[41] Lacritz LH, Dewey R Jr, Giller C, et al. Cognitive functioning in individuals with "benign" essential tremor. J Int Neuropsychol Soc 2002;8:125–9.

[42] Vermilion K, Stone A, Duane D. Cognition and affect in idiopathic essential tremor. Mov Disord 2001;16:S30.

[43] Duane DD, Vermilion KJ. Cognitive deficits in patients with essential tremor. Neurology 2002;58:1706.

[44] Benito-Leon J, Louis ED, Bermejo-Pareja F. Population-based case-control study of cognitive function in essential tremor. Neurology 2006;66:69–74.

[45] Chatterjee A, Jurewicz EC, Applegate LM, et al. Personality in essential tremor. J Neurol Neurosurg Psychiatry 2004;75:958–61.

[46] Louis ED, Jurewicz EC. Olfaction in essential tremor patients with and without isolated rest tremor. Mov Disord 2003;18:1387–9.

[47] Louis ED, Bromley SM, Jurewicz EC, et al. Olfactory dysfunction in essential tremor: a deficit unrelated to disease duration or severity. Neurology 2002;59:1631–3.

[48] Applegate LM, Louis ED. Essential tremor: mild olfactory dysfunction in a cerebellar disorder. Parkinsonism Relat Disord 2005;11:399–402.

[49] Herskovitz E, Blackwood W. Essential (familial, hereditary) tremor: a case report. J Neurol Neurosurg Psychiatry 1969;32:509–11.

[50] Mylle G, Van Bogaert L. Du tremblement essentiel non familial. Monatsschr Psychiatr Neurol 1948;115:80–90.

[51] Hassler R. Zur pathologischen anatomie des senilen und des parkinsonistischen Tremor. J Psychol Neurol 1939;49:193–230.

[52] Mylle G, Van Bogaert L. Etudes anatomo-cliniques de syndromes hypercinetiques complexes. I. Sur le tremblement familial. Monatsschr Psychiatr Neurol 1940;103:28–43.

[53] Bergamasco I. Intorno ad un caso di tremore essenziale simulant in parte il quadro della sclerosi multipla. Riv Pat Nerv Ment 1907;115:80–90.

[54] Lapresle J, Rondot P, Said G. Tremblement idopathique de repos, d'attitude et d'action. Etude anatomo-clinique d'une observation. Rev Neurol 1974;130:343–8.

[55] Frankl-Hochwart. La degenerescence hepato-lenticulaire (maladie de Wilson, pseudosclerose). Paris: Masson et Cie; 1903.

[56] Boockvar J, Telfeian A, Baltuch GH. Long-term deep brain stimulation in a patient with essential tremor: clinical response and postmortem correlation with stimulator termination sites in ventral thalamus. J Neurosurg 2000;93:140–4.

[57] Louis ED, Honig LS, Vonsattel JPG, et al. Essential tremor associated with focal nonnigral Lewy bodies: a clinical-pathological study. Arch Neurol 2005;62:1004–7.

[58] Louis ED, Vonsattel JPG, Honig LS, et al. Neuropathological findings in essential tremor. Neurology 2006;66:1756–9.

[59] Louis ED, Vonsattel JPG, Honig LS, et al. Essential tremor pathology: a case-control study from the Essential Tremor Centralized Brain Repository. Mov Disord 2005;20:1241.

[60] Constantino AEA, Louis ED. Unilateral disappearance of essential tremor after cerebral hemispheric infarct. J Neurol 2003;250:354–5.

[61] Koller WC, Vetere-Overfield B, Barter R. Tremors in early Parkinson disease. Clin Neuropharmacol 1989;12:293–7.

[62] Louis ED, Ford B, Barnes LF. Clinical subtypes of essential tremor. Arch Neurol 2000;57:1194–8.

[63] Higgins JJ, Pho LT, Nee LE. A gene (ETM) for essential tremor maps to chromosome 2p22-p25. Mov Disord 1997;12:859–64.

[64] Louis ED. Essential tremor. N Engl J Med 2001;345:887–91.

[65] Jankovic J, Schwartz KS, Ondo W. Re-emergent tremor of Parkinson's disease. J Neurol Neurosurg Psychiatry 1999;67:646–50.

[66] Louis ED, Klatka LA, Lui Y, et al. Comparison of extrapyramidal features in 31 pathologically confirmed cases of diffuse Lewy body disease and 34 pathologically confirmed cases of
Parkinson disease. Neurology 1997;48:376–80.

[67] Benamer TS, Patterson J, Grosset DG, et al. Accurate differentiation of parkinsonism
and essential tremor using visual assessment of [123I]-FP-CIT SPECT imaging: the
[123I]-FP-CIT study group. Mov Disord 2000;15:503–10.

[68] Antonini A, Moresco RM, Gobbo C, et al. The status of dopamine nerve terminals in Parkinson's disease and essential tremor: a PET study with the tracer [11-C]FE-CIT. Neurol
Sci 2001;22:47–8.

[69] Louis ED. Essential tremor. Lancet Neurol 2005;4:100–10.

[70] Zesiewcz TA, Elble R, Louis ED, et al. Practice parameter: therapies for essential tremor.
Report of the Quality Standards Subcommittee of the American Academy of Neurology.
Neurology 2005;64:2008–20.

[71] Rincon F, Louis ED. Benefits and risks of pharmacological and surgical treatments for
essential tremor: disease mechanisms and current management. Expert Opin Drug Saf
2005;4:899–913.

[72] Jefferson D, Jenner P, Marsden CD. B-Adrenoreceptor antagonists in essential tremor.
J Neurol Neurosurg Psychiatry 1979;42:904–9.

[73] Tolosa ES, Loewenson RB. Essential tremor: treatment with propranolol. Neurology 1975;
25:1041–4.

[74] Packer M, Cohn JN, Abraham WT, et al. Consensus recommendations for the management of chronic heart failure. Am J Cardiol 1999;83:1A–38A.

[75] Lee KS, Kim JS, et al. A multicenter randomized crossover multiple-dose comparison study
of arotinolol and propranolol in essential tremor. Parkinsonism Relat Disord 2003;9:341–7.

[76] Cleeves L, Findley LJ. Propranolol and propranolol-LA in essential tremor: a double blind
comparative study. J Neurol Neurosurg Psychiatry 1988;51:379–84.

[77] Findley LJ, Cleeves L, Calzetti S. Primidone in essential tremor of the hands and head:
a double blind controlled clinical study. J Neurol Neurosurg Psychiatry 1985;48:911–5.

[78] Sasso E, Perucca E, Fava R, et al. Primidone in the long-term treatment of essential tremor:
a prospective study with computerized quantitative analysis. Clin Neuropharm 1990;13:
67–76.

[79] Gorman WP, Cooper R, Pocock P, et al. A comparison of primidone, propranolol, and placebo in essential tremor, using quantitative analysis. J Neurol Neurosurg Psychiatry 1986;
49:64–8.

[80] Sasso E, Perucca E, Calzetti S. Double-blind comparison of primidone and phenobarbital
in essential tremor. Neurology 1988;38:808–10.

[81] O'Suilleabhain P, Dewey RB Jr. Randomized trial comparing primidone initiation schedules for treating essential tremor. Mov Disord 2002;17:382–6.

[82] Koller WC, Royse VL. Efficacy of primidone in essential tremor. Neurology 1986;36:121–4.

[83] Koller WC, Vetere-Overfield B. Acute and chronic effects of propranolol and primidone in
essential tremor. Neurology 1989;39:1587–8.

[84] Gironell A, Kulisevsky J, Barbanoj M, et al. A randomized placebo-controlled comparative
trial of gabapentin and propranolol in essential tremor. Arch Neurol 1999;56:475–80.

[85] Pahwa R, Lyons K, Hubble JP, et al. Double-blind controlled trial of gabapentin in essential tremor. Mov Disord 1998;13:465–7.

[86] Ondo W, Hunter C, Dat Vuong K, et al. Gabapentin for essential tremor: a multiple-dose,
double-blind, placebo-controlled trial. Mov Disord 2000;15:678–82.

[87] Connor GS. Efficacy of topiramate in treatment of essential tremor: a randomized, double-
blind, placebo-controlled, cross-over study. Ann Neurol 2000;48:486.

[88] Ondo WG, Jankovic J, Connor GS, et al. Topiramate in essential tremor. A double-blind,
placebo-controlled trial. Neurology 2006; In press.

[89] Huber SJ, Paulson GW. Efficacy of alprazolam for essential tremor. Neurology 1988;38:
241–3.

[90] Thompson C, Lang A, Parkes JD, et al. A double-blind trial of clonazepam in benign essential tremor. Clin Neuroparm 1984;7:83–8.

[91] Biary N, Koller W. Kinetic predominant essential tremor: successful treatment with clonazepam. Neurology 1987;37:471–4.

[92] Curran T, Lang AE. Flunarizine in essential tremor. Clin Neuropharm 1993;16:460–3.

[93] Biary N, Bahou Y, Sofi MA, et al. The effect of nimodipine on essential tremor. Neurology 1995;45:1523–5.

[94] Ceravolo R, Salvetti S, Piccini P, et al. Acute and chronic effects of clozapine in essential tremor. Mov Disord 1999;14:468–72.

[95] Mortia S, Miwa H, Kondo T. Effect of zonisamide on essential tremor: a pilot crossover study in comparison with arotinolol. Parkinsonism Relat Disord 2005;11:101–3.

[96] Bushara KO, Malik T, Exconde RE. The effect of levetiracetam on essential tremor. Neurology 2005;64:1078–80.

[97] Jankovic J, Schwartz K, Clemence W, et al. A randomized, double-blind, placebo-controlled study to evaluate botulinum toxin type A in essential hand tremor. Mov Disord 1996;11:250–6.

[98] Schuurman PR, Bosch DA, Bossuyt PMM, et al. A comparison of continuous thalamic stimulation and thalamotomy for suppression of severe tremor. N Engl J Med 2000;432:461–8.

[99] Hariz GM, Lindberg M, Bergenheim AT. Impact of thalamic deep brain stimulation on disability and health-related quality of life in patients with essential tremor. J Neurol Neurosurg Psychiatry 2002;72:47–52.

[100] Niranjan A, Kondziolka D, Baser S, et al. Functional outcomes after gamma knife thalamotomy for essential tremor and MS-related tremor. Neurology 2000;55:443–6.

[101] Young RF, Jacques K, Mark R, et al. Gamma knife thalamotomy for treatment of tremor: long-term results. J Neursurg 2000;93:128–35.

[102] Growden JH, Shahani BT, Young RR. The effect of alcohol on essential tremor. Neurology 1975;25:259–62.

[103] Koller WC, Biary N. Effect of alcohol on tremors: comparison with propranolol. Neurology 1984;34:221–2.

[104] Bushara KO, Goldstein SR, Grimes GJ Jr, et al. Pilot trial of 1-octanol in essential tremor. Neurology 2004;62:122–4.

ELSEVIER
SAUNDERS

Clin Geriatr Med 22 (2006) 859–877

CLINICS IN
GERIATRIC
MEDICINE

Ataxias

Susan L. Perlman, MD

*Division of Neurogenetics, Department of Neurology, David Geffen School
of Medicine at University of California, Los Angeles, 300 UCLA
Medical Plaza, Suite B200, Los Angeles, CA 90095, USA*

Gait disorders in elderly individuals are a major cause of falls and their attendant morbidities. Ataxia is one neurologic component of fall risk, as are inattention or confusion; visual impairment; vestibular impairment; subcortical white matter disease; parkinsonism; weakness; sensory loss; orthostasis or arrhythmia with alterations in blood pressure; pain; medication use; and environmental hazards. Ataxia in the geriatric population has many causes. Correctly identifying them can improve clinicians' ability to offer treatment and management strategies to patients and their families. The goals should be safe mobility and preserved activities of daily living.

Clinical symptoms of ataxia

Ataxia is incoordination or clumsiness of movement that is not the result of muscle weakness. It is caused by cerebellar, vestibular, or proprioceptive sensory (large fiber/posterior column) dysfunction. Cerebellar ataxia is produced by lesions of the cerebellum or its afferent or efferent connections in the cerebellar peduncles, red nucleus, pons, medulla, or spinal cord. Crossed connections between the frontal cerebral cortex and the cerebellum may allow unilateral frontal disease to mimic a contralateral cerebellar problem.

Cerebellar ataxia causes irregularities in the rate, rhythm, amplitude, and force of voluntary movements, especially at initiation and termination of motion, resulting in jerky trajectories (dyssynergia), terminal tremor, and overshoot (dysmetria) in limbs. Speech can become dysrhythmic (scanning dysarthria) and articulation slurred, with irregular breath control. Difficulty swallowing or frank choking may also be present. Similar changes can be seen in control of eye movement, with jerky (saccadic) pursuit, gaze-evoked nystagmus, and overshoot. Muscle tone is decreased, resulting in defective posture maintenance and reduced ability to check excessive movement

---

E-mail address: sperlman@ucla.edu

(rebound or sway). Truncal movement is unsteady, feet are held wider apart during standing and walking, and the ability to stand on one foot or with feet together or to walk a straight line is diminished. Altered cerebellar connections to brainstem oculomotor and vestibular nuclei may result in sensations of dizziness or environmental movement (oscillopsia). Vestibular ataxia has prominent vertigo (directional spinning sensations) and spares the limbs and speech. Sensory ataxia has no vertigo or dizziness, also spares speech, worsens when the eyes are closed (positive Romberg sign), and is accompanied by decreased vibration and joint position sense.

Cerebellar influence is ipsilateral (the right hemisphere controls the right side of the body), and within the cerebellum are regions responsible for particular functions (midline: gait, head and trunk control, eye movement control; superior vermis: gait; hemispheres: limb tone and control, eye movement control, speech). Cerebellar signs on the neurologic examination can help determine whether a process is unilateral or involves the entire cerebellum and whether a particular region of the cerebellum has been targeted (eg, vermis, outflow tracts). Certain causes may then become more likely.

The genetically mediated ataxias typically have insidious onset and slow (months to years) symmetrical progression, affecting both sides of the body and moving from the legs to the arms to speech or from midline (gait/trunk) to hemispheric (limb) structures to deep outflow pathways (increasing tremor). Acquired ataxias may have more sudden or subacute onset and progression (weeks to months) and be asymmetrical or frankly focal in presentation. Acute onset with no progression suggests a monophasic insult (eg, injury, vascular event or hemorrhage, anoxia). Subacute onset with progression suggests infectious/inflammatory/immune processes, metabolic or toxic derangements, neoplastic/mass effects, or normal-pressure hydrocephalus.

The neurologic history may provide clues to possible cause related to associated illnesses, medication use, or lifestyle/environmental exposures. The neurologic examination can be supplemented by neural imaging (brain or spine MRI or CT) and electrophysiologic studies (eg, electromyogram and nerve conduction; evoked potential testing, including visual evoked response, brainstem auditory evoked response, and somatosensory evoked response; electronystagmography of oculomotor and vestibular pathways; electroencephalogram) to confirm the anatomic localization of the process and often the actual cause (eg, mass lesion of a specific type, stroke or hemorrhage, inflammation/infection or vasculitis, demyelination, characteristic regional atrophy). Additional laboratory studies can also be ordered (eg, blood, urine, spinal fluid, biopsy of muscle, nerve, or brain). The presence of a known genetic disorder does not rule out the presence of additional acquired insults that might alter the presentation and course of the symptoms of ataxia and may warrant further investigation.

Similarly, the absence of a clear family history does not rule out the role of genetic factors in an apparently sporadic disorder. No family history may exist because the history wasn't taken or the information is unavailable (eg, adoption, loss of contact, noncooperation, paternity issues), because of non-dominant inheritance patterns (eg, recessive, X-linked, maternal), or because of specific genetic processes (eg, anticipation, incomplete penetrance, mosaicism) that modify disease presentation in the pedigree. Genetic studies of large groups of older patients who have sporadic ataxia have shown that 4% to 29% have one of the dominantly inherited triplet repeat disorders (most commonly spinocerebellar ataxia [SCA] 6) and 2% to 11% have Friedreich's ataxia [1–14]. Recessively inherited inborn errors of metabolism may also occur in patients older than 25 years [15]. Fragile X tremor ataxia syndrome has most recently been described as a cause of ataxia, tremor, and dementia in older men (and occasionally female carriers) who have the fragile X permutation [16], occurring in up to 4% of individuals with later-onset, sporadic cerebellar ataxia. Table 1 outlines the genetic causes of adult-onset cerebellar ataxia.

Research is ongoing in identifying genetic susceptibility factors or genes that may participate in multifactorial pathologic processes affecting the cerebellum [17–20].

Box 1 summarizes the workup of patients who have symptoms of cerebellar ataxia. In older patients, multiple factors usually contribute to ataxic symptoms.

Causes of ataxia

Congenital

Congenital ataxic syndromes (without other features, such as mental retardation and spasticity) are rare, but patients who have these conditions may survive into adulthood and the associated ataxic symptoms may worsen with aging. Progressive early-onset cerebellar diseases are typically genetically determined (eg, inborn errors of metabolism, X-linked or maternal disorders, early-onset dominant disorders). Children who have these conditions may not survive into adulthood.

Congenital nonprogressive syndromes are also frequently genetic and include cerebellar/vermian agenesis and hypoplasia (which may be minimally symptomatic), more complex cerebellar dysgenesis disorders (eg, Joubert's syndrome, pontoneocerebellar hypoplasia, granule cell layer hypoplasia, Gillespie's syndrome, Paine syndrome, disequilibrium syndrome), and the congenital malformations. The congenital conditions may have contributory genetic factors or environmental causes of developmental disruption. They include the Chiari's malformations (types I–IV, of increasing severity of displacement of the cerebellar tonsils, inferior vermis, and associated brainstem regions below the foramen magnum) and the cystic posterior fossa malformations (eg, Dandy-Walker and variants; megacisterna magna; Blake's pouch cyst). These may require surgical intervention to decompress the posterior fossa structures and treat associated dysraphism, meningomyelocele,

Table 1
The inherited ataxias—prioritizing genetic testing, as tests continue to become available[a]

Characteristic feature	Genetic syndromes to consider
Pure cerebellar phenotype and MRI	SCA5, 6, 8, 10, 11, 14, 15, 16, 22, 26
Complex phenotype, but pure cerebellar atrophy on MRI	SCA4, 18, 21, 23, 25, 27
Brainstem involvement or atrophy on MRI	SCA1, 2, 3, 7, 13, DRPLA
Pyramidal involvement, hyperreflexia	SCA1, 3, 4, 7, 8, 11, 12, 23, 28
Extrapyramidal involvement	SCA1, 2, 3, 12, 21, 27, DRPLA
Peripheral nerve involvement or hyporeflexia on the basis of spinal long tract changes	SCA1, 2, 3, 4, 8, 12, 18, 19, 21, 22, 25, 27 Friedreich's ataxia
Supratentorial features or MRI findings	Cerebral atrophy: SCA2, 12, 17, 19 Subcortical white matter changes: DRPLA Dementia: SCA2, 7, 13, 17, 19, 21, DRPLA, FXTAS; or milder cognitive defects: SCA1, 2, 3, 6, 12 Mental retardation: SCA13, 21, 27 Seizures: SCA7, 10, 17; EA types 5 and 6; DRPLA Psychosis: SCA3, 17, 27; DRPLA
Ocular features	Slow saccades: SCA1, 2, 3, 7, 17, 23, 28 Downbeat nystagmus: SCA6, EA2 Maculopathy: SCA7
Prominent postural/action tremor	SCA2, 8, 12, 16, 19, 21, 27; FXTAS Palatal tremor: SCA20 (dentate calcification) Myoclonus: SCA1, 2, 3, 6, 7, 14, 19; DRPLA
Episodic features	EA1-6, SCA6
Early-onset (<20 years)	Childhood: SCA2, 7, 13, 25, 27; DRPLA
Most can have rare cases with early-onset	Young adult: SCA1, 2, 3, 21
Late-onset (>50 years)	SCA6, FXTAS, Friedreich's ataxia
Most can have rare cases with late-onset	Multiple system atrophy (nongenetic)
Rapid progression (death in <10 years) (Average progression is 5–10 years to disability, and 10–20 years to death)	Early-onset SCA2, 3, 7; DRPLA
Slow progression over decades	SCA4, 5, 8, 11, 13, 14, 15, 16, 18, 20, 21, 22, 23, 26, 27, 28 Normal lifespan: SCA5, 6, 11, 18, 26, 27, 28
Anticipation/intergenerational DNA instability (usually paternal more than maternal; maternal more than paternal indicated by (m))	SCA1, 2, 3, 4, 5 (m), 6 (not because of repeat size), 7, 8 (m), 10, ?19, 20, ?21, 22; DRPLA
Variable phenotype	SCA2, 3, 4, 5, 7, 14, 15, 17; GSS
Cerebellar ataxia, parkinsonism, and autonomic instability	SCA3 Multiple system atrophy (nongenetic)

Abbreviations: DRPLA, dentatorubropallidoluysian atrophy; EA, episodic ataxia; FXTAS, fragile X tremor ataxia syndrome; GSS, glutathione synthetase; ?, anticipation suspected, but not proven.

[a] SCAs now number 28. Test availability can be found at www.geneclinics.org.

and hydrocephalus. With proper treatment, children who have these conditions survive into adulthood, albeit with significant disability.

The most common acquired, nonprogressive, congenital cerebellar syndromes are caused by perinatal trauma and hypercoagulable or hemorrhagic vascular events (ataxic cerebral palsy) [21–23]. Aging patients who have cerebral palsy may experience worsening of neurologic symptoms caused by progressive loss of reserve or co-occurrence of other neurologic illnesses, and are at greater risk for other medical conditions because of the lifelong disability [24].

Traumatic

Open or closed head injury, with traumatic brain injury, is a leading cause of death in children and adults [25]. Among survivors, 100,000 per year will have long-term disabling residua and 2% will live in a persistent vegetative state. Head injury is most often a result of car or motorcycle accidents (49%), often complicated by alcohol intake [26]. Accidental falls in elderly individuals account for 29% of cases of head injury. Major injuries within the posterior fossa are seen in 3.3% of all head trauma [27], usually intra-axial brainstem (36%) or cerebellar (25%) parenchymal damage, and less commonly epidural (25%) or subdural (14%) hematomas and subarachnoid hemorrhage. Bleeding complications are more likely to occur in individuals taking anticoagulant medication. Balance difficulties from any cause in elderly individuals may lead to falls, which may cause brain injury that predisposes to future falls.

Acute treatment of traumatic brain injury centers on support of vital functions, control of increased intracranial pressure, and surgical intervention for space-occupying lesions (evacuation of hematomas and decompression for diffuse brain swelling). Ultimately, treatment focuses on intensive rehabilitation to enhance plastic neuronal change and outcome. Long-term complications of cerebellar injury include delayed-onset tremor from reorganization of outflow pathways [28], segmental myoclonus (eg, palatal myoclonus) from disruption of the dentate–rubro–olivary pathway and olivary hypertrophy [29], and superficial siderosis (deposition of hemosiderin from hemorrhage on the leptomeninges), which can lead to cerebellar signs and hearing loss [30].

Vascular

Cerebellar stroke can be ischemic (arterial embolic or atherosclerotic thrombosis), hemorrhagic (10%), mixed (ischemia with secondary bleed, hemorrhage with vasospasm), or caused by thrombosis of cerebellar venous structures that results in symptoms and signs in the vascular territory affected. The posterior inferior cerebellar artery arises from the vertebral artery and supplies the posterior and caudal cerebellum. Deficits in its distribution include the lateral medullary syndrome, ipsilateral impairment of facial

Box 1. Workup for patients who have ataxia and no family history

MRI brain and spinal cord, with and without contrast, with diffusion weighted imaging sequences
Electroencephalogram
Evoked potentials (visual, auditory, somatosensory)
Electronystagmogram
Electromyogram with nerve conduction studies
Chest radiograph
First-line blood studies
- Complete blood count
- Chemistry panel
- Hgb A1c
- Fasting lipids
- Erythrocyte sedimentation rate
- Antinuclear antibody index
- Rapid plasma regain
- Thyroid stimulating hormone
- Vitamin E
- Folic acid
- Vitamin B_{12}
- Methylmalonic acid
- Homocysteine
- Urine heavy metals
Second-line blood studies
- Creatine phosphokinase
- Serum protein electrophoresis
- Postprandial lactate-pyruvate-ammonia
- Ketones
- Copper
- Ceruloplasmin
- Zinc
- Angiotensin-converting enzyme
- Lyme titers
- Human T-lymphotropic virus 1 and 2
- HIV
- Antithyroid antibodies
- Antigliadin antibodies (and antiendomysial/antitransglutaminase antibodies)
- Antiglutamate decarboxylase antibodies (and antiamphiphysin antibodies)

Spinal fluid studies
- Cell count
- Glucose
- Lactate
- Protein
- Veneral disease research laboratory slide test
- Gram stain
- Cultures as appropriate
- Cryptococcal antigen
- 14-3-3 Protein
- Neuron specific enolase
- Prion protein studies
- Neurotransmitter levels as appropriate
- Myelin basic protein
- Oligoclonal bands
- IgG synthesis (process-specific)
- Polymerase chain reaction (pathogen-specific)

Third-line blood studies
- Very long chain fatty acids/phytanic acid
- Plasma or urine amino acids
- Urine organic acids
- Lysosomal hydrolase screen, including hexosaminidase A
- Coenzyme Q10 levels
- Glutathione levels
- Prion protein gene analysis

Magnetic resonance spectroscopy
Positron emission tomography (PET) scan/dopa-PET scan
Biopsies
- Conjunctival
- Muscle/nerve
- Gastrointestinal tract
- Bone marrow
- Brain

Paraneoplastic workup
- Appropriate imaging
- α-Fetoprotein
- Paraneoplastic antibodies (Yo, Hu, Ri, CV2, MaTa, Zic4, and others as available)

Genetic workup[a]

---

[a] Occasionally positive gene tests for SCA6, SCA3, SCA1, Friedreich's ataxia, and fragile X-tremor-ataxia syndrome may be seen in patients older than 50 years. Inborn errors of metabolism may also occur in patients older than 25 years.

sensation, ipsilateral limb incoordination and tremor, ataxia of gait, trouble swallowing, vertigo, and eye movement abnormalities. The anterior inferior cerebellar artery arises from the first third of the basilar artery and supplies the pons, middle cerebellar peduncle, and the flocculus. Stroke in these areas causes ipsilateral impairment of facial sensation and strength, ipsilateral limb incoordination, altered speech and swallowing, vertigo and tinnitus, ataxia of gait, and impaired sensation of the contralateral body. The superior cerebellar artery arises from the top of the basilar artery and supplies the superior cerebellum. Loss of its blood supply causes primarily ipsilateral limb incoordination and tremor, ataxia of gait, altered speech, and some eye movement abnormalities. Stroke in the distribution of the superior cerebellar artery is most likely to result in later onset of palatal or jaw myoclonus [31]. Thrombosis of the veins draining from the cerebellar surface into the transverse sinus or of the superior vermian vein into the vein of Galen causes bilateral cerebellar signs and is seen in patients in hypercoagulable states (eg, pregnancy, during oral contraceptive use, diabetes in the hyperosmolar state), with infections near the base of the skull, and as a complication of intracranial surgery [32].

Cerebellar infarction may also lead to regional cerebellar edema with increased posterior fossa pressures and delayed loss of consciousness. A risk for potentially lethal brainstem compression, tonsillar herniation, and acute hydrocephalus is seen in 20% to 25% of patients [33].

As with cerebellar trauma, treatment is supportive, including close monitoring for complications and the use of intensive rehabilitation to ensure optimal recovery. Thrombolytic therapy for acute ischemic stroke increases reperfusion and may improve the ability of patients to survive stroke without disability [34]. Risk factors for recurrent stroke (eg, hypertension, hyperlipidemia, diabetes, hypercoagulable factors, cigarette smoking, vascular stenosis, embolic sites) must be identified and addressed and the use of antiplatelet agents considered.

Risk factors for hemorrhage include complications of anticoagulation therapy, other coagulation disorders, trauma, brain metastases, and vascular defects (eg, aneurysm, arteriovenous malformation, angioma, hemangioblastoma), some of which may be familial (eg, Von Hippel-Lindau disease) and require genetic consultation and counseling, and possible surgical intervention.

Infectious

Infectious agents of all classes can target the central nervous system (CNS) directly or through exotoxins (eg, pertussis [35,36]), through delayed antigen–antibody reactions involving molecular mimicry (eg, antigens of infectious agents and epitopes in the cerebellum), through mechanisms not completely understood (eg, cerebellar degeneration associated with HIV infection [37]), and possibly from the deleterious effects of high fever on cerebellar neurons [38]. Causative organisms can usually be identified through visualization or culture from spinal fluid samples. Antibodies specific for the infectious agent can also be detected. Evidence may exist for increased synthesis of immunoglobulins in the CNS (elevated cerebrospinal fluid IgG synthesis rates), although this is also seen in some noninfectious CNS inflammatory conditions. Rarely brain biopsy will be necessary to establish an infectious cause. Treatment uses appropriate antimicrobial regimens (with broad coverage often starting before the culture results are ready, then modified for the specific agent found), and supportive measures, steroids for associated brain edema, and, when necessary, surgical intervention (eg, decompression, shunting).

Bacteria typically gain access to the brain by colonizing and locally invading the mucous membranes of the nasopharynx, then traveling hematogenously to the subarachnoid space and meninges, where the resultant inflammatory reaction promotes blood–brain barrier permeability, vasogenic edema, altered blood flow/stroke, and possible direct neuronal toxicity. Direct bacterial invasion of the brain occurs rarely. Typical early symptoms can be fever, confusion, headache, vomiting, and neck stiffness, followed by focal neurologic signs. Bacteria may also enter the nervous system through anatomic defects in the skull or parameningeal sites, such as the paranasal sinuses or middle ear. Individuals who have a history of head trauma, prior neurosurgery, alcoholism, tuberculosis, cancer, or immunodeficiency are at greater risk for developing infection [39].

The most common bacterial pathogens are enteric Streptococcal species, *Escherichia coli*, and *Listeria monocytogenes* in infants; *Neisseria meningitides* (meningococcus), *Streptococcus pneumoniae* (pneumococcus), and *Haemophilus influenzae* in children and young adults; and *S pneumoniae*, *L monocytogenes*, and gram-negative bacilli in older adults and individuals who have impaired cellular immunity. Immunization is available against *H influenzae* for children; against *N meningitides* for military recruits, college students, and those in areas of ongoing epidemics; and against *S pneumoniae* for older adults and patients who have undergone splenectomy. Patients who have experienced head injury, undergone neurosurgery, or a cerebrospinal fluid shunt are more likely to develop staphylococcal and gram-negative bacilli infections [40].

Tuberculous granulomas affecting the basal meninges and arteries (causing cranial neuropathies and stroke) usually result from reactivation of earlier latent infection that seeded the meninges and surface of the brain. Individuals who have a history of pulmonary tuberculosis, alcoholism, steroid treatment, HIV infection, or other conditions that impair the immune response are at greatest risk.

Tropheryma whippelii, an actinomycete (filamentous bacterial class, which also includes *Nocardia*) and the causative bacterium of Whipple's disease, leads to granulomatous infection of the small intestine, regional lymph nodes, liver, heart, lungs, and CNS, preferentially the deep brain structures and cerebellum. Gastrointestinal and joint symptoms are prominent, with associated cerebellar ataxia, myoclonus/myorrhythmia (classically affecting visual convergence, jaw, tongue, and neck muscles), dementia, seizures, insomnia, hyperphagia, and polydipsia [41]. Accurate diagnosis may require duodenal or brain biopsy, with polymerase chain reaction assay for *T whippelii*–specific DNA sequences [42]. Aggressive and lengthy antibiotic treatment (up to 2 years) may stop progression of neurologic signs, but cerebellar deficits may remain disabling. Disease can recur in one third of cases [43].

Spirochetal infections (eg, Lyme disease, syphilis) typically manifest neurologic signs weeks to years after the primary infection, in both central (eg, meningitis, meningoencephalitis, cranial neuropathies) and peripheral (eg, spinal radiculopathies, peripheral neuropathies) locations. The ataxia of syphilis (eg, tabes dorsalis) is sensory in origin, caused by involvement of dorsal root ganglia and posterior columns.

Systemic fungal infections may invade the CNS hematogenously from internal organ or skin sites or through direct extension from parameningeal sites (eg, orbits, paranasal sinuses), causing meningitis, focal abscess, parenchymal granulomas, infarction caused by vasculitis, or communicating hydrocephalus. Their clinical presentation can resemble that of tuberculosis. Diabetes, carcinoma, hematologic malignancy, AIDS, organ transplantation, steroid or cytotoxic drug treatment, prolonged antibiotic therapy, and intravenous drug use predispose individuals to these often opportunistic infections, which include *Cryptococcus, Coccidioides, Candida, Aspergillus, Mucor, Histoplasma*, and *Blastomyces*. Antifungal therapy has frequent complications, may require long-term maintenance regimens, and may not prevent neurologic residua.

Parasitic infections, including protozoal (malaria, *Toxoplasma, Naegleria, Acanthamoeba*), helminthic (eg, cysticercosis, *Angiostrongylus*), and rickettsial (eg, Rocky Mountain spotted fever), are also more common in patients who are immunocompromised, and cause meningoencephalitic symptoms (eg, altered mental status, seizures, myoclonus, ataxia) or focal mass lesions.

Viral and viral-associated cerebellar syndromes can present as a straightforward cerebellitis or a more complicated illness with extracerebellar features (eg, dystonia, myoclonus, brainstem signs, seizures, altered mental status). They can occur within hours of the acute infection or develop slowly over a month, implying both direct infectious or toxic mechanisms and delayed, postinfectious, immune-mediated demyelination. Many infectious agents have been documented to precede an acute/subacute cerebellitis. In children, the most common viruses are varicella (1 in 1000 cases of varicella infection will develop ataxia), measles, mumps, rubella, infectious mononucleosis, human parvovirus B19, and hepatitis A. Rubella infection contracted in utero may also cause a chronic progressive panencephalitis with prominent ataxia, similar to subacute sclerosing panencephalitis that may follow measles infection. Cerebellitis has also been seen after vaccination for diphtheria, tetanus, and pertussis; mumps, measles, and rubella; varicella; influenza; and hepatitis B [44,45].

In adults, Epstein-Barr virus, influenza, parainfluenza, the enteroviruses (eg, polio, Coxsackie, echo), herpes simplex virus, varicella zoster virus, cytomegalovirus, adenovirus, HIV-1, and mumps are reported, but the causative agent cannot be identified in up to 35% of cases [46].

Children and young adults who have acute cerebellitis have an 80% to 90% chance for good functional recovery within 7 to 8 months, with minimal residua in 10% to 40% and rare cerebellar atrophy [47]. Older patients may not recover as favorably as those younger than 40 years, and are more likely to sustain permanent cerebellar disability and cerebellar atrophy.

Antiviral agents (eg, acyclovir) started within the first few days of a viral infection (eg, varicella) can reduce the duration and severity of the acute illness, but may not interfere with the subsequent immunologic response [48]. The effect of steroids on modifying the outcome of viral-mediated cerebellitis is also not confirmed, although adrenocorticotrophic hormone reduces symptoms in up to 85% of children who have postviral opsoclonus–myoclonus syndrome ("dancing eyes–dancing feet"). Plasmapheresis and high-dose intravenous immunoglobulin therapy have been used to try to stop the progression of ataxia in the Miller Fisher variant of Guillain-Barré syndrome, a postinfectious disorder that may include ataxia, ophthalmoplegia, and areflexia [49] and is associated with IgG antibodies directed against GQ1b or GT1b ganglioside [50].

Individuals who have altered cell-mediated immunity (eg, AIDS, lymphoma, inherited immunodeficiency syndromes) are at risk for developing progressive multifocal leukoencephalopathy, a severe demyelinating disease of the CNS. It begins focally, usually in the parieto-occipital white matter, and progresses over weeks to months, causing altered mental status, visual deficits, and motor weakness. The cerebellum is affected in 13% [51]. It is caused by a neurotropic papovavirus (JC virus) that is transported from the kidney by infected B lymphocytes to the brain, where it may persist as a latent infection of oligodendroglia until it is reactivated during the immunosuppressed state [52].

Sporadic Creutzfeldt-Jakob disease, the most common of the human prion disorders (transmissible spongiform encephalopathies), typically presents in the seventh decade as a rapidly progressive dementia with myoclonus, but may also have an ataxic form. An incubation period of months to years may occur after exposure (eg, dietary exposure, corneal transplantation or dura mater grafting of infected tissues, treatment with cadaveric human growth hormone). Variant Creutzfeldt-Jakob disease has earlier onset (third decade) and prominent psychiatric and ataxic features, and may relate to human exposure to bovine spongiform encephalopathy (mad cow disease). Diagnosis may be difficult clinically, but electroencephalography, brain magnetic resonance scanning with diffusion-weighted imaging, and specialized spinal fluid studies can be helpful. Brain biopsy may be necessary to confirm this diagnosis [53]. The National Prion Disease Pathology Surveillance Center (from the Division of Neuropathology, Case Western Reserve University, http://www.cjdsurveillance.com) assists in evaluating suspected cases of prion disease.

Neoplastic

Primary or metastatic neoplasms, complications of antineoplastic therapy (eg, surgery, radiation, chemotherapy), delayed-onset superficial siderosis, secondary vascular and infectious lesions, and the remote effects of cancer (most often felt to be immune-mediated) can all affect the cerebellum.

Space-occupying lesions of the posterior fossa can directly damage regions of the cerebellum or cause mass effects (eg, herniations, obstructive hydrocephalus, increased intracranial pressure) manifesting initially as headache, vomiting, and papilledema, and progressing to focal brainstem deficits, altered level of consciousness, cardiorespiratory instability, and death.

Cerebellar medulloblastomas represent 20% of pediatric primary brain tumors and are also associated with certain inherited disorders (eg, ataxia-telangiectasia, basal cell nevus syndrome). Cerebellar astrocytomas (10%–20%) and fourth-ventricle ependymomas (10% to 20%) and brainstem gliomas (10% to 20%) are also more common in children [54]. Metastatic disease to the cerebellum and extrinsic meningiomas and schwannomas are more common in adults [55]. Meningiomas and schwannomas may present before age 20 in patients who have neurofibromatosis type 1 or 2 (von Recklinghausen's disease). Rarer tumors are the cerebellar hemangioblastomas (a common manifestation in the dominantly inherited Von Hippel-Lindau disease), the congenital ectodermally-derived epidermoid and dermoid cysts, primary CNS lymphomas, and the quasi-neoplasm syndromes, Lhermitte-Duclos disease (dysplastic cerebellar gangliocytoma), and Langerhans' cell histiocytosis (eosinophilic granuloma, causing ataxia with diabetes insipidus).

The paraneoplastic cerebellar syndromes evolve slowly over weeks to months, may present up to 5 years before an occult carcinoma manifests itself, and can be identified in approximately 50% of patients through antibodies in serum or cerebrospinal fluid. Anti-Yo antibodies are associated with ovarian and breast cancer and target certain Purkinje cell cytoplasmic 34- and 62-kD proteins [56,57]. Anti-Ri antibodies are also associated with breast and gynecologic tumors, but target 55- and 80-kD proteins found in all neuronal nuclei and cause a specific syndrome of opsoclonus and myoclonus, distinct from the syndrome seen with small cell lung cancer and neuroblastoma. Anti-Hu (small cell lung cancer; targeting a 35- to 40-kD neuronal nuclear protein), anti-CV2 (small cell lung cancer, uterine sarcoma, malignant thymoma; targeting a 66-kD oligodendrocyte cytoplasmic protein), anti-Tr (Hodgkin's lymphoma; targeting Purkinje cell body and dendrites), and anti-Ma1 (parotid, breast, and colon cancer; targeting a 37-kD neuronal protein) cause cerebellar degeneration similar to the anti-Yo syndrome. Diagnostic evaluation should include a brain MRI study, serum or cerebrospinal fluid studies for paraneoplastic antibodies, and an aggressive evaluation for occult neoplasm if the source is not already known. Treatment consists of removing the source of the antibody (the underlying tumor) and suppressing the immune response using methods such as plasmapheresis; intravenous immunoglobulin infusion; anti–T- and B-cell drugs (eg, tacrolimus, mycophenolate mofetil); or other immunosuppressant agents (eg, corticosteroids, cyclophosphamide) [58]. Recovery depends on stopping the cerebellar disease process before significant loss of Purkinje cells occurs [59].

Autoimmune

Autoantibodies directed against the cerebellum have been found in other cerebellar syndromes not related to prior viral infection or underlying carcinoma.

Gluten enteropathy (celiac sprue) is associated with immune-mediated neurologic disease caused by cross-reacting antibodies produced in response to the gluten-sensitive small bowel disorder. Antigliadin antibodies target the Purkinje cell and can be seen in individuals who have no gastrointestinal symptoms or the tissue transglutaminase and endomysial antibodies associated with the gut disease. These antibodies are reported to occur in up to 27% of individuals who have sporadic ataxia and 37% of patients who have dominantly inherited ataxia, possibly resulting from Purkinje cell degeneration and antigen release. The pathologic role of these antibodies and the effect of the gluten-free diet or immunomodulating therapy is under investigation in this syndrome [60–62].

In insulin-dependent diabetes, antibodies directed against glutamic acid decarboxylase in the spinal cord are known to cause stiff-person syndrome and, in rare cases, cerebellar ataxia [63,64]. This outcome is suspected to be caused by a functional decline in γ-aminobutyric acid neurons in the spinal cord and cerebellum resulting from presynaptic impairment of inhibitory synapses [65], and may be steroid-responsive [66].

Endocrine

Several acquired endocrine disorders are associated with cerebellar ataxia, usually related to thyroid dysfunction or a disturbance of calcium/parathyroid metabolism. These conditions will typically show signs of endocrine and neurologic disease.

Hypothyroidism in adults manifests a slowly progressive superior vermian syndrome, with gait instability and truncal titubation and less common involvement of eye movement and arms. Cognitive dysfunction, seizures, myoclonus, deep tendon reflex changes, and myopathy may also be present [67]. Hyperthyroidism (eg, as seen in Hashimoto's thyroiditis) may cause postural tremor and episodic gait ataxia, and motor unit fasciculations, choreoathetosis, seizures, confusion, and psychiatric symptoms. Although the deficits in Hashimoto's are believed to be immune-mediated and may respond to steroids, the hyperthyroid-related reduction of low-density lipoproteins and associated reduction in vitamin E levels (as also seen in abetalipoproteinemia and hypobetalipoproteinemia) may also contribute to the cerebellar dysfunction [68]. Amiodarone treatment can interfere with thyroid function and may contribute to ataxia on that basis.

Hypo- and hyperparathyroidism (primary, secondary, and pseudo) are associated with cerebellar dysfunction, but the mechanism is not fully understood.

Toxic

Many toxic exposures can target the cerebellum, the most common being ethanol consumption, which has been found to affect the structure and function of granule and Purkinje cells in animals. Of individuals who have alcoholism, 27% to 47% will develop cerebellar degeneration [69], primarily in the superior vermis, but frequently affecting other parts of the neuraxis [70]. Anticonvulsant medication (eg, phenytoin, carbamazepine, barbiturates, gabapentin, lamotrigine, topiramate, vigabatrin), antineoplastics (eg, cytosine arabinoside, 5-fluorouracil, methotrexate), and other agents (eg, amiodarone, bismuth, bromides, cimetidine, cyclosporin, isoniazid, lindane, lithium, mefloquine, perhexiline maleate) can cause cerebellar dysfunction, either acutely or with chronic use. Heavy metal intoxication (eg, germanium, lead, manganese, mercury, methylmercury, thallium), exposure to benzene or toluene derivatives, insecticide/herbicide poisoning (eg, carbon disulfide, chlordecone, phosphine), and recreational drug use (eg, cocaine, heroin, phencyclidine) can all cause irreversible cerebellar damage. Purkinje cells are extremely sensitive to hyperthermic damage, anoxia (including carbon monoxide poisoning), and any process that interferes with oxidative metabolism (eg, acute and chronic B-vitamin deficiencies, such as thiamine, vitamin B_{12}; cyanide poisoning; certain shellfish neurotoxins, such as saxitoxin from *Mylius*) [71].

Nongenetic ataxias of unknown origin

In a study of 112 patients who had sporadic ataxia [72], onset after age 20 (median age 56 years), and no identifiable family history or other cause, 29% met criteria for possible or probable multiple system atrophy, 13% had an unexpected genetically mediated ataxia (6% SCA6, 3% SCA3, 1% SCA2, 4% Friedreich's ataxia), and 58% remained with unknown origin. Of these unknowns, 15% tested positive for antigliadin antibodies (none had antiglutamate decarboxylase antibodies), but 9% of those who had inherited ataxias also tested positive.

Currently, more than half of adults presenting with late-onset, sporadic cerebellar ataxia will not be able to be given a specific diagnosis or prognosis. Some will progress rapidly, others indolently. All will suffer some disability. Approximately one third will develop multiple system atrophy, with its severe morbidity and mortality [73]. Some will ultimately be found to suffer from unknown processes related to the immune system or environmental factors or cerebellar homeostasis.

Treatment of ataxia in elderly individuals

The treatment of cerebellar ataxia [74,75] remains primarily a neurorehabilitation challenge. Potentially helpful treatment modalities include physical, occupational, and speech/swallowing therapy; adaptive equipment implementation; driver safety training; and nutritional counseling. Modest additional gains may be made with the use of medications that can improve imbalance, incoordination, or dysarthria (eg, amantadine, buspirone, acetazolamide); cerebellar tremor (eg, clonazepam, propranolol); and cerebellar or central vestibular nystagmus (eg, gabapentin, baclofen, clonazepam).

Many of the progressive cerebellar syndromes have associated features in other neurologic systems, including spasticity, dystonia/rigidity, resting or rubral tremor, chorea, motor unit weakness or fatigue, autonomic dysfunction, peripheral or posterior column sensory loss, neuropathic pain or cramping, bowel/bladder/sexual dysfunction, double vision, vision and hearing loss, and dementia, and can impede the treatment of the ataxic symptoms or can worsen with the use of certain drugs for ataxia. Treatment of the associated features themselves may in turn worsen the ataxia, either directly (side-effects of medication) or indirectly (relaxation of lower limb spasticity that was acting as a stabilizer for an ataxic gait).

Secondary complications of progressive ataxia can include deconditioning/immobility, weight loss or gain, skin breakdown, recurrent pulmonary and urinary tract infections, aspiration, occult respiratory failure, and obstructive sleep apnea, all of which can be life-threatening. The authors have found depression to be common in patients and their family members.

Although no cures are available for most of the causes of cerebellar ataxia and no proven ways exist to protect neurons from premature cell death or to restore neuronal populations that have been lost, symptomatic treatment can greatly improve the quality of life of these patients and prevent complications that could hasten death. Supportive interventions should always be offered, such as education about the disease itself, genetic counseling, individual and family counseling, referral to support groups and advocacy groups, and guidance to online resources (Appendix). Misinformation, fear, depression, hopelessness, isolation, and financial and interpersonal stress can often cause more harm to patients and their families or caregivers than the ataxia itself.

Appendix

Medline, PubMed: www.ncbi.nlm.nih.gov
Online Mendelian Inheritance in Man/OMIM: www.ncbi.nlm.nih.gov
GeneReviews/University of Washington: www.geneclinics.org
Neuromuscular web page at Washington University: www.neuro.
    wustl.edu/neuromuscular
National Ataxia Foundation: www.ataxia.org

References

[1] Moseley ML, Benzow KA, Schut LJ, et al. Incidence of dominant spinocerebellar and Friedreich triplet repeats among 361 ataxia families. Neurology 1998;51(6):1666–71.
[2] Jardim LB, Silveira I, Pereira ML, et al. A survey of spinocerebellar ataxia in South Brazil—
66 new cases with Machado-Joseph disease, SCA7, SCA8, or unidentified disease-causing
mutations. J Neurol 2001;248(10):870–6.
[3] Leggo J, Dalton A, Morrison PJ, et al. Analysis of spinocerebellar ataxia types 1, 2, 3, and 6,
dentatorubral-pallidoluysian atrophy, and Friedreich's ataxia genes in spinocerebellar
ataxia patients in the UK. J Med Genet 1997;34(12):982–5.
[4] Schols L, Gispert S, Vorgerd M, et al. Spinocerebellar ataxia type 2. Genotype and phenotype in German kindreds. Arch Neurol 1997;54(9):1073–80.
[5] Schols L, Kruger R, Amoiridis G, et al. Spinocerebellar ataxia type 6: genotype and phenotype in German kindreds. J Neurol Neurosurg Psychiatry 1998;64(1):67–73.
[6] Schols L, Szymanski S, Peters S, et al. Genetic background of apparently idiopathic sporadic
cerebellar ataxia. Hum Genet 2000;107(2):132–7.
[7] Giuffrida S, Saponara R, Trovato Salinaro A, et al. Identification of SCA2 mutation in cases
of spinocerebellar ataxia with no family history in mid-eastern Sicily. Ital J Neurol Sci 1999;
20(4):217–21.
[8] Pujana MA, Corral J, Gratacos M, et al. Spinocerebellar ataxias in Spanish patients: genetic
analysis of familial and sporadic cases. The Ataxia Study Group. Hum Genet 1999;104(6):
516–22.
[9] Ramesar RS, Bardien S, Beighton P, et al. Expanded CAG repeats in spinocerebellar ataxia
(SCA1) segregate with distinct haplotypes in South African families. Hum Genet 1997;
100(1):131–7.
[10] Futamura N, Matsumura R, Fujimoto Y, et al. CAG repeat expansions in patients with sporadic cerebellar ataxia. Acta Neurol Scand 1998;98(1):55–9.
[11] Hsieh M, Lin SJ, Chen JF, et al. Identification of the spinocerebellar ataxia type 7 mutation
in Taiwan: application of PCR-based Southern blot. J Neurol 2000;247(8):623–9.
[12] Soong BW, Lu YC, Choo KB, et al. Frequency analysis of autosomal dominant cerebellar
ataxias in Taiwanese patients and clinical and molecular characterization of spinocerebellar
ataxia type 6. Arch Neurol 2001;58(7):1105–9.
[13] Storey E, du Sart D, Shaw JH, et al. Frequency of spinocerebellar ataxia types 1, 2, 3, 6, and 7
in Australian patients with spinocerebellar ataxia. Am J Med Genet 2000;95(4):351–7.
[14] Maruyama H, Izumi Y, Morino H, et al. Difference in disease-free survival curve and regional distribution according to subtype of spinocerebellar ataxia: a study of 1,286 Japanese
patients. Am J Med Genet 2002;114(5):578–83.
[15] Gray RG, Preece MA, Green SH, et al. Inborn errors of metabolism as a cause of neurological disease in adults: an approach to investigation. J Neurol Neurosurg Psychiatry 2000;
69(1):5–12.
[16] Jacquemont S, Hagerman RJ, Leehey MA, et al. Penetrance of the fragile X-associated
tremor/ataxia syndrome in a premutation carrier population. JAMA 2004;291(4):460–9.

[17] Sun G, Gargus JJ, Ta DT, et al. Identification of a novel candidate gene in the iron-sulfur pathway implicated in ataxia-susceptibility: human gene encoding HscB, a J-type co-chaperone. J Hum Genet 2003;48(8):415–9.

[18] Chataway J, Sawcer S, Coraddu F, et al. Evidence that allelic variants of the spinocerebellar ataxia type 2 gene influence susceptibility to multiple sclerosis. Neurogenetics 1999;2(2): 91–6.

[19] Jardim L, Silveira I, Pereira ML, et al. Searching for modulating effects of SCA2, SCA6 and DRPLA CAG tracts on the Machado-Joseph disease (SCA3) phenotype. Acta Neurol Scand 2003;107(3):211–4.

[20] Li YJ, Oliveira SA, Xu P, et al. Glutathione S-transferase omega-1 modifiesage-at-onset of Alzheimer disease and Parkinson disease. Hum Mol Genet 2003;12(24):3259–67.

[21] Mercuri E, He J, Curati WL, et al. Cerebellar infarction and atrophy in infants and children with a history of premature birth. Pediatr Radiol 1997;27(2):139–43.

[22] Nelson KB, Lynch JK. Stroke in newborn infants. Lancet Neurol 2004;3(3):150–8.

[23] Ozduman K, Pober BR, Barnes P, et al. Fetal stroke. Pediatr Neurol 2004;30(3):151–62.

[24] Kinne S, Patrick DL, Doyle DL. Prevalence of secondary conditions among people with disabilities. Am J Public Health 2004;94(3):443–5.

[25] Goldstein M. Traumatic brain injury: a silent epidemic. Ann Neurol 1990;27(3):327.

[26] Kraus JF, Morgenstern H, Fife D, et al. Blood alcohol tests, prevalence of involvement, and outcomes following brain injury. Am J Public Health 1989;79(3):294–9.

[27] Tsai FY, Teal JS, Itabashi HH, et al. Computed tomography of posterior fossa trauma. J Comput Assist Tomogr 1980;4(3):291–305.

[28] Louis ED, Lynch T, Ford B, et al. Delayed-onset cerebellar syndrome. Arch Neurol 1996; 53(5):450–4.

[29] Kawata Y, Suzuki T, Kagaya H, et al. An MRI analysis of brain-stem and cerebellar lesions and olivary hypertrophy. Neuroradiology 1996;38(5):441–3.

[30] Bracchi M, Savoiardo M, Triulzi F, et al. Superficial siderosis of the CNS: MR diagnosis and clinical findings. AJNR Am J Neuroradiol 1993;14(1):227–36.

[31] Freeman W, Jaffe D. Occlusion of superior cerebellar artery: report of a case with necropsy. Arch. Neurol. Psychiatry 1941;46:115–26.

[32] Andeweg J. Consequences of the anatomy of deep venous outflow from the brain. Neuroradiology 1999;41(4):233–41.

[33] Amarenco P. The spectrum of cerebellar infarctions. Neurology 1991;41(7):973–9.

[34] Hacke W, Zeumer H, Ferbert A, et al. Intra-arterial thrombolytic therapy improves outcome in patients with acute vertebrobasilar occlusive disease. Stroke 1988;19(10):1216–22.

[35] Askelof P, Gillenius P. Effect of lymphocytosis-promoting factor from Bordetella pertussis on cerebellar cyclic GMP levels. Infect Immun 1982;36(3):958–61.

[36] Setta F, Baecke M, Jacquy J, et al. Cerebellar ataxia following whooping cough. Clin Neurol Neurosurg 1999;101(1):56–61.

[37] Tagliati M, Simpson D, Morgello S, et al. Cerebellar degeneration associated with human immunodeficiency virus infection. Neurology 1998;50(1):244–51.

[38] Yaqub BA, Daif AK, Panayiotopoulos CP. Pancerebellar syndrome in heat stroke: clinical course and CT scan findings. Neuroradiology 1987;29(3):294–6.

[39] Garvey G. Current concepts of bacterial infections of the central nervous system. Bacterial meningitis and bacterial brain abscess. J Neurosurg 1983;59(5):735–44.

[40] Quagliarello VJ, Scheld WM. Treatment of bacterial meningitis. N Engl J Med 1997;336(10): 708–16.

[41] Perkin GD, Murray-Lyon I. Neurology and the gastrointestinal system. J Neurol Neurosurg Psychiatry 1998;65(3):291–300.

[42] Lynch T, Odel J, Fredericks DN, et al. Polymerase chain reaction-based detection of Tropheryma whippelii in central nervous system Whipple's disease. Ann Neurol 1997;42(1): 120–4.

[43] Singer R. Diagnosis and treatment of Whipple's disease. Drugs 1998;55(5):699–704.

[44] Mancini J, Chabrol B, Moulene E, et al. Relapsing acute encephalopathy: a complication of diphtheria-tetanus-poliomyelitis immunization in a young boy. Eur J Pediatr 1996;155(2): 136–8.

[45] Sunaga Y, Hikima A, Ostuka T, et al. Acute cerebellar ataxia with abnormal MRI lesions after varicella vaccination. Pediatr Neurol 1995;13(4):340–2.

[46] Klockgether T, Doller G, Wullner U, et al. Cerebellar encephalitis in adults. J Neurol 1993; 240(1):17–20.

[47] Hayakawa H, Katoh T. Severe cerebellar atrophy following acute cerebellitis. Pediatr Neurol 1995;12(2):159–61.

[48] Dangond F, Engle E, Yessayan L, et al. Pre-eruptive varicella cerebellitis confirmed by PCR. Pediatr Neurol 1993;9(6):491–3.

[49] Zifko U, Drlicek M, Senautka G, et al. High dose immunoglobulin therapy is effective in the Miller Fisher syndrome. J Neurol 1994;241(3):178–9.

[50] Nagashima T, Koga M, Odaka M, et al. Clinical correlates of serum anti-GT1a IgG antibodies. J Neurol Sci 2004;219(1–2):139–45.

[51] Jones HR Jr, Hedley-Whyte ET, Friedberg SR, et al. Primary cerebellopontine multifocal leucoencephalopathy diagnosed premortem by cerebellar biopsy. Ann Neurol 1982;11: 199–202.

[52] Brink NS, Miller RF. Clinical presentation, diagnosis, and therapy of progressive multifocal leukoencephalopathy. J Infect 1996;32:97–102.

[53] Will RG. Acquired prion disease: iatrogenic CJD, variant CJD, kuru. Br Med Bull 2003;66: 255–65.

[54] Ullrich NJ, Pomeroy SL. Pediatric brain tumors. Neurol Clin 2003;21(4):897–913.

[55] Zabek M. Primary posterior fossa tumours in adult patients. Folia Neuropathol 2003;41(4): 231–6.

[56] Furneaux HM, Rosenblum MK, Dalmau J, et al. Selective expression of Purkinje-cell antigens in tumor tissue from patients with paraneoplastic cerebellar degeneration. N Engl J Med 1990;322(26):1844–51.

[57] Drlicek M, Bianchi G, Bogliun G, et al. Antibodies of the anti-Yo and anti-Ri type in the absence of paraneoplastic neurological syndromes: a long-term survey of ovarian cancer patients. J Neurol 1997;244(2):85–9.

[58] Darnell RB, Posner JB. Paraneoplastic syndromes involving the nervous system. N Engl J Med 2003;349(16):1543–54.

[59] Graus F, Vega F, Delattre JY, et al. Plasmapheresis and antineoplastic treatment in CNS paraneoplastic syndromes with antineuronal autoantibodies. Neurology 1992;42(3 Pt 1): 536–40.

[60] Bushara KO, Goebel SU, Shill H, et al. Gluten sensitivity in sporadic and hereditary cerebellar ataxia. Ann Neurol 2001;49(4):540–3.

[61] Hadjivassiliou M, Davies-Jones GA, Sanders DS, et al. Dietary treatment of gluten ataxia. J Neurol Neurosurg Psychiatry 2003;74(9):1221–4.

[62] Hadjivassiliou M, Grunewald R, Sharrack B, et al. Gluten ataxia in perspective: epidemiology, genetic susceptibility and clinical characteristics. Brain 2003;126(Pt 3):685–91.

[63] Kono S, Miyajima H, Sugimoto M, et al. Stiff-person syndrome associated with cerebellar ataxia and high glutamic acid decarboxylase antibody titer. Intern Med 2001;40(9):968–71.

[64] Iwasaki H, Sato R, Shichiri M, et al. A patient with type 1 diabetes mellitus and cerebellar ataxia associated with high titer of circulating anti-glutamic acid decarboxylase antibodies. Endocr J 2001;48(2):261–8.

[65] Mitoma H, Song SY, Ishida K, et al. Presynaptic impairment of cerebellar inhibitory synapses by an autoantibody to glutamate decarboxylase. J Neurol Sci 2000;175(1):40–4.

[66] Lauria G, Pareyson D, Pitzolu MG, et al. Excellent response to steroid treatment in anti-GAD cerebellar ataxia. Lancet Neurol 2003;2(10):634–5.

[67] Harayama H, Ohno T, Miyatake T. Quantitative analysis of stance in ataxic myxoedema. J Neurol Neurosurg Psychiatry 1983;46(6):579–81.

[68] Asayama K, Dobashi K, Hayashibe H, et al. Vitamin E protects against thyroxine-induced acceleration of lipid peroxidation in cardiac and skeletal muscles in rats. J Nutr Sci Vitaminol (Tokyo) 1989;35(5):407–18.

[69] Torvik A. Brain lesions in alcoholics: neuropathological observations. Acta Med Scand Suppl 1987;717:47–54.

[70] Fadda F, Rossetti ZL. Chronic ethanol consumption: from neuroadaptation to neurodegeneration. Prog Neurobiol 1998;56(4):385–431.

[71] Manto MU, Jacquy J. Other cerebellotoxic agents. In: Pandolfo M, editor. The Cerebellum and its Disorders. Cambridge: Cambridge University Press; 2002. p. 342–66.

[72] Abele M, Burk K, Schols L, et al. The aetiology of sporadic adult-onset ataxia. Brain 2002; 125(Pt 5):961–8.

[73] Gilman S, Little R, Johanns J, et al. Evolution of sporadic olivopontocerebellar atrophy into multiple system atrophy. Neurology 2000;55(4):527–32.

[74] Perlman SL. Cerebellar ataxia. Curr Treat Options Neurol 2000;2(3):215–24.

[75] Perlman SL. Symptomatic and disease-modifying therapy for the progressive ataxias. Neurologist 2004;10(5):275–89.

ELSEVIER
SAUNDERS

CLINICS IN
GERIATRIC
MEDICINE

Clin Geriatr Med 22 (2006) 879–897

Geriatric Chorea

Matthew T. Lorincz, MD, PhD

*Department of Neurology, University of Michigan, 200 Zina Pitcher, 4412 Kresge III,
Ann Arbor, MI 48109-0585, USA*

The word chorea is derived from the Greek verb meaning "to dance," and in Homer's *Iliad* it is used to describe a Greek circle dance accompanied by singing. Chorea falls into the category of hyperkinetic movement disorders and is characterized by involuntary, irregular, rapid movements of the face, head, trunk, and extremities that are superimposed on and interrupt normal movement. The movements can flow from one body part to another in a nonstereotyped manner. The spectrum of chorea ranges from small twitches to large jerks that can be generalized, affect one half of the body (hemichorea), or occur focally in any body part. Choreic movements can be subtle and small, resembling piano playing movements when occurring distally in the fingers; they may also resemble fidgetiness and be incorporated into apparently purposeful movements. In an extreme form, they can manifest as disabling, uncontrolled, flailing movements of the extremities, termed ballism. Chorea can exist independently and be the sole type of abnormal movement, or it can be one of many movements in a single patient. Chorea is frequently accompanied by athetosis, a slow, writhing movement of the limbs, trunk, or neck, and this combination is referred to as choreoathetosis.

The mechanisms causing chorea are not known, but it is generally thought to result from dysfunction of the basal ganglia and their connections. The basal ganglia are generally believed to modulate motor and cognitive programs by means of parallel circuits that initiate in the cortex, pass through the basal ganglia to the thalamus, and return to the cortex [1]. The major components of the basal ganglia are a group of subcortical nuclei composed of the striatum, globus pallidus, subthalamic nuclei, and the substantia nigra. The basal ganglia are at least partially organized into two pathways, the direct and indirect pathways, whose outputs act to balance

Supported by NS 045180.

E-mail address: lorincz@umich.edu

doi:10.1016/j.cger.2006.06.005
geriatric.theclinics.com

each other. The normal net effect of the direct pathway is to increase output from the thalamus to the cortex, whereas the normal net effect of the indirect loop is to inhibit cortical activity [1]. Two classic examples of indirect loop lesions causing choreic movements are ballism caused by subthalamic nuclei lesions and chorea caused by preferential early indirect loop neuron degeneration in Huntington's disease. It is interesting to note that some acute lesions of the subthalamic nuclei causing ballism (large flailing movements) have been described as progressing to chorea as they resolve, suggesting that chorea and ballism may be on a continuum, with ballism being more severe and chorea less severe. It is consistent with this suggestion that some patients who have acute subthalamic lesions manifest chorea.

Chorea may be seen secondary to an exhaustive list of neurodegenerative disorders, medical conditions, medication side effects, and toxins [2]. The purpose of this article is to provide a practical approach to chorea as a main manifestation in patients of geriatric age. In some instances, rare but treatable causes are considered.

Few modern studies look prospectively at the incidence or prevalence of chorea, and fewer still focus on late-onset chorea [3–7]. In one study of patients of any age admitted to the neurology service at two hospitals over approximately 3 years, 23 cases of sporadic chorea were identified out of 7829 neurology admissions (0.3% or 2.94 per 1000 admissions). Fourteen of the 23 (61%) were older than 55 years at onset. Another study from the same group, including some of the same patients, identified 51 consecutive patients who had sporadic chorea admitted to a hospital [7]. In this cohort the average onset was 60.5 years, and 31 of 46 cases (67%) of nonhereditary chorea occurred in those older than 55 years. In this series, the most frequent causes of chorea in those older than 55 years were vascular (68%), drug-related (13%), metabolic (9.6%), AIDS-related (3.2%), vasculitis-related (3.2%), and undetermined (3.2%). Of the 51 total cases, five (9.8%) had "late-onset" Huntington's disease (HD). This study is most likely an underestimation of chorea, because for the requirement of hospitalization. It is likely that a larger number of patients would have been identified in an outpatient population, because chorea often does not limit activity. In a 3-year prospective series from a movement disorder clinic, 12 patients who had "sporadic and 'senile' chorea" aged 50 to 89 were identified [5]. The total number of patients from which these 12 were identified is not provided. Of these 12 cases, six (50%) had late-onset HD, two (17%) had anti-phospholipid syndrome, one (8.3%) had hypocalcemia, one (8.3%) had basal ganglia calcifications, one (8.3%) had tardive chorea (see article in this issue by Chou and Friedman), and one (8.3%) had an undetermined cause with a family history of chorea. Another study identified 21 of 3084 (0.7%) outpatients to a tertiary referral center over approximately 11 years as having hemiballism-hemichorea [3]. Of the 21, 10 were older than 55 (48%), and nine of these (90%) had a vascular cause; one patient older than 55 had only chorea. Taken together, these investigations suggest that geriatric chorea severe enough to seek medical evaluation is rare and heterogeneous in causation. Table 1 delineates the causes of late-onset chorea and serves as an outline for this article.

Cerebrovascular causes

Based on the case reports summarized earlier, a vascular etiology may be the most frequent cause of geriatric chorea, but chorea as a result of a stroke is rare. In a study of 2500 patients presenting with first stroke, 29 (1%) developed hyperkinetic movement disorders, and 11 (0.4%) developed hemichorea-hemiballism [8]. In this study, hemichorea was found contralateral to infarcts in the lenticular nuclei (globus pallidus and putamen), thalamus, caudate, parieto-occipital area, internal capsule, and subcortical white matter. Ischemia was concluded to be the cause of hemichorea-hemiballism in 9 of 11 patients, hemorrhage in 1 of 11, and no detected lesion in 1 of 11. Two thirds of the lesions were small infarcts, implicating small vessel disease with hypertension as the leading risk factor. In 83% of patients, hyperkinetic movement disorders had an acute onset that occurred with other deficits, such as hemiparesis (91%) or sensory loss (27%). The symptoms were transient, lasting less than 2 weeks, with spontaneous remission in 58% and responsiveness to haloperidol (1.5 to 9 mg/d) in all five treated patients. One person who had hemichorea-hemiballism had persistent symptoms. Over the same period, in the same 2500 patients, the authors reported 536 ischemic or hemorrhagic infarcts involving a large part of the basal ganglia, without subsequent movement disorders. This finding indicates that only 29 of the 536 basal ganglia lesions (5.4%) caused a movement disorder, and only 2% caused chorea.

Another group used a meta-analysis approach to investigate the consequences of focal lesions in the basal ganglia [9]. These authors identified 240 cases of neurologic deficits caused by focal basal ganglia lesions in the literature to 1992 and found that chorea was uncommon (18/240; 8%). The most common lesion location was the caudate or the caudate and

Table 1
Causes of late-onset chorea

Cerebrovascular	Ischemic and hemorrhagic
Medications and toxins	See Table 2
Hereditary	Huntington's disease and neuroacanthocytosis
Autoimmune	SLE, lupus-like or probable SLE, primary antiphospholipid syndrome, and paraneoplastic
Metabolic	Hyperthyroidism, hyperglycemia, and hypocalcemia
Infectious	AIDS and CJD
Other	Polycythemia vera, senile chorea, and basal ganglion mineralization

Abbreviations: CJD, Creutzfeldt-Jakob disease; SLE, systemic lupus erythematosus.

lentiform nuclei. Unilateral lesions were most common, causing contralateral chorea. Three patients had generalized chorea as a result of bilateral caudate and lentiform lesions. Isolated lesions of the putamen, globus pallidus, or lentiform nuclei were found to cause contralateral chorea in one patient. Small, isolated caudate lesions causing chorea were not found to have associated signs, such as hemiparesis or sensory loss. Most lesions were infarcts (63%), followed by hemorrhages (28%).

Based on these studies, it is clear that, although vascular causes of geriatric chorea are common, stroke is a rare cause of chorea in the general geriatric population. When basal ganglia strokes do occur, they rarely cause chorea. The most likely causative locations of strokes are the caudate, lentiform nuclei, or caudate plus lentiform nuclei, but strokes in other areas infrequently cause chorea, including the thalamus, subthalamic nuclei, and subcortical white matter. Although rare, strokes of the subthalamic nuclei frequently cause hemichorea-hemiballism. Cerebrovascular chorea is predominantly unilateral, transient, and responsive to dopaminergic blockade or depletion. It is somewhat surprising that such a small percentage of basal ganglia lesions result in chorea, given the prominence of chorea in other basal ganglion disorders such as HD. The reason for this disparity is not known. It may be that gross acute basal ganglion lesions, perhaps with equal involvement of the direct and indirect pathways, rarely cause chorea, whereas diseases with gradual degeneration of the indirect pathway, such as HD, cause prominent chorea.

Medications and toxins

Although the list of medications that can cause chorea is extensive and growing, the frequency of medication-induced chorea is unclear. In the series of hemidystonia-hemichorea reported by Dewey and Jankovic [3], none of the 21 cases were caused by medications. In the series of sporadic late-onset chorea reported by Warren and colleagues [5], one case of tardive chorea in a 73-year-old man is described of their 12 cases (8%). Piccolo and colleagues [6], found medication to be the second most frequent cause of chorea, in 6 of 51 sporadic chorea patients (12%); four of these six patients were older than 55 years. Although not described in any case series of sporadic or late-onset chorea, choreic dyskinesias observed as a treatment consequence in Parkinson's disease (PD) are undoubtedly the most common form of geriatric chorea. The epidemiology, course, cause, and treatment of dyskinesias in PD are areas of extensive investigation and are not further considered here [10].

Drug-induced movement disorders can be divided into movement disorders that occur acutely while one is taking the offending medications and those that occur following long-term use or after discontinuation of medications (tardive disorders). The list of medications that have been reported to cause chorea is extensive; a partial version is provided in Table 2.

Table 2
Medications and toxins reported to cause chorea

Antiparkinsonian medications	Levodopa, pramipexole, ropinirole, bromocriptine, pergolide, amantadine
Anticonvulsants	Phenytoin, carbamazepine, valproic acid, lamotragine, gabapentin
Stimulants	Amphetamines, methyphenidate, methamphetamine, theophylline, caffeine
Psychiatric	Tricyclic antidepressants, fluoxetine, paroxetine, lithium, risperidone, phenothiazines, amoxapine
Steroids	Oral contraceptives, hormone replacement therapy, anabolic steroids
Opiates	Methadone
Other	Levofloxacin, ciprofloxacin, amoxapine, antihistamines, cimetidine, ranitidine, metoclopramide, digoxin, isoniazide, reserpine, triazolam, cyclosporine, propofol, sulfasalazine, cyproheptadine
Toxins	Ethanol/ethanol withdrawal, carbon monoxide, manganese, mercury, thallium, toluene, organophosphate poisoning

Data from Shoulson I. On chorea. Clin Neuropharmacol 1986;9(Suppl 2):S85–99; Cardoso F. Chorea: non-genetic causes. Curr Opin Neurol 2004;17:433–6; Janavs JL, Aminoff MJ. Dystonia and chorea in acquired systemic disorders. J Neurol Neurosurg Psychiatry 1998;65:436–45.

Medication-induced chorea can occur in isolation or, more frequently, in combination with other abnormal movements. Table 2 also contains a short list of toxins reported to cause chorea, all of which have been reported infrequently.

Tardive dyskinesias are abnormal movements that occur following long-term treatment with dopamine antagonists [11]. The most common classes of medication causing tardive dyskinesia are antipsychotics, antidepressants, and antiemetic medications that block dopamine receptors. Neuroleptics are historically the most common offending antipsychotic medications. Amoxapine is an example of an antidepressant that partially antagonizes dopamine receptors. Trimethobenzamide, prochlorperazine, and metoclopramide are antiemetic medications that can cause tardive dyskinesias. The incidence of tardive dyskinesia of any kind is estimated to be approximately 5%; the risk for occurrence increases with age and female gender [11–13]. The most common movements are repetitive facial movements (oro-buccal-lingual dyskinesias; 78%), dystonia (75%), akathisia (31%), tremor (5%), and chorea (3%) [11].

Hereditary causes

Huntington's disease

HD is a progressive neurodegenerative disorder with clinical manifestations that are traditionally divided into motor, cognitive, and behavioral disturbances. Of its first modern description in 1872, by the then 21-year-old

George Huntington, William Osler says that there are "few instances in the history of medicine in which a disease has been more accurately, more graphically, or more briefly described" [14]. Disease progression is variable and is characterized by loss of saccadic eye movements, chorea, athetosis, dystonia, dyskinesia, dysarthria, dysphagia, cognitive decline, emotional lability, psychosis, depression, and generalized wasting despite a normal appetite. The prevalence in populations of European descent is approximately 10 per 100,000. Age at onset is usually between 30 and 50 but ranges from 2 to 80 years. Symptoms progress over 15 to 20 years, with death at an average age of 54, often secondary to infection [15,16]. Pathologically, preferential degeneration of striatal medium spiny γ-aminobutyric acid–ergic projection neurons with preservation of striatal interneurons leads to gross bilateral progressive reduction in the size of the striata. Widespread degeneration of cortical neurons, primarily cortical projection neurons from layers 5 and 6, leads to generalized brain atrophy [17].

HD occurs when a cytosine, adenine, guanine (CAG) repeat in the HD gene is larger than 36 repeats. Positional cloning linked HD to the telomeric region of chromosome 4p in 1983 [18]. In 1993, the HD gene, IT15, was identified. It has 67 exons spanning 180 kb that encode a widely expressed 10- to 11-kb transcript that is translated into the 350-kDa huntington protein [19,20]. HD is one of nine neurodegenerative disorders caused by expanded CAG alleles that are translated into polyglutamine tracts. The other CAG repeat disorders are spinal and bulbar muscular atrophy, dentatorubral-pallidoluysian atrophy (DRPLA), and the spinocerebellar ataxias (SCA) 1 through 3, 6, 7, and 17 [21,22]. CAG repeat disorders are progressive fatal neurodegenerative diseases with typical onset in midlife. Pathologically, these disorders produce characteristic patterns of regionally selective neurodegeneration, despite widespread gene expression both within and outside the central nervous system [17]. Disease occurs when the CAG repeat size is greater than approximately 40. As repeat size increases, there is increased neuropathologic and clinical overlap among the disorders, suggesting that common molecular mechanisms may be involved [16,23,24]. The polymorphic CAG repeat in HD has a normal allele size of 9 to 35 (median 17 repeats); HD occurs when the CAG repeat is expanded beyond 36 (median 45 repeats) [25,26]. Paternal intergenerational CAG repeat expansion is associated with an earlier onset and a more severe phenotype in subsequent generations (anticipation) [27]. Although there is an inverse correlation between disease onset and repeat size in HD, a small number of individuals with fewer than 42 CAG repeats never develop symptoms, even into the eighth decade [28]. How the expanded CAG repeat causes HD is not known, but a multitude of potential mechanisms are experimentally supported, including transcriptional dysregulation, abnormal axonal transport, altered calcium homeostasis, and aberrant protein processing [29,30].

How commonly does HD present in the geriatric years? Before definitive HD genetic testing, it is likely that a large proportion of sporadic late-onset chorea and senile chorea may have been late-onset HD. Case series reports of late-onset nonhereditary chorea that include HD genetic testing indicate that HD is the cause in 10% to 50% of patients [4,5,7]. Between 10% and 25% of patients who have HD develop symptoms after age 50, and 3% to 12% do so after age 60 [31,32]. If late-onset HD is considered separately, the mean age at symptom onset is 58, and mean age at diagnosis is 63 [31]. Chorea is a prominent early motor manifestation of HD, particularly with adult onset. Chorea has often been a prerequisite for diagnosis of HD, so its frequency as the sole manifestation of late-onset HD is not known [31–35].

Chorea can be the sole manifestation of late-onset HD [35], but more commonly it is accompanied by cognitive decline [31,32]. Cognitive and behavioral deficits frequently precede motor symptoms and are heterogeneous. Early cognitive decline is characterized as a subcortical dementia with impaired executive function. This type of cognitive deficit is manifest as a decreased ability to plan, sequence, and carry out complex tasks, with slow thinking; it differs from cortical deficits such as aphasia, apraxia, and agnosia [36]. Common early behavioral deficits include depression, apathy, and impulsivity. The disease course in late-onset HD is generally less severe, with some patients remaining stable for years and many maintaining daily activities after a disease duration of 7 years [31]. Although it might be expected that smaller CAG repeats would be responsible for late-onset HD, this is only true when HD patients older than 50 years are considered. For those older than 60 years who have late-onset HD, no significant association between expanded repeat size and age at onset was found [32].

Two other CAG repeat disorders can have clinical presentations similar to that of HD, namely SCA17 and DRPLA. In addition to dementia and chorea, patients who have SCA17 also typically exhibit ataxia. Although onset after 50 years of age has been reported for SCA17, none of these patients had chorea [37,38]. DRPLA is most frequent in those of Japanese descent, with an estimated prevalence of 0.2 to 0.7 per 100,000 [39], but it has now been described in other ethnicities [40]. Haw River syndrome is a clinical variant of DRPLA, in a North Carolina kindred of African descent that can exhibit prominent centrum semiovale demyelination and MRI T2 hyperintensities [41]. DRPLA has a wide range of onset ages, from 1 to 62 years, with approximately 16% having onset after age 50 [40,42,43]. The heterogeneous clinical features of DRPLA include ataxia, epilepsy, dementia, psychosis, chorea, myoclonus, dystonia, and parkinsonism. In those who have juvenile onset, before 20 years of age, the most common features are ataxia, epilepsy, dementia, and myoclonus. Those who have onset after 40 years of age infrequently have epilepsy and typically exhibit ataxia, dementia, and choreoathetosis [40,42,43]. In those who are older than 40 years at onset, ataxia precedes chorea; isolated chorea is not described, but chorea is present during the course of the illness in 80% [39]. Ataxia may be quite mild; in such cases the presentation has been confused with HD.

Neuroacanthocytosis

Neuroacanthocytosis refers to a group of neurologic diseases that occur with an abnormal red cell morphology, acanthocytes [44,45]. Acanthocytes are abnormal red blood cells with irregularly spaced, thorny surface projections that are associated with at least five neurodegenerative disorders: chorea-acanthocytosis, McLeod syndrome, pantothenate kinase–associated neurodegeneration (PANK2), Huntington's disease like–2 (HDL2), and abetalipoproteinemia (Bassen-Kornzweig syndrome). PANK2 is also known as neurodegeneration with brain iron accumulation (NBIA-1) and was formerly known as Hallervorden-Spatz syndrome. Of these disorders, chorea-acanthocytosis, McLeod syndrome, HDL2, and PANK2 can occur with chorea as a predominant feature, although typically all have associated features [44,45].

Chorea-acanthocytosis is an autosomal-recessive disease characterized by chorea, tics, dystonia, dementia, an axonal peripheral neuropathy, and acanthocytes. As the disease progresses, a parkinsonian phenotype can result. The average age at onset is 35 years, but 5% to 10% present after age 50 [44]. The clinical picture can be much like that of HD but with the addition of an axonal peripheral neuropathy and acanthocytes. The overall prevalence is not known, but it is rare. Caudate and generalized brain atrophy are identified on neuroimaging and at autopsy. Chorea-acanthocytosis is caused by multiple mutations in a large gene of unknown function called chorein. How mutations in chorein cause acanthocytes and other disease manifestations is not known. A wet preparation of the peripheral blood smear is preferred to evaluate acanthocytes. Echinocytes are spiculated, normally occurring red blood cells (RBCs) that may be confused with acanthocytes and can compose 3% of RBCs. To make a diagnosis, it has been suggested that acanthocytes must be present at a rate of greater than 3% in repeat samplings. The acanthocyte percentage is variable between 5% and 50% in chorea-acanthocytosis and is not correlated to clinical severity. Creatine kinase (CK) and liver functions are elevated, with reduced haptoglobin in the majority of patients [44,45].

McLeod syndrome is a rare X-linked disorder similar to chorea-acanthocytosis. Clinically it manifests as chorea, axonal peripheral neuropathy, myopathy, cardiomyopathy, and hemolysis. It is a slowly progressive disorder, with approximately 60% of individuals diagnosed after 50 years of age. Atrophy of the caudate is seen on neuroimaging. Multiple responsible mutations have been identified in the XK gene, which normally encodes a precursor substance to the Kell blood group antigen. Patients who have McLeod lack the Kx antigen, and Kell antigens are severely reduced. How mutations in the XK gene cause the McLeod phenotype is not known. Acanthocyte levels range from 3% to 40%, and CK is elevated [44,45].

PANK2 is an autosomal recessive disorder with typical childhood onset dystonia, chorea, rigidity, and dysarthria. Rarer adult onset cases have parkinsonism and dementia. Recently, a case with autopsy confirmed that PANK2 presented at age 76 with chorea [46]. Acanthocytes occur in 8%

of individuals who have PANK2 [44,45]. The clinical presentation of HDL2 is that of typical HD, and although the full clinical spectrum is not known, onset after age 50 has not been described [47].

Autoimmune causes

The best-known immune cause of chorea was first described in 1686 by Thomas Sydenham as St. Vitus's Dance and is now referred to as Sydenham's chorea. It is widely accepted to be caused by an immune reaction to group A β-hemolytic streptococcal infection, but it is a disease not described in those older than 50 years, with a mean age at onset of 8 to 9 years [48].

Chorea is known to occur in systemic lupus erythematosus (SLE), but it is not clear whether the chorea is secondary to vascular insult or antibody-induced neuronal dysfunction. Frequently no ischemic lesion can be identified, so chorea associated with SLE and its related disorders is considered here [49]. SLE is a chronic heterogeneous autoimmune disorder that can involve multiple organ systems; four or more of 11 specific criteria must be present to make a diagnosis. SLE can occur in any age group but is primarily a disease of young women, with a mean age at onset of 32 years. There is a 5:1 female/male ratio, with disease in males having a mean onset at age 40. Prevalence estimates range from 15 to 51 per 100,000 [50]. One of the 11 diagnostic criteria for SLE is a neurologic disorder. The complete spectrum of neurologic involvement is debated, but studies indicate that central nervous system involvement in SLE is common, occurring in 18% to 69% [51]. Chorea occurs in approximately 1% to 4% of those who have SLE, but it appears to be uncommon in SLE patients older than 60 years. In one literature review of 50 patients who had chorea secondary to SLE or SLE-related disorders, only two (4%) were older than 60 [52]. These data suggest that SLE is a rare cause of geriatric chorea.

Chorea can be an initial manifestation of SLE, occurring as a single episode or less frequently recurring. In approximately half of the cases, chorea is bilateral. CT imaging is normal in 76% of patients, whereas 38% have normal brain MRIs. Lesions are rarely found in areas likely to be causative of chorea (the caudate or caudate and lentiform nuclei), suggesting a nonvascular causation [52]. Chorea in SLE is generally responsive to treatment, but it is unclear whether the response is due to dopamine antagonism, immune suppression, or anticoagulation [53].

The cause of chorea in SLE is not known, but evidence supports an association with antiphospholipid (aPL) antibodies [49,51,54]. aPL antibodies are a group of autoantibodies directed against negatively charged phospholipids, first described in SLE. aPL antibodies can also be found in disorders not completely fulfilling criteria for SLE, the so-called "SLE-like" disorders or probable SLE, and independently of SLE in primary antiphospholipid syndrome [53]. Chorea is also seen in probable SLE and primary aPL syndrome. A history of thrombotic events, such as deep vein thrombosis with or without pulmonary embolism, or of fetal loss should raise suspicion for aPL antibodies.

Paraneoplastic syndromes

Paraneoplastic disorders are caused by remote immune-mediated effects of a malignant neoplasm. Paraneoplastic syndromes affect 0.01% of patients who have cancer. Chorea is a rare paraneoplastic complication seen most frequently in association with small-cell lung carcinoma [55]. Paraneoplastic chorea has also been reported much less frequently in renal carcinoma and non-Hodgkin's lymphoma. Chorea may be seen in isolation but more frequently is seen in combination with visual loss, peripheral neuropathy, ataxia, and subacute dementia (limbic encephalitis) [56,57]. The chorea is usually subacute at onset, bilateral or generalized, but it can also be unilateral [58]. MRI can demonstrate bilateral basal ganglia T2 hyperintensities. Studies indicate that a novel autoantibody directed against collapsing response-mediating protein–5 (CRMP-5) may be highly associated with paraneoplastic chorea. Anti-CRMP-5 is believed to be the same antibody as anti-CV-2, which has also been associated with paraneoplastic chorea [56,58]. In case series reporting anti-CRMP-5–associated paraneoplastic syndromes, 36 of 39 patients were older than 55 years [56,58]. It is estimated that anti-CRMP-5 may be the second most common paraneoplastic autoantibody, with anti-Hu (ANNA1) being the most common. CRMP-5 and anti-Hu may be seen in combination, and reported cases of anti-Hu–associated chorea may in fact be CRMP-5 associated [58]. In 80% to 90% of patients, chorea preceded cancer diagnosis, emphasizing the importance of identifying paraneoplastic chorea. Treatment of the underlying neoplasm has been associated with chorea remission in approximately 50% [56,58].

Metabolic causes

Late-onset chorea as a consequence of metabolic abnormalities appears to be extremely rare. In the series reported by Piccolo and colleagues [7], two cases each of chorea secondary to hyperglycemia and hyponatremia were reported. None of these four patients were older than 50 years [7]. Hyperthyroidism as a cause of chorea has a long history but infrequent occurrence [59]. It was first described by Gowers in 1893 and again by Southerland in 1903; since that time, scattered case reports exist. When present, chorea may be unilateral, bilateral in the upper extremities, generalized, or paroxysmal, and it resolves with treatment of the hyperthyroidism. Hashimoto's thyroiditis has also infrequently been reported to cause a steroid-responsive chorea [60].

Nonketotic hyperglycemia with glucose between 300 and 1000 mg/dL has been reported to cause primarily unilateral, transient chorea in some cases, with high T1 MRI signal in the contralateral striatum [61,62]. The majority of the reported patients are older than 50 years. Chorea generally abates within days to weeks of normalized glucose but has also been described as persistent [63]. The causative agent of chorea and the associated high T1 MRI signal secondary to hyperglycemia is not known.

Hypocalcemia, typically in the setting of hypoparathyroidism, has been associated with unilateral, generalized, or paroxysmal chorea. The chorea is generally responsive to treatment of hypocalcemia, indicating that the basal ganglion calcifications frequently associated with hypoparathyroidism, which do not diminish, are not the cause of chorea [64,65].

Infectious causes

A number of infections have been described as causing chorea, primarily by local vasculitic or structural involvement of the basal ganglion [65]. In the series reported by Piccolo and colleagues [7], 7 of the 51 cases (14%) were of infectious origin, but only one patient (2%) was older than 50: a patient who had progressive multifocal leukoencephalopathy secondary to AIDS. Toxoplasmosis abscesses in the basal ganglion have been reported in those older than 50 who have AIDS or who are otherwise immunocompromised [66]. As patients who have AIDS survive into older age in larger numbers, this may become a more frequent cause of late-onset chorea. Other infections reported to cause late-onset chorea include mycoplasma pneumonia and legionella pneumophila [65].

Creutzfeldt-Jakob disease (CJD) is a devastating subacute neurodegenerative disorder, typified by dementia, myoclonus, and characteristic electroencephalographic changes, with average onset age of 62. Chorea is rare and has not been reported in isolation. New-variant CJD is clinically distinct, with a typical onset at younger than 30 years, a longer course, psychiatric symptoms, sensory complaints, ataxia, cognitive impairment, and involuntary movements, including chorea reported in 57% of patients. Chorea was not seen in isolation or as a presenting symptom in a series of new-variant CJD patients [67], but it has been described in isolated cases [68]. Because approximately 6% of those who have new-variant CJD survive past age 50, it could be a rare cause of chorea in this age group.

Other causes

Polycythemia vera

The polycythemias are a group of primary or secondary disorders characterized by an increased number of RBCs. Polycythemia vera (PV) is the most common primary polycythemia and results from clonal expansion of a hematopoietic stem cell, resulting in increased RBC mass [69]. It is estimated that the incidence of PV is 1.9 per 100,000 per year [70]. Although

PV can occur in any age group, the median age at diagnosis is 60 years. PV is more common in men (1.5–2:1), with the highest incidence in men aged 70 to 79 (24 per 100,000 per year) [70]. Chorea has been reported as the presenting symptom and occurs more frequently in women (5:2) after the age of 50. It is estimated that 1% to 1.5% of those who have PV develop chorea [71,72]. Chorea in PV can be acute or gradually progressive, asymmetric or generalized, but it tends to be most severe in the face, head, and neck regions. The cause of polycythemic chorea is unknown, but sluggish basal ganglion blood flow and dopamine receptor hypersensitivity have been proposed [66]. The degree of chorea is not highly correlated with RBC counts, but treatment of PV typically improves or abolishes chorea [71,72].

Senile chorea

Senile chorea has been defined as late-onset generalized chorea, without a family history or other neurologic manifestations. Until HD gene testing became available, it was suggested that senile chorea did not exist but was actually late-onset HD. Examination of the HD CAG repeat in those fulfilling the diagnosis of senile chorea indicates that a significant proportion, approximately 50%, do carry the HD mutation and have late-onset HD [4,73]. This finding also demonstrates that senile chorea is a rare disease entity separate from HD. Others suggest that PV is a leading candidate for the cause of senile chorea [66]. The chorea is typically of gradual onset and generalized, appearing in the sixth to eighth decades [4,73,74]. The majority of MRI and CT scans are normal, but a minority demonstrate mild generalized atrophy or nonspecific T2 hyperintensities [4,73]. This diagnosis is one of exclusion in which no other cause of chorea can be identified.

Basal ganglion mineralization

Apparent basal ganglion calcification (BGC) on CT scans is found in 0.6% to 1.2% of normal brains and is much more common in those older than 50 years [75–77]. This entity has been referred to by a number of names, including Fahr's disease, striopallidiodentatal calcification, bilateral striopallidiodentate calcinosis, and basal ganglion mineralization [75–78]. Early pre–CT scan reports of a frequent correlation between BGC and movement disorders, including chorea, have given way to the view that the majority of BGCs are asymptomatic incidental findings [76,77]. Although some studies have found that 7% of those who had apparent BGC on CT scan had a clinical disorder that could be referred to the basal ganglion [75,79], none had chorea. When the condition is symptomatic, onset is in the fourth to sixth decades, with parkinsonism, dystonia, ataxia, seizures, cognitive decline, and, rarely, chorea that usually occur in combination with other symptoms. Autosomal-dominant inheritance has been described in some families [78]. The most common cause of BGC is hypoparathyroidism, with 70% having BGC [80–82]. Hypoparathyroidism is also associated with neurologic manifestations, including chorea, seizures, parkinsonism, and tetany. The relationship of BGC and hypoparathyroid-related neurologic symptoms is unclear, but basal ganglion fluoro-dopa positron emission tomography signal was not found to be abnormal in one case, arguing against basal ganglion dysfunction as a cause [78].

Investigations into the cause of late-onset chorea

The work-up of apparently sporadic late-onset chorea can be extensive and unrevealing. It is reasonable to proceed with a staged work-up, first obtaining imaging and basic serologies and then proceeding to investigations of more rare causes (Table 3). It would also be reasonable to refer affected patients to a movement disorder neurologist. Medications known to cause chorea may be tapered if this is medically possible. Gadolinium-enhanced brain MRI can identify cerebrovascular causes, focal caudate atrophy, T1-weighted high signal associated with hyperglycemia, BGC, and other structural causes. Complete blood count should be performed to look for elevated hemoglobin in PV and a wet smear performed to identify acanthocytes. The presence of acanthocytes can be missed if not evaluated properly. The preferred method calls for a 1:1 dilution of whole blood and heparinized saline to be incubated for 30 to 120 minutes at room temperature and a wet preparation viewed under a phase contrast microscope [45]. Aspartate aminotransferase, alanine aminotransferase, lactate dehydrogenase, and CK can also be elevated in neuroacanthocytosis. A complete blood count can also identify SLE-related thrombocytopenia, leucopenia, or lymphopenia. Both hyperthyroidism and hyperglycemia are treatable causes of chorea, and thyroid-stimulating hormone T4 and glucose should be checked.

When medication withdrawal is not successful and initial work-up unrevealing, one should proceed to less likely causes. The implications of

Table 3
Imaging and serologic investigations of late-onset chorea

Initial work-up	Subsequent work-up
Gadolinium-enhanced brain MRI	HD gene test
Complete blood cell count[a]	CRMP-5 and anti-Hu antibodies. Chest, abdomen, and pelvis CT or MRI scan with contrast or positron emission tomography scan
Erythrocyte sedimentation rate	Antiphospholipid antibodies (IgG and IgM), lupus anticoagulant, β-2-glycoprotein I, antinuclear antibody, and extractable nuclear antigens[b]
Thyroid-stimulating hormone, T4	Calcium, phosphorous, and parathyroid hormone levels[c]

[a] It is reasonable to have a routine wet smear examined for acanthocytes because there is little added expense or discomfort.

[b] If there is a history of venous thrombosis or fetal loss, these tests can be part of the initial work-up.

[c] If basal ganglion calcifications are observed on neuroimaging.

a positive HD gene test should be discussed and genetic counseling offered to asymptomatic family members. An anticardiolipin panel for IgG and IgM antiphospholipid antibody titers should be obtained. High IgG titers are generally more significant. Lupus anticoagulant screening, including a tissue thromboplastin inhibition test and dilute Russell's viper venom test (which can be abnormal in the presence of antiphospholipids), may be obtained. β-2-glycoprotein I elevations have also been reported in patients who have antiphospholipid syndrome, and these may also be drawn. Elevated erythrocyte sedimentation rate, antinuclear antibodies, extractable nuclear antibodies, and low complement are frequently present in SLE, but their relationship to chorea is not clear. A paraneoplastic cause should be investigated, even in the absence of systemic manifestations, by looking for anti-CRMP-5 and anti-Hu antibodies. If suspicion is high, chest, abdomen, and pelvis CT, MRI, or positron emission tomography scans may identify a primary tumor. Although BGC rarely causes chorea, if this is identified on neuroimaging, serum calcium and parathyroid levels may be evaluated.

Treatment

Most treatments of chorea have not been evaluated in a rigorous manner. When a medication is believed to be causative and may be safely discontinued, a trial off the medication is reasonable. When a primary medical condition is identified, it should be treated. Frequently, choreic movements are neither disabling nor obstructive to activities of daily living, so treatment may not be necessary.

In general, medications that deplete or antagonize dopamine are considered most effective, but they cause orthostatic hypotension, parkinsonism, and depression. Tetrabenazine and reserpine deplete dopamine by blocking its transport into presynaptic vesicles. The peripheral blockade of monoamines by reserpine mediates its antihypertensive effect but also causes postural hypotension. The side effects of reserpine may be diminished by starting with 0.125 to 0.25 mg per day and increasing the dose by 0.125 to 0.25 mg weekly with blood pressure monitoring. Reserpine doses as high as 6 mg/d may be required [11,83]. Tetrabenazine has higher central nervous system specificity than reserpine and, unlike those of reserpine, its effects are reversible within hours. Tetrabenazine is not currently available in the United States, but a recent prospective double-blind, placebo-controlled study showed that as much as 100 mg of tetrabenazine daily significantly improved chorea in HD [84]. Beginning at 25 mg/d for the first day, proceeding with 25 mg twice daily for the remainder of the first week, and increasing by 25 mg per week to a maximum of 50 mg twice a day was well tolerated [84].

No controlled clinical data exist to evaluate the effectiveness of atypical neuroleptics on chorea, but they are widely used as first-line agents. Neuroleptics have a large number of side effects, including parkinsonism, imbalance, acute dystonic reactions, tardive dyskinesias, apathy, and neuroleptic malignant syndrome. If neuroleptics are initiated, patients should be closely monitored. Haloperidol given at bedtime in low doses can be quite effective (1–10 mg/d). Risperdone and quetiapine may also be effective but have less anecdotal support [85]. Modest efficacy in chorea reduction has been obtained in HD with remacemide and riluzole [86,87], but efficacy in other choreas is not known. The effects of amantadine have been mixed, but a double-blind study in HD did not show benefit on chorea [88]. It is important to recall that many types of sporadic chorea have spontaneous remission, so long-term treatment may not be necessary. Withdrawal of treatment that has eliminated the movements for 2 to 3 months should be considered.

Summary

Late-onset chorea is rare and has a heterogeneous causation. It is remarkable that such a wide range of conditions cause chorea. A systematic approach to geriatric chorea greatly enhances a correct diagnosis. An accurate diagnosis is important because many causes of chorea are treatable or, when heritable, may have significant implications for subsequent generations. Most late-onset chorea is either nonlimiting, requiring no treatment, has a spontaneous remission, or responds to medication. In a minority of patients, chorea is medically refractory or a manifestation of an untreatable disorder.

Acknowledgments

The author would like to thank Malorie Sprunger and Virginia Zawistowski for assistance in manuscript preparation.

References

[1] Albin RL, Young AB, Penney JB. The functional anatomy of basal ganglia disorders. Trends Neurosci 1989;12(10):366–75.
[2] Shoulson I. On chorea. Clin Neuropharmacol 1986;9(Suppl 2):S85–99.
[3] Dewey RB Jr, Jankovic J. Hemiballism-hemichorea. Clinical and pharmacologic findings in 21 patients. Arch Neurol 1989;46(8):862–7.
[4] Garcia Ruiz PJ, Gomez-Tortosa E, del Barrio A, et al. Senile chorea: a multicenter prospective study. Acta Neurol Scand 1997;95(3):180–3.
[5] Warren JD, Firgaira F, Thompson EM, et al. The causes of sporadic and 'senile' chorea. Aust N Z J Med 1998;28(4):429–31.
[6] Piccolo I, Sterzi R, Thiella G, et al. Sporadic choreas: analysis of a general hospital series. Eur Neurol 1999;41(3):143–9.
[7] Piccolo I, Defanti CA, Soliveri P, et al. Cause and course in a series of patients with sporadic chorea. J Neurol 2003;250(4):429–35.
[8] Ghika-Schmid F, Ghika J, Regli F, et al. Hyperkinetic movement disorders during and after acute stroke: the Lausanne Stroke Registry. J Neurol Sci 1997;146(2):109–16.

[9] Bhatia KP, Marsden CD. The behavioural and motor consequences of focal lesions of the basal ganglia in man. Brain 1994;117(Pt 4):859–76.

[10] Fahn S. The spectrum of levodopa-induced dyskinesias. Ann Neurol 2000;47(4 Suppl. 1): S2–9 [discussion: S9–11].

[11] Stacy M, Cardoso F, Jankovic J. Tardive stereotypy and other movement disorders in tardive dyskinesias. Neurology 1993;43(5):937–41.

[12] Smith JM, Oswald WT, Kucharski LT, et al. Tardive dyskinesia: age and sex differences in hospitalized schizophrenics. Psychopharmacology (Berl) 1978;58(2):207–11.

[13] Chouinard G, Annable L, Ross-Chouinard A, et al. A 5-year prospective longitudinal study of tardive dyskinesia: factors predicting appearance of new cases. J Clin Psychopharmacol 1988;8(4 Suppl):21S–6S.

[14] Goetz CG, Chmura TA, Lanska DJ. History of movement disorders as a neurological specialty: Part 14 of the MDS-sponsored History of Movement Disorders exhibit, Barcelona, June 2000. Mov Disord 2001;16(5):954–9.

[15] Folstein SE. Huntington's disease. Baltimore (MD): Johns Hopkins University Press; 1989.

[16] Nance MA. Clinical aspects of CAG repeat diseases. Brain Pathol 1997;7(3):881–900.

[17] Robitaille Y, Lopes-Cendes I, Becher M, et al. The neuropathology of CAG repeat diseases: review and update of genetic and molecular features. Brain Pathol 1997;7(3):901–26.

[18] Gusella JF, Wexler NS, Conneally PM, et al. A polymorphic DNA marker genetically linked to Huntington's disease. Nature 1983;306(5940):234–8.

[19] The Huntington's Disease Collaborative Research Group. A novel gene containing a trinucleotide repeat that is expanded and unstable on Huntington's disease chromosomes. Cell 1993;72(6):971–83.

[20] Li SH, Schilling G, Young WS III, et al. Huntington's disease gene (IT15) is widely expressed in human and rat tissues. Neuron 1993;11(5):985–93.

[21] Zoghbi HY, Orr HT. Glutamine repeats and neurodegeneration. Annu Rev Neurosci 2000; 23:217–47.

[22] Nakamura K, Jeong SY, Uchihara T, et al. SCA17, a novel autosomal dominant cerebellar ataxia caused by an expanded polyglutamine in TATA-binding protein. Hum Mol Genet 2001;10(14):1441–8.

[23] Cummings CJ, Zoghbi HY. Trinucleotide repeats: mechanisms and pathophysiology. Annu Rev Genomics Hum Genet 2000;1:281–328.

[24] Luthi-Carter R, Strand AD, Hanson SA, et al. Polyglutamine and transcription: gene expression changes shared by DRPLA and Huntington's disease mouse models reveal context-independent effects. Hum Mol Genet 2002;11(17):1927–37.

[25] American College of Medical Genetics/American Society of Human Genetics Huntington Disease Genetic Testing Working Group. Laboratory guidelines for Huntington disease genetic testing. Am J Hum Genet 1998;62:1243–7.

[26] Wexler NS, Lorimer J, Porter J, et al. Venezuelan kindreds reveal that genetic and environmental factors modulate Huntington's disease age of onset. Proc Natl Acad Sci U S A 2004; 101(10):3498–503.

[27] Goldberg YP, Kremer B, Andrew SE, et al. Molecular analysis of new mutations for Huntington's disease: intermediate alleles and sex of origin effects. Nat Genet 1993;5(2): 174–9.

[28] Langbehn DR, Brinkman RR, Falush D, et al. A new model for prediction of the age of onset and penetrance for Huntington's disease based on CAG length. Clin Genet 2004;65(4): 267–77.

[29] Harjes P, Wanker EE. The hunt for Huntington function: interaction partners tell many different stories. Trends Biochem Sci 2003;28(8):425–33.

[30] Sugars KL, Rubinsztein DC. Transcriptional abnormalities in Huntington disease. Trends Genet 2003;19(5):233–8.

[31] Myers RH, Sax DS, Schoenfeld M, et al. Late onset of Huntington's disease. J Neurol Neurosurg Psychiatry 1985;48(6):530–4.

[32] Kremer B, Squitieri F, Telenius H, et al. Molecular analysis of late onset Huntington's disease. J Med Genet 1993;30(12):991–5.

[33] Young AB, Shoulson I, Penney JB, et al. Huntington's disease in Venezuela: neurologic features and functional decline. Neurology 1986;36(2):244–9.

[34] Penney JB Jr, Young AB, Shoulson I, et al. Huntington's disease in Venezuela: 7 years of follow-up on symptomatic and asymptomatic individuals. Mov Disord 1990;5(2):93–9.

[35] Britton JW, Uitti RJ, Ahlskog JE, et al. Hereditary late-onset chorea without significant dementia: genetic evidence for substantial phenotypic variation in Huntington's disease. Neurology 1995;45(3 Pt 1):443–7.

[36] Bamford KA, Caine ED, Kido DK, et al. A prospective evaluation of cognitive decline in early Huntington's disease: functional and radiographic correlates. Neurology 1995; 45(10):1867–73.

[37] Bauer P, Laccone F, Rolfs A, et al. Trinucleotide repeat expansion in SCA17/TBP in white patients with Huntington's disease–like phenotype. J Med Genet 2004;41(3):230–2.

[38] Fujigasaki H, Martin JJ, De Deyn PP, et al. CAG repeat expansion in the TATA box-binding protein gene causes autosomal dominant cerebellar ataxia. Brain 2001;124(Pt 10): 1939–47.

[39] Ikeuchi T, Koide R, Tanaka H, et al. Dentatorubral-pallidoluysian atrophy: clinical features are closely related to unstable expansions of trinucleotide (CAG) repeat. Ann Neurol 1995; 37(6):769–75.

[40] Warner TT, Williams LD, Walker RW, et al. A clinical and molecular genetic study of dentatorubropallidoluysian atrophy in four European families. Ann Neurol 1995;37(4):452–9.

[41] Burke JR, Wingfield MS, Lewis KE, et al. The Haw River syndrome: dentatorubropallidoluysian atrophy (DRPLA) in an African-American family. Nat Genet 1994;7(4):521–4.

[42] Ikeuchi T, Onodera O, Oyake M, et al. Dentatorubral-pallidoluysian atrophy (DRPLA): close correlation of CAG repeat expansions with the wide spectrum of clinical presentations and prominent anticipation. Semin Cell Biol 1995;6(1):37–44.

[43] Komure O, Sano A, Nishino N, et al. DNA analysis in hereditary dentatorubral-pallidoluysian atrophy: correlation between CAG repeat length and phenotypic variation and the molecular basis of anticipation. Neurology 1995;45(1):143–9.

[44] Rampoldi L, Danek A, Monaco AP. Clinical features and molecular bases of neuroacanthocytosis. J Mol Med 2002;80(8):475–91.

[45] Danek A, Jung HH, Melone MA, et al. Neuroacanthocytosis: new developments in a neglected group of dementing disorders. J Neurol Sci 2005;229–230:171–86.

[46] Grimes DA, Lang AE, Bergeron C. Late onset chorea with typical pathology of Hallervorden-Spatz syndrome. J Neurol Neurosurg Psychiatry 2006;69:392–5.

[47] Holmes SE, O'Hearn E, Rosenblatt A, et al. A repeat expansion in the gene encoding junctophilin-3 is associated with Huntington disease–like 2. Nat Genet 2001;29(4):377–8.

[48] Marques-Dias MJ, Mercadante MT, Tucker D, et al. Sydenham's chorea. Psychiatr Clin North Am 1997;20(4):809–20.

[49] Sanna G, Bertolaccini ML, Cuadrado MJ, et al. Neuropsychiatric manifestations in systemic lupus erythematosus: prevalence and association with antiphospholipid antibodies. J Rheumatol 2003;30(5):985–92.

[50] Jennekens FG, Kater L. The central nervous system in systemic lupus erythematosus. Part 1. Clinical syndromes: a literature investigation. Rheumatology (Oxford) 2002;41(6):605–18.

[51] Jennekens FG, Kater L. The central nervous system in systemic lupus erythematosus. Part 2. Pathogenetic mechanisms of clinical syndromes: a literature investigation. Rheumatology (Oxford) 2002;41(6):619–30.

[52] Cervera R, Asherson RA, Font J, et al. Chorea in the antiphospholipid syndrome. Clinical, radiologic, and immunologic characteristics of 50 patients from our clinics and the recent literature. Medicine (Baltimore) 1997;76(3):203–12.

[53] Sanna G, Bertolaccini ML, Cuadrado MJ, et al. Central nervous system involvement in the antiphospholipid (Hughes) syndrome. Rheumatology (Oxford) 2003;42(2):200–13.

[54] Toubi E, Khamashta MA, Panarra A, et al. Association of antiphospholipid antibodies with central nervous system disease in systemic lupus erythematosus. Am J Med 1995;99(4): 397–401.

[55] Albin RL, Bromberg MB, Penney JB, et al. Chorea and dystonia: a remote effect of carcinoma. Mov Disord 1988;3(2):162–9.

[56] Rogemond V, Honnorat J. Anti-CV2 autoantibodies and paraneoplastic neurological syndromes. Clin Rev Allergy Immunol 2000;19(1):51–9.

[57] Yu Z, Kryzer TJ, Griesmann GE, et al. CRMP-5 neuronal autoantibody: marker of lung cancer and thymoma-related autoimmunity. Ann Neurol 2001;49(2):146–54.

[58] Vernino S, Tuite P, Adler CH, et al. Paraneoplastic chorea associated with CRMP-5 neuronal antibody and lung carcinoma. Ann Neurol 2002;51(5):625–30.

[59] Shahar E, Shapiro MS, Shenkman L. Hyperthyroid-induced chorea. Case report and review of the literature. Isr J Med Sci 1988;24(4–5):264–6.

[60] Shaw PJ, Walls TJ, Newman PK, et al. Hashimoto's encephalopathy: a steroid-responsive disorder associated with high anti-thyroid antibody titers—report of 5 cases. Neurology 1991;41(2 Pt 1):228–33.

[61] Lin JJ, Chang MK. Hemiballism-hemichorea and non-ketotic hyperglycaemia. J Neurol Neurosurg Psychiatry 1994;57(6):748–50.

[62] Linazasoro G, Urtasun M, Poza JJ, et al. Generalized chorea induced by nonketotic hyperglycemia. Mov Disord 1993;8(1):119–20.

[63] Ahlskog JE, Nishino H, Evidente VG, et al. Persistent chorea triggered by hyperglycemic crisis in diabetics. Mov Disord 2001;16(5):890–8.

[64] Christiansen NJ, Hansen PF. Choreiform movements in hypoparathyroidism. N Engl J Med 1972;287(11):569–70.

[65] Janavs JL, Aminoff MJ. Dystonia and chorea in acquired systemic disorders. J Neurol Neurosurg Psychiatry 1998;65(4):436–45.

[66] Nath A, Hobson DE, Russell A. Movement disorders with cerebral toxoplasmosis and AIDS. Mov Disord 1993;8(1):107–12.

[67] Will RG, Zeidler M, Stewart GE, et al. Diagnosis of new variant Creutzfeldt-Jakob disease. Ann Neurol 2000;47(5):575–82.

[68] McKee D, Talbot P. Chorea as a presenting feature of variant Creutzfeldt-Jakob disease. Mov Disord 2003;18(7):837–8.

[69] Prchal JT. Classification and molecular biology of polycythemias (erythrocytoses) and thrombocytosis. Hematol Oncol Clin North Am 2003;17(5):1151–8, vi.

[70] Ania BJ, Suman VJ, Sobell JL, et al. Trends in the incidence of polycythemia vera among Olmsted County, Minnesota residents, 1935–1989. Am J Hematol 1994;47(2):89–93.

[71] Bruyn GW, Padberg G. Chorea and polycythaemia. Eur Neurol 1984;23(1):26–33.

[72] Mas JL, Gueguen B, Bouche P, et al. Chorea and polycythaemia. J Neurol 1985;232(3): 169–71.

[73] Shinotoh H, Calne DB, Snow B, et al. Normal CAG repeat length in the Huntington's disease gene in senile chorea. Neurology 1994;44(11):2183–4.

[74] Friedman JH, Ambler M. A case of senile chorea. Mov Disord 1990;5(3):251–3.

[75] Murphy MJ. Clinical correlations of CT scan–detected calcifications of the basal ganglia. Ann Neurol 1979;6(6):507–11.

[76] Harrington MG, Macpherson P, McIntosh WB, et al. The significance of the incidental finding of basal ganglia calcification on computed tomography. J Neurol Neurosurg Psychiatry 1981;44(12):1168–70.

[77] Forstl H, Krumm B, Eden S, et al. Neurological disorders in 166 patients with basal ganglia calcification: a statistical evaluation. J Neurol 1992;239(1):36–8.

[78] Manyam BV, Bhatt MH, Moore WD, et al. Bilateral striopallidodentate calcinosis: cerebrospinal fluid, imaging, and electrophysiological studies. Ann Neurol 1992;31(4):379–84.

[79] Brannan TS, Burger AA, Chaudhary MY. Bilateral basal ganglia calcifications visualised on CT scan. J Neurol Neurosurg Psychiatry 1980;43(5):403–6.

[80] Okada J, Takeuchi K, Ohkado M, et al. Familial basal ganglia calcifications visualized by computerized tomography. Acta Neurol Scand 1981;64(4):273–9.

[81] Illum F, Dupont E. Prevalences of CT-detected calcification in the basal ganglia in idiopathic hypoparathyroidism and pseudohypoparathyroidism. Neuroradiology 1985;27(1):32–7.

[82] Sachs C, Sjoberg HE, Ericson K. Basal ganglia calcifications on CT: relation to hypoparathyroidism. Neurology 1982;32(7):779–82.

[83] Lang AE, Marsden CD. Alpha methylparatyrosine and tetrabenazine in movement disorders. Clin Neuropharmacol 1982;5(4):375–87.

[84] Huntington Study Group. Tetrabenazine as antichorea therapy in Huntington disease: a randomized controlled trial. Neurology 2006;66(3):366–72.

[85] Bonelli RM, Hofmann P. A review of the treatment options for Huntington's disease. Expert Opin Pharmacother 2004;5(4):767–76.

[86] Huntington Study Group. A randomized, placebo-controlled trial of coenzyme Q10 and remacemide in Huntington's disease. Neurology 2001;57(3):397–404.

[87] Huntington Study Group. Dosage effects of riluzole in Huntington's disease: a multicenter placebo-controlled study. Neurology 2003;61(11):1551–6.

[88] O'Suilleabhain P, Dewey RB Jr. A randomized trial of amantadine in Huntington disease. Arch Neurol 2003;60(7):996–8.

ELSEVIER
SAUNDERS

CLINICS IN
GERIATRIC
MEDICINE

Clin Geriatr Med 22 (2006) 899–914

Dystonia

Ninith Kartha, MD

Department of Neurology, University of Michigan Medical Center,
1500 Medical Center Drive, 1324 Taubman Center, Ann Arbor, MI 48109-0322, USA

Dystonia is a disorder of involuntary sustained muscle contractions, often resulting in twisting and repetitive movements or abnormal postures [1]. When the duration of contractions is short, dystonic movements can appear rapid, resembling myoclonus. When these movements exhibit a rhythmic or jerky quality, the term *dystonic tremor* has been applied [2]. Involvement can be restricted to a single body part (focal dystonia) or encompass multiple body regions (segmental, multifocal, or generalized dystonia). Dystonic contractions may be present only with voluntary activity; dystonia that is present at rest often is exacerbated by activity. When dystonia is limited to one type of action only, it is considered task-specific (ie, writer's cramp or occupational dystonia). Dystonia is not a diagnosis in itself, but rather a symptom or feature of several disorders of various etiologies.

Classification

Dystonic disorders typically are classified by age of onset, distribution of involvement, or etiology (Box 1). Identifying age of onset helps to point toward an etiology and can guide diagnostic workup and treatment. Placing the dividing age between early-onset and late-onset dystonia at age 26 has been a useful guideline in determining who should undergo genetic testing because early-onset cases are more likely to carry a mutation in the *DYT1* gene locus causing primary torsion dystonia (PTD) [3]. PTD, in which dystonia is the only neurologic sign, is usually due to an inherited disorder in early-onset cases. Late-onset PTD is often sporadic, although as more information is accumulated about etiology, it is recognized that many forms of late-onset PTD also may have a genetic basis [4]. Early-onset PTD typically

E-mail address: nkartha@umich.edu

Box 1. Classification of dystonia

By age of onset
Early (<26 years)
Late

By distribution
Focal (single body region)
Segmental (contiguous regions)
Multifocal (noncontiguous regions)
Hemi (a type of multifocal—ipsilateral arm and leg)
Generalized (leg + trunk + one other region or both legs +/−
    trunk + one other region)

By cause
Primary—dystonia is only sign except tremor, and no acquired
    or exogenous cause or degenerative disorder
Secondary
    Due to inherited or degenerative disorders—signs other
        than dystonia or brain degeneration distinguish from
        primary dytonia
    Due to acquired or exogenous causes

Dystonia as a feature of another neurologic disorder (eg, tics,
    paroxysmal dyskinesias)
Pseudodystonia (eg, Sandifer's syndrome, psychogenic)

From Bressman SB. Dystonia genotypes, phenotypes, and classification. Adv
Neurol 2004;94:101–107; with permission.

---

starts in a lower limb and progresses to become generalized. Late-onset PTD
most often affects the cranial musculature or upper extremities and remains
focal [5].

A second method of classification is by distribution of body involvement.
In focal dystonia, a single body region is affected. This single area could be
a limb, such as the arm in writer's cramp, or axial musculature, such as the
neck in spasmodic torticollis. Segmental dystonia involves two or more contiguous body areas, whereas multifocal dystonia involves two or more noncontiguous areas. In generalized dystonia, multiple regions are affected,
including the legs and one other region or one leg, the trunk, and one other
region [6]. Hemidystonia often is associated with a structural lesion or degenerative disorders, and this finding should prompt evaluation for secondary causes [7,8].

A third method of classification is by etiology. A common system divides
causes of dystonia into two groups—primary and secondary. In primary

disorders, dystonia is the only abnormal sign, although tremor if associated with dystonia also can be present. Other criteria include absence of clinical history, laboratory findings, or imaging findings that suggest a secondary cause and lack of response to levodopa [6]. The most common cause of PTD in childhood, or Oppenheim dystonia, is a mutation in the *DYT1* gene locus located on chromosome 9 [9,10]. Approximately 90% of early-onset dystonia in the Ashkenazi Jewish population is due to *DYT1* mutation. This mutation accounts for 40% to 65% of early-onset dystonia in the non-Jewish population [3,11].

Secondary dystonia comprises dystonia plus syndromes, heredodegenerative disorders, dystonia associated with parkinsonism, and acquired causes of dystonia. In dystonia plus, dystonia is accompanied by other neurologic abnormalities, such as ataxia, myoclonus, or parkinsonism; however, these disorders are often nondegenerative, and brain imaging studies are negative for identifiable structural abnormalities [11]. The classic example is dopa-responsive dystonia (DRD), or Segawa's syndrome, which is a childhood-onset dystonia and parkinsonism that shows a dramatic response to low doses of levodopa [12,13]. Heredodegenerative diseases that cause dystonia are inherited disorders associated with progressive neurodegeneration. Examples include Huntington's disease, spinocerebellar ataxia type 3 (Machado-Joseph disease) and Wilson's disease. Parkinsonian disorders have complex etiologies and are likely due to a combination of inherited and environmental factors. This includes idiopathic Parkinson's disease and the Parkinson-plus syndromes of multiple system atrophy, progressive supranuclear palsy, and corticobasal ganglionic degeneration.

Acquired dystonias include disorders caused by structural damage to the brain and iatrogenic causes. Structural abnormality can be caused by congenital malformations, head trauma, stroke, and tumor. Dystonia also can be caused by hypoxia, demyelination (multiple sclerosis), infection (encephalitis, tuberculosis, syphilis), and inflammatory disorders affecting the brain (lupus, antiphospholipid antibody syndrome). Medications most likely to cause secondary dystonia include dopamine-stimulating agents (dopamine agonists and levodopa), dopamine D_2 receptor blocking agents (antipsychotics and antiemetics), antiepileptic agents, selective serotonin reuptake inhibitors, and monoamine oxidase inhibitors. Spinal cord and peripheral nerve injury also have been reported to cause dystonia [11].

Some classification systems also include categories for dystonia when it is a feature of another neurologic disorder and for pseudodystonia. Sustained postures can be seen in tic disorders (dystonic tics) or paroxysmal dyskinesias (paroxysmal dystonia) [4]. Pseudodystonia refers to disorders that can be mistaken for dystonia because of sustained or twisting postures. Examples include Sandifer syndrome and stiff-person syndrome. Finally, some systems also include psychogenic causes as a separate etiology. A comprehensive listing of etiologies of dystonia is beyond the scope of this article; however, several lists have been developed that provide a sense of the extensive variety of disorders that can be associated with this symptom [4,11].

Epidemiology

Prevalence estimates of primary dystonia vary widely. A review by Defazio and colleagues [14] of 14 epidemiologic studies showed that prevalence estimates for early-onset dystonia range from 2 to 50 cases per 1 million, and for late onset (focal) dystonia from 30 to 7320 per 1 million. This variation is likely due to differences in study design and study populations and variations in allele prevalence. Several studies have shown that mild forms of dystonia are likely to be misdiagnosed or undiagnosed [15–17]. The prevalence rate of secondary dystonia is even more difficult to determine because disorders in which dystonia is not the main feature may be underrepresented in epidemiologic studies. A study of medical records in Rochester, Minnesota, found the prevalence of primary generalized dystonia to be 3.4 per 100,000, and that of focal dystonia to be 29.5 per 100,000 [18]. A study by a European collaborative group found the prevalence of focal dystonia in eight European countries to be 11.7 per 100,000; however, this was a clinic-based study with subjects recruited through neurology or botulinum toxin (BTX) clinics, possibly leading to underestimation [19]. A population-based study by Muller and coworkers [17] of subjects older than age 50 found a prevalence of focal dystonia of 732 per 100,000. Cervical dystonia was found to be the most common focal dystonia [18–21]. There also seems to be a female predominance in most forms of focal dystonia, including spasmodic torticollis, blepharospasm, and laryngeal dystonia, although limb dystonia seems to have an equal male-to-female ratio or slight preponderance in men [22].

Pathophysiology

The neural mechanisms underlying dystonia are complex and incompletely understood, although multiple levels of the central nervous system clearly are involved. Neurophysiologic studies indicate that dystonic postures are produced by the cocontraction of agonist and antagonist muscles. Voluntary movement leads to abnormally prolonged bursts of muscle activity on electromyography (EMG) [23]. Superimposed tremor or myoclonus is represented by shorter bursts of EMG activity occurring on top of the underlying spasm [2,24]. In patients with focal hand dystonia, EMG studies show a lack of selectivity when attempts are made to perform individual finger movements, with overflow into unrelated muscles of the arm and impairment of appropriate agonist muscle activation [25]. Abnormal cocontraction is thought to be due to reduced reciprocal inhibition of opposing muscle groups; this can be seen by examining spinal reflexes in dystonic patients in whom stimulation of extensor muscle afferents in the forearm produced a reduced amount of inhibition of flexor muscle groups [26,27]. Brainstem involvement is indicated by the enhanced blink reflex recovery cycle in subjects with blepharospasm and in subjects with spasmodic torticollis and spasmodic dysphonia even without eyelid involvement [28,29].

The abnormalities of spinal and brainstem interneuronal circuits leading to reduced reciprocal inhibition are likely to originate in higher brain centers. Although no consistent structural pathology has been found in primary dystonia, abnormality of basal ganglia output has been suggested by studies of hemidystonia associated with lesions of contralateral putamen and globus pallidus [8] and the symptomatic improvement seen in subjects with dystonia after pallidotomy and deep brain stimulation [30]. Positron emission tomography and functional MRI studies have shown abnormal activity in the motor cortex, supplementary motor areas, cerebellum, and basal ganglia in *DYT1* gene carriers [31,32]. Transcranial magnetic stimulation studies indicate that abnormal cortical motor excitability in dystonic subjects results in reduced cortical inhibition, leading to abnormal movements [23,33].

Sensory system involvement is suggested clinically by the phenomenon of *geste antagoniste,* or sensory trick in which light touch to an affected body region can reduce the severity of dystonia. There are several indications that dystonia may be related to impaired sensorimotor integration secondary to improper processing of sensory input [34]. Peripheral nerve injury may lead to dystonia by causing an alteration of sensory input [35,36]. A study investigating the regional cerebral blood flow response to vibration in the hand in subjects with writer's cramp showed diminished response in the supplementary motor cortex and primary sensory cortex in subjects compared with normals [37]. Another study shows that finger representation in the primary sensory cortex in subjects with hand dystonia is abnormally organized [38].

The manner in which basal ganglia output affects cortical inhibition in dystonia is not fully understood. A simplified model suggests that decreased and disordered activity of basal ganglia output structures leads to thalamic and cortical disinhibition, which results in disinhibition at the brainstem and spinal level [34]. This abnormality of output could be a result of a structural lesion or could result from a deficit in dopamine as in the case of DRD. In *DYT1* dystonia, abnormal dopamine transmission has been implicated as an etiology for the resultant symptoms [39].

Genetics

There are currently 14 genetic forms of dystonia identified, designated *DYT1* through *DYT14* [6]. These disorders are transmitted in an autosomal dominant pattern except for *DYT2* (autosomal recessive), *DYT3* (X-linked recessive), and some instances of *DYT5* (autosomal recessive). *DYT1, DYT2, DYT4, DYT6, DYT7,* and *DYT13* are associated with primary dystonias, whereas the others are associated with dystonia plus syndromes. *DYT1* dystonia is associated with a three base pair deletion (GAG) in the *TOR1A* gene and is associated with early-onset generalized dystonia [10]. Although the function of the encoded protein torsin A is unknown, it is expressed in substantia nigra pars compacta dopamine neurons, suggesting its role in impaired dopamine transmission [40,41]. Owing to variable penetrance, severity of symptoms can range from asymptomatic to focal or segmental dystonia to severe generalized cases [42]. The increased frequency of *DYT1* dystonia in the Ashkenazi Jewish population is thought to be due to a founder mutation [15]. Mutations in the *DYT6* and *DYT13* gene loci result in a mixed-onset (late childhood or adolescent) dystonia, with prominent involvement of the cranial, cervical, and upper limb musculature [43,44].

A mutation in the *DYT7* locus located on chromosome 18p was discovered in a German family, resulting in late-onset focal or multifocal dystonia. Areas of involvement included the neck, vocal cord, or upper extremity (writer's cramp), and the average age of onset of symptoms was 43 [45]. Although other genetic loci for adult-onset focal dystonia have yet to be discovered, it is likely that many cases that are apparently sporadic do have a genetic basis as indicated by studies describing familial cases of various focal dystonias [46,47].

DYT5 gene locus mutation produces DRD, or Segawa's syndrome. A characteristic of DRD is diurnal fluctuation, in which symptoms are more severe in the evening and better on awakening in the morning or after a nap. *DYT5* has been associated with mutations in the guanosine triphosphate cyclohydrolase I region of chromosome 14 and the tyrosine hydroxylase region on chromosome 11 [48,49]. The former produces an autosomal dominant and the latter an autosomal recessive disorder. More recently, a mutation in another region of chromosome 14 (*DYT14*) has been shown to produce a similar syndrome with autosomal dominant transmission [50]. Myoclonus-dystonia, associated with the *DYT11* region, is manifested by myoclonus with dystonic features. Myoclonus is the more prominent symptom, and dystonia may be present only infrequently [51]. Symptoms typically respond well to low doses of alcohol [52]. *DYT12* dystonia causes rapid-onset dystonia-parkinsonism, and the mutation has been localized to a gene on chromosome 19 encoding the Na^+/K^+-ATPase $\alpha 3$ subunit [53]. The other identified *DYT* loci include *DYT2* causing an early-onset dystonia, *DYT3* causing dystonia parkinsonism, *DYT4* producing whispering dysphonia, and *DYT8* through *DYT10* producing paroxysmal dystonias [54].

Clinical features

The main features distinguishing a dystonic contraction are that the movement is sustained, has a consistent direction, and involves the same body region or regions in a predictable manner. Dystonia often has a rotatory or torsional component. The movement can be slow and sinuous or rapid, and the posture may be sustained for only a second before release. Dystonia typically occurs with voluntary movement of a body region (action dystonia), but with increasing severity, it can occur with movement of other body regions (overflow) and eventually at rest. Dystonia at rest typically is worsened by voluntary activity. Some forms of dystonia occur only with specific activities, such as handwriting in writer's cramp; however, with increasing severity, task-specific dystonias, too, can evolve to occur with other activities or at rest. As with several movement disorders, dystonia is usually worse with stress, anxiety, or fatigue and improved with rest or relaxation. A unique characteristic of dystonia is the phenomenon of the sensory trick in which tactile or proprioceptive stimulation can relieve or reduce the abnormal contraction. This is seen most commonly in cervical dystonia, in which lightly touching the cheek or chin can reduce head rotation [55]. With increasing severity, dystonia can result in fixed postures. Permanent contractures can occur if untreated.

Dystonia sometimes can be difficult to distinguish from other movement disorders. When dystonic contractions are rapid and only briefly sustained, the movements can resemble myoclonus. EMG needle examination typically shows prolonged bursts of muscle activity, rather than the short bursts seen in myoclonus [24]. Repetitive and rhythmic dystonic contractions can resemble tremor. Dystonic tremor typically can be distinguished from essential tremor by a directional preponderance, irregularity, or worsening of the tremor when the affected body part is moved in the opposite direction of pull [2]. In some cases, tremor can precede the clinical onset of dystonia, causing errors in diagnosis [56].

Primary dystonia

Early-onset PTD typically affects a leg first, initially only with action, but then progressing to affect the leg at rest [9]. A typical early symptom is inversion posturing of the foot with walking or running. In most cases, symptoms subsequently become generalized. Initial manifestation in the arm also can occur, but is more common in late childhood onset cases (12–14 years) and is less likely to be associated with subsequent generalization [5]. The average age of onset of dystonia in individuals with the *DYT1* mutation is 14, and most cases (65%) are generalized. Although limbs are most commonly involved, the trunk and neck is affected in 25% to 35% of cases, and cranial musculature is affected in less than 15% [3,6]. Symptom onset has occurred as late as age 64 in rare isolated cases [42].

Late-onset primary dystonia is typically focal or segmental and rarely generalizes. Most cases are considered sporadic. Table 1 lists typical focal dystonia syndromes and affected muscles. In a retrospective study of subjects with adult-onset dystonia, the mean age of onset of symptoms ranged from 38 for arm dystonia to 44 for laryngeal dystonia and spasmodic

Table 1
Focal dystonias

Focal dystonia	Region of involvement
Blepharospasm	Periocular muscles
Oromandibular dystonia	Lower facial, masticatory, lingual, or pharyngeal muscles
Meige syndrome	Periocular muscles plus lower facial, masticatory, pharyngeal, or lingual muscles
Spasmodic dysphonia (laryngeal dystonia)	Laryngeal muscles
Cervical dystonia (spasmodic torticollis)	Cervical and shoulder muscles
Limb dystonia, occupational dystonia, writer's cramp	Upper or lower extremity muscles

torticollis to 54 for blepharospasm [5]. In this study, two thirds of subjects with blepharospasm and torticollis were women, whereas 52% with laryngeal dystonia and 34% with arm dystonia were women. In a separate retrospective study, the female-to-male ratio in different types of focal dystonia ranged from 1.6:1 to 3.3:1 except for writer's cramp, which had a ratio of 1:2 [57]. The typical course of symptoms consists of slow progression for the initial few years with spread to contiguous regions (segmental dystonia) in 15% to 30% and eventual stabilization [5]. Subjects with spasmodic torticollis are the most likely to experience spontaneous remission of their symptoms, usually occurring within 1 year of symptom onset and lasting transiently. In two retrospective studies, spontaneous remissions occurred in 9% and 12% of subjects [5,58].

Blepharospasm is involuntary bilateral eye closure resulting from sustained contractions of orbicularis oculi muscles. Symptoms initially can affect only one eye. Patients may complain of excessive eye blinking, twitching, or irritation. Eye closure may be prolonged or present as rapid blinking. In some patients, the eyes simply may be closed without pronounced contraction. Symptoms typically worsen with bright light or activity such as reading and may be improved with sensory trick, such as light touch near the eyes or by opening the mouth, chewing, or yawning. Patients may have functional blindness owing to inability to open the eyes [59,60]. Oromandibular dystonia affects the lower face, including the jaw and mouth. Symptoms can include involuntary jaw opening or closing, jaw deviation, bruxism, lip pursing or retraction, tongue protrusion, and platysmal contractions. Patients may present with jaw pain, dysarthria, or difficulty chewing, but also may observe improvement of symptoms with chewing, talking, or light touch near the affected region. When upper and lower facial dystonia is present, the disorder is called Meige syndrome [59,61].

Spasmodic dysphonia, or laryngeal dystonia, is due to abnormal contraction of the laryngeal muscles causing hoarse or strained speech production. The adductor type of spasmodic dysphonia, which is the more common type, is caused by excessive adduction of the vocal cords, whereas the abductor type is caused by vocal cord hyperabduction. The former produces strained and strangled speech, whereas the latter results in breathy or whispery speech production [62].

Cervical dystonia affects the cervical musculature and results in abnormal head rotation (torticollis), lateral flexion (laterocollis), forward flexion (anterocollis), or posterior extension (retrocollis). Head deviation can be intermittent or constant and can be accompanied by dystonic tremor. Shoulder elevation is a common accompanying finding. Neck, shoulder, or arm pain is common. Symptoms typically are improved by light touch to the face or neck or by relaxing the head against a headrest [46,63].

Limb dystonia can affect the upper or lower extremity, the former more commonly in primary adult-onset focal dystonias. Upper limb dystonia is commonly task-specific, and the most common form is writer's cramp. Affected individuals frequently have difficulty describing the problem other than complaining of a slowly progressive inability to write legibly. Some subjects may complain of difficulty gripping the pen properly, usually describing an excessively forceful grip, commonly causing the writing utensil to slip into the palm. In some cases, the problem may be hyperextension of the fingers. The wrist also can be hyperflexed or hyperextended. Abnormal grip can begin immediately on writing or may develop after prolonged writing and may cause pain or discomfort. Writing sometimes can be stabilized by using a thicker pen or by touching the fingers or palm with the contralateral finger or hand [64]. With progression, posturing can occur with activities other than writing. Some cases are associated with a tremor that occurs only with writing [65]. Task-specific, or occupational, dystonias have been described in several professions, typically those associated with repetitive movements. Musician's dystonia has been described in individuals who play many types of instruments, but particularly the piano. Oral muscles can be involved in trumpet players [66,67]. Athletes also can experience dystonia. A commonly described dystonia occurs in golfers, called the "yips," in which the hand jerks suddenly, particularly when putting [68].

Secondary dystonia

Clinical features that may suggest dystonia is due to a secondary cause include historical, examination, and imaging findings. A history of perinatal injury, head trauma, peripheral trauma in an affected limb, encephalitis, or drug or toxin exposure points toward an acquired dystonia. The presence of other neurologic abnormalities, such as dementia, ataxia, weakness, or parkinsonism, on examination also suggests a secondary cause. Hemidystonia strongly suggests a structural lesion, although degenerative disorders such as Parkinson's disease or Parkinson plus syndromes can manifest with hemidystonia as well. Other features include onset at rest, rapid progression, atypical site of onset (the lower extremity in an adult or cranial muscles in children), abnormal brain imaging findings, or abnormal laboratory findings [55]. Clues that dystonia may be psychogenic in origin include other signs that are obviously psychogenic, such as false weakness or sensory findings, movements that are inconsistent or incongruent with organic dystonia, the presence of multiple somatic symptoms, and the improvement of symptoms with suggestion or psychotherapy [69].

Diagnosis

Evaluation of a patient with dystonia begins with a thorough history and physical examination. In addition to eliciting any information regarding prior head or peripheral trauma, encephalitis, or developmental disorders, patients should be asked about all current or recent medication use, with particular focus on antipsychotic, antidepressant, or antiemetic agents with dopamine receptor blocking activity. Examination should be focused on eliciting other neurologic signs that may suggest a heredodegenerative or dystonia plus disorder. In adult-onset dystonia, further workup may be guided by distribution of symptoms. Patients with a focal dystonia affecting the craniocervical or limb musculature and nothing to suggest a secondary cause may not require further workup. The author screens for Wilson's disease in individuals younger than 40 with liver enzymes and a serum ceruloplasmin. Because ceruloplasmin is not a particularly sensitive test for Wilson's disease, in patients in whom there is a strong suspicion of the disorder, a 24-hour urine copper evaluation is warranted. In adults with focal dystonia of lower limb musculature, further head and spine MRI studies may be indicated even in the absence of other neurologic signs. MRI of the brain and cervical spine should be performed in cases of hemidystonia to exclude a structural, ischemic, or demyelinating cause. In early-onset cases, MRI and Wilson's disease testing, including serum ceruloplasmin, 24-hour urine copper, and slit-lamp evaluation for Kayser-Fleischer rings, are almost always indicated, unless strong evidence of an alternative cause is present.

Further diagnostic testing is guided by accompanying symptoms, examination findings, and history. Other laboratory evaluations to consider include blood smear for acanthocytes, creatine phosphokinase, lactate and pyruvate levels, serum and urine amino acids, urine organic acids, antiphospholipid antibodies, α-fetoprotein, lysosomal enzymes, HIV, cerebrospinal fluid analysis, and DNA analysis for heredodegenerative disorders such as Huntington's disease or mitochondrial disorders. EMG and nerve conduction study can be useful in evaluating for a peripheral nerve lesion or differentiating dystonia from other movement disorders or to evaluate for pseudodystonia. In adults with a strong family history, particularly if there is a family member with early-onset generalized dystonia, *DYT1* genetic testing may be warranted in focal and generalized cases. In early-onset cases with primary dystonia, *DYT1* testing is advised. Genetic counseling should accompany genetic analysis in affected individuals and unaffected at-risk relatives who seek testing [3]. In early-onset dystonia, a therapeutic challenge with levodopa is recommended; genetic analysis for *DYT5* mutations generally is not recommended because sensitivity is low [70].

Treatment

There are three options for the treatment of primary dystonia: oral medication, BTX therapy, and surgical management. All three options are geared toward symptomatic and not curative improvement; treatment typically must be individualized to the distribution of symptoms and level of disability. Treatment of some forms of secondary dystonia can be directed toward the underlying disorder (eg, Wilson's disease and dystonia associated with Parkinson's disease). All patients with early-onset dystonia should be given a trial of levodopa to assess for possible DRD. Patients typically respond to low doses of levodopa (<300 mg/d) combined with carbidopa [55]. Dopaminergic therapy is rarely effective in other forms of dystonia.

Oral agents used to treat primary dystonia include anticholinergic agents, baclofen and other muscle relaxants, clonazepam, and dopamine-depleting agents. The most commonly encountered difficulty with oral agents is the side effects that occur with the high doses needed for clinical improvement. The anticholinergic agent trihexyphenidyl (Artane) was shown to be effective in a double-blind, placebo-controlled trial [71]. More than 40% of patients treated showed a long-term response with 70% showing initial improvement. Doses usually start at 1 to 2 mg/d and can be titrated up slowly to 60 to 100 mg/d. Very high doses are rarely tolerated because typical side effects include cognitive slowing and memory loss, sedation, blurry vision, dry mouth, and urinary retention. Anticholinergics are especially poorly tolerated by patients older than age 70. Trihexyphenidyl is typically still the first-line oral agent used for cervical, task-specific, and generalized dystonias. Other anticholinergic medications used for dystonia include diphenhydramine (Benadryl) and benztropine (Cogentin), although benefit is less well documented.

Baclofen (Lioresal) is a γ-aminobutyric acid receptor agonist that has been helpful in some patients, particularly patients with oromandibular dystonia [72]. Doses titrated to 40 to 80 mg can be attempted in patients who have failed trihexyphenidyl or if there is concern regarding anticholinergic side effects. Possible side effects include sedation, cognitive changes, and muscle weakness. Limited benefit has been seen with tizanidine (Zanaflex) and cyclobenzaprine (Flexeril) in some patients. The efficacy of intrathecal baclofen has been reported in individual cases [73,74], and this agent is a treatment consideration for generalized dystonia unresponsive to oral medications or dystonia associated with pain and spasticity. Clonazepam has been shown in uncontrolled studies to improve symptoms in approximately 20% of patients [72]. Blepharospasm and myoclonic dystonia are typically more responsive than other forms of dystonia. Tetrabenazine is a dopamine-depleting agent available in Europe and Canada, but not the United States. It can be used in generalized dystonia unresponsive to other more readily available agents and is particularly useful for tardive dystonia. Its most favorable aspect is that it does not cause tardive dyskinesia. Limiting side effects include depression and parkinsonism [75]. Dopamine-blocking drugs, although they can improve dystonia, are generally discouraged because of potential development of tardive dyskinesia; however, clozapine has been shown to be effective in a small open-label trial [76]. Other medications that have been used for symptomatic treatment include reserpine, carbamazepine, and other benzodiazepines.

BTX is an effective agent for dystonia and is now the treatment of choice for several focal dystonias. Although side effects of local irritation and pain at injection site, weakness, and dysphagia can occur, these are usually transient and self-limited. BTX has been approved by the Food and Drug Administration for use in cervical dystonia and blepharospasm, but is often used in an off-label manner for spasmodic dysphonia, oromandibular dystonia, and limb dystonia, including writer's cramp. Its mechanism of action is the blocking of acetylcholine release at the neuromuscular junction, causing localized muscle weakness. Clinically available forms of BTX include BTX-A (Botox) and BTX-B (Myobloc). Many open-label and controlled trials of BTX in cervical dystonia report approximately 90% of subjects experience improvement in involuntary movement and pain [77,78]. Onset of improvement occurs 1 to 14 days after injection, and improvement typically lasts 3 to 4 months, with most patients getting repeat injections every 3 to 6 months. Dysphagia and neck weakness can occur at higher doses (>300 U), but rarely last longer than 2 weeks. After long-term use, particularly at high doses, some patients develop antibodies against BTX, leading to clinical resistance.

Surgical treatment for dystonia is used only in severe cases that have showed insufficient response to medical management. Peripheral surgeries for cervical dystonia include posterior cervical ramisectomy and myotomy, anterior rhizotomy, and microvascular decompression of the spinal accessory nerve. Although several uncontrolled studies have reported symptomatic benefit of neck control and pain, these procedures are limited by potential side effects of weakness, neck instability, and dysphagia [79]. These surgeries have been performed less frequently since the advent of BTX therapy. Central surgeries for dystonia are aimed at affecting basal ganglia outflow. Open studies of subjects undergoing thalamotomy and pallidotomy for generalized dystonia have reported improvement in involuntary postures and functional disability [80,81]. Deep brain stimulation procedures are directed at altering the pattern of discharge of the globus pallidus internum and have been more effective than thalamic deep brain stimulation in improving symptoms of dystonia [82]. Further investigations into the benefit of these interventions continue.

Summary

Dystonia is a disorder of sustained muscle contractions that can affect almost any muscle group and arises from various etiologies. Current treatment of primary dystonia is aimed at symptomatic relief. The complex pathophysiology of dystonia is yet to be fully elucidated; it is hoped that further understanding of this disorder will guide the development of new treatments.

References

[1] Fahn S. Concept and classification of dystonia. Adv Neurol 1988;50:1–8.
[2] Jedynak CP, Bennet AM, Agid Y. Tremor and idiopathic dystonia. Mov Disord 1991;6: 230–6.
[3] Bressman SB, Sabatti C, Raymond D, et al. The DYT1 phenotype and guidelines for diagnostic testing. Neurology 2000;54:1746–52.
[4] Fahn S, Bressman SB, Marsden CD. Classification of dystonia. Adv Neurol 1998;78:1–10.
[5] Greene P, Kang UJ, Fahn S. Spread of symptoms in idiopathic torsion dystonia. Mov Disord 1995;10:143–52.
[6] Bressman SB. Dystonia genotypes, phenotypes and classification. Adv Neurol 2004;94: 101–7.
[7] Pettigrew LC, Jankovic J. Hemidystonia: a report of 22 patients and a review of the literature. J Neurol Neurosurg Psychiatry 1985;48:650–7.
[8] Marsden CD, Obeso JA, Zarranz JJ, et al. The anatomical basis of symptomatic hemidystonia. Brain 1985;108:463–83.
[9] Bressman SB, de Leon D, Brin MF, et al. Idiopathic torsion dystonia among Ashkenazi Jews: evidence for autosomal dominant inheritance. Ann Neurol 1989;26:612–20.
[10] Ozelius L, Kramer PL, Maskowitz CB, et al. Human gene for torsion dystonia located on chromosome 9q32–34. Neuron 1989;2:1427–34.
[11] Friedman J, Standaert DG. Dystonia and its disorders. Neurol Clin 2001;19:681–705.
[12] Segawa M, Hosaka A, Miyagawa F, et al. Hereditary progressive dystonia with marked diurnal fluctuation. Adv Neurol 1976;14:215–33.
[13] Nygaard TG, Marsden CD, Fahn S. Dopa-responsive dystonia: long-term treatment response and prognosis. Neurology 1991;41:174–81.
[14] Defazio G, Abbruzzese G, Livrea P, et al. Epidemiology of primary dystonia. Lancet Neurol 2004;3:673–8.
[15] Risch N, de Leon D, Ozelius L, et al. Genetic analysis of idiopathic torsion dystonia in Ashkenazi Jews and their recent descent from a small founder population. Nat Genet 1995;9: 152–9.
[16] Leube B, Kessler KR, Goecke T, et al. Frequency of familial inheritance among 488 index patients with idiopathic focal dystonia and clinical variability in a large family. Mov Disord 1997;12:1000–6.
[17] Muller J, Kiechl S, Wenning GK, et al. The prevalence of primary dystonia in the general community. Neurology 2002;59:941–3.
[18] Nutt JG, Muenter MD, Aronson A, et al. Epidemiology of focal and generalized dystonia in Rochester, MN. Mov Disord 1988;3:188–94.
[19] Warner T, Camfield L, Marsden CD, et al. A prevalence study of primary dystonia in eight European countries. J Neurol 2000;247:787–92.
[20] Nakashima K, Kusumi M, Inoue Y, et al. Prevalence of focal dystonias in the western area of Tottori prefecture in Japan. Mov Disord 1995;10:440–3.
[21] Dung Le K, Niulsen B, Dietrichs E. Prevalence of primary focal and segmental dystonia in Oslo. Neurology 2003;61:1294–6.

[22] Warner T, Camfield L, Marsden CD, et al. Sex-related influences on the frequency and age of onset of primary dystonia. Neurology 1999;53:1871–4.

[23] Berardelli A, Rothwell JC, Hallett M, et al. The pathophysiology of primary dystonia. Brain 1998;121:1195–212.

[24] Obeso JA, Rothwell JC, Lang AE, et al. Myoclonic dystonia. Neurology 1983;33:825–30.

[25] Cohen LG, Hallett M. Hand cramps: clinical features and electromyographic patterns in focal dystonia. Neurology 1988;38:1005–12.

[26] Panizza ME, Hallett M, Nilsson J. Reciprocal inhibition in patients with hand cramps. Neurology 1989;39:85–9.

[27] Chen RS, Tsai CH, Lu CS. Reciprocal inhibition in writer's cramp. Mov Disord 1995;10: 556–61.

[28] Berardelli A, Rothwell JC, Day BL, et al. Pathophysiology of blepharospasm and oromandibular dystonia. Brain 1985;108:593–608.

[29] Cohen LG, Ludlow CL, Warden M, et al. Blink reflex excitability recovery curves in patients with spasmodic dysphonia. Neurology 1989;39:572–7.

[30] Lozano AM, Kumar R, Gross RE, et al. Globus pallidus internus pallidotomy for generalized dystonia. Mov Disord 1997;12:865–70.

[31] Eidelberg D, Moeller JR, Ishikawa T, et al. The metabolic topography of idiopathic torsion dystonia. Brain 1995;118:1473–84.

[32] Eidelberg D, Moeller JR, Antonini A, et al. Functional brain networks in DYT1 dystonia. Ann Neurol 1998;44:303–12.

[33] Ikoma K, Samii A, Mercuri B, et al. Abnormal cortical motor excitability in dsytonia. Neurology 1996;46:1371–6.

[34] Trost M. Dystonia update. Curr Opin Neurol 2003;16(4):495–500.

[35] Hallett M. Physiology of dystonia. Adv Neurol 1998;78:11–8.

[36] Jankovic J. Post-traumatic movement disorders: central and peripheral mechanisms. Neurology 1994;44:2006–14.

[37] Tempel LW, Perlmutter JS. Abnormal cortical responses in patients with writer's cramp. Neurology 1993;43:2252–7.

[38] Bara-Jiminez W, Catalan MJ, Hallett M, et al. Abnormal sensory homunculus in dystonia of the hand. Ann Neurol 1998;44:828–31.

[39] Augood SJ, Hollingsworth Z, Albers DS, et al. Dopamine transmission in DYT1 dystonia: a biochemical and autoradiographical study. Neurology 2002;59:445–8.

[40] Augood SJ, Penney JB Jr, Friberg IK, et al. Expression of the early-onset torsion dystonia gene (DYT1) in human brain. Ann Neurol 1998;43:669–73.

[41] Klein C, Ozelius L. Dystonia: clinical features, genetics, and treatment. Curr Opin Neurol 2002;15:491–7.

[42] Opal P, Tintner R, Jankovic J, et al. Intrafamilial phenotypic variability of the DYT1 dystonia: from asymptomatic TOR1A gene carrier status to dystonic storm. Mov Disord 2002;17:339–45.

[43] Almasy L, Bressman SB, Raymond D, et al. Idiopathic torsion dystonia linked to chromosome 8 in two Mennonite families. Ann Neurol 1997;42:670–3.

[44] Valente EM, Bentivoglio AR, Cassetta E, et al. DYT13, a novel primary torsion dystonia locus, maps to chromosome 1p36.13–36.32 in an Italian family with cranial-cervical or upper limb onset. Ann Neurol 2001;49:363–4.

[45] Leube B, Doda R, Ratzlaff T. Idiopathic torsion dystonia: assignment of a gene to chromosome 18p in a German family with adult onset, autosomal inheritance and purely focal distribution. Hum Mol Genet 1996;5:1673–7.

[46] Chan J, Brin MF, Fahn S. Idiopathic cervical dystonia: clinical characteristics. Mov Disord 1991;6:119–26.

[47] Waddy HM, Fletcher NA, Harding AE, et al. A genetic study of idiopathic focal dystonias. Ann Neurol 1991;29:320–4.

[48] Ichinose H, Ohye T, Takahashi E, et al. Hereditary progressive dystonia with marked diurnal fluctuation caused by mutations in the GTP cyclohyrdrolase I gene. Nat Genet 1994;8:236–42.

[49] Ludecke B, Dworniczak B, Bartholome K. A point mutation in the tyrosine hydroxylase gene associated with Segawa's syndrome. Hum Genet 1995;95:123–5.

[50] Grotzsch H, Pizzolato G-P, Ghika J, et al. Neuropathology of a case of dopa-responsive dystonia associated with a new genetic locus, DYT 14. Neurology 2002;58:1839–42.

[51] Gasser T. Inherited myoclonus-dystonia syndrome. Adv Neurol 1998;78:325–34.

[52] Quinn NP. Essential myoclonus and myoclonic dystonia. Mov Disord 1996;11:119–24.

[53] de Carvalho Aguiar P, Sweadner KJ, Penniston JT, et al. Mutations in the Na+/K+-ATPase alpha3 gene ATP1A3 are associated with rapid-onset dystonia parkinsonism. Neuron 2004; 43(2):169–75.

[54] Klein C, Breakefield XO, Ozelius L. Genetics of primary dystonia. Semin Neurol 1999;3: 271–80.

[55] Bressman SB. Dystonia update. Clin Neuroharmacol 2000;23:239–51.

[56] Rivest J, Marsden CD. Trunk and head tremor as isolated manifestation of dystonia. Mov Disord 1990;5:60–5.

[57] Soland VL, Bhatia KP, Marsden CD. Sex prevalence of focal dystonias. J Neurol Neurosurg Psychiatry 1996;60:204–5.

[58] Friedman A, Fahn S. Spontaneous remissions in spasmodic torticollis. Neurology 1986;36: 398–400.

[59] Tolosa E, Marti MJ. Blepharospasm-oromandibular dystonia syndrome (Meige's syndrome): clinical aspects. Adv Neurol 1988;49:73–84.

[60] Elston JS. A new variant of blepharospasm. J Neurol Neurosurg Psychiatry 1992;55:369–71.

[61] Marsden CD. Blepharospasm-oromandibular dystonia syndrome (Brueghel's syndrome): a variant of adult-onset torsion dystonia? J Neurol Neurosurg Psychiatry 1976;39:1204–9.

[62] Rosenfield DB. Spasmodic dysphonia. Adv Neurol 1988;49:317–28.

[63] Jankovic J, Leder S, Warner D, et al. Cervical dystonia: clinical findings and associated movement disorders. Neurology 1991;41:1088–91.

[64] Sheehy MP, Marsden CD. Writer's cramp: a focal dystonia. Brain 1982;105:462–80.

[65] Rothwell JC, Traub MM, Marsden CD. Primary writing tremor. J Neurol Neurosurg Psychiatry 1979;42:1106–14.

[66] Lockwood AH. Medical problems in musicians. N Engl J Med 1989;320:221–7.

[67] Frucht SJ, Fahn S, Greene PE, et al. The natural history of embouchure dystonia. Mov Disord 2001;16:899–906.

[68] McDaniel KD, Cummings JL, Shain S. The "yips": a focal dystonia in golfers. Neurology 1989;39:192–5.

[69] Fahn S, Williams DT. Psychogenic dystonia. Adv Neurol 1988;50:431–55.

[70] Furukawa Y, Kish SJ. Dopa-responsive dystonia: recent advances and remaining issues to be addressed. Mov Disord 1999;14:709–15.

[71] Burke R, Fahn S, Marsden CD. Torsion dystonia: a double blind, prospective trial of high-dosage trihexyphenidyl. Neurology 1986;36:160–4.

[72] Greene P, Shale H, Fahn S. Experience with high dosages of anticholinergic and other drugs in the treatment of torsion dystonia. Adv Neurol 1988;50:547–56.

[73] Narayan RK, Loubser PG, Jankovic J, et al. Intrathecal baclofen for intractable axial dystonia. Neurology 1991;41:1141–2.

[74] Walker RH, Danisi FO, Swope DM, et al. Intrathecal baclofen for dystonia: benefits and complications during six years of experience. Mov Disord 2000;15:1242–7.

[75] Jankovic J, Beach J. Long-term effects of tetrabenazine in hyperkinetic movement disorders. Neurology 1997;48:358–62.

[76] Karp BI, Goldstein SR, Chen R, et al. An open trial of clozapine for dystonia. Mov Disord 1999;14:652–7.

[77] Jankovic J, Orman J. Botulinum A toxin for cranial-cervical dystonia: a double-blind, placebo-controlled study. Neurology 1987;37:616–23.

[78] Jankovic J. Dystonia: medical therapy and botulinum toxin. Adv Neurol 2004;94:275–86.

[79] Lang AE. Surgical treatment of dystonia. Adv Neurol 1998;78:185–98.

[80] Cardoso F, Jankovic J, Grossman R, et al. Outcome after stereotactic thalamotomy for dys-
      tonia and hemiballismus. Neurosurgery 1995;36:501–8.
[81] Ondo WG, Desaloms M, Jankovic J, et al. Surgical pallidotomy for the treatment of gener-
      alized dystonia. Mov Disord 1998;13:693–8.
[82] Vercueil L, Pollack P, Fraix V, et al. Deep brain stimulation in the treatment of severe dys-
      tonia. J Neurol 2001;248:695–700.

ELSEVIER
SAUNDERS

Clin Geriatr Med 22 (2006) 915–933

CLINICS IN
GERIATRIC
MEDICINE

Tardive Syndromes in the Elderly

Kelvin L. Chou, MD[a,b],*, Joseph H. Friedman, MD[a,b]

[a]*Department of Clinical Neurosciences, Brown Medical School, 227 Centerville Road, Warwick, RI 02886, USA*
[b]*NeuroHealth Parkinson's Disease and Movement Disorders Center, 227 Centerville Road, Warwick, RI 02886, USA*

Tardive syndromes are a group of disorders characterized by the presence of abnormal involuntary movements caused by prolonged exposure to drugs that block dopamine receptors. The tardive disorders were once among the most feared side effects of the drug-induced movement disorders. The advent of the second-generation antipsychotic drugs, the atypical antipsychotics, has reduced the incidence of tardive syndromes, thereby lessening the concern. However, the number of elderly patients receiving antipsychotic drugs has been increasing. More than 20% of people in nursing homes are now prescribed antipsychotic drugs [1,2], mainly for behavioral disturbances due to dementia. Thus, tardive movement disorders are still a problem, and because they may be severe and permanent, a proper understanding is important.

Definitions

The word *tardive* shares the same root as *tardy*, meaning *late*. Neuroleptic induced tardive dyskinesia (TD) is defined in the *Diagnostic and Statistical Manual of Mental Disorders, Fourth Edition, Text Revision* (DSM IV-TR; ICD 9 code 333.82) as "involuntary choreiform, athetoid, or rhythmic movements (lasting at least a few weeks) of the tongue, jaw, or extremities developing in association with the use of neuroleptic medication for at least a few months (may be for shorter period of time in elderly persons)." The research criteria for TD, as listed in the appendix of the DSM IV-TR, call for an exposure of 30 days or more in people older than age 60, and 3 months or more in those younger than age 60 [3].

---

* Corresponding author.
E-mail address: Kelvin_Chou@brown.edu (K.L. Chou).

0749-0690/06/$ - see front matter © 2006 Elsevier Inc. All rights reserved.
doi:10.1016/j.cger.2006.06.008   *geriatric.theclinics.com*

Other definitions are used, but all center on the development of a movement disorder that was not present before the use of a dopamine receptor antagonist (DRA), and emerges only after patients have been taking the drug for a sustained period. The movement disorder may emerge after the DRA is stopped, or may develop while it is still being used. The phenomenology and severity of the movements are not clearly specified. Tremor is excluded, however, because of the possible confusion with drug-induced parkinsonism.

Some experts on movement disorders believe a permanent movement disorder can develop after a single exposure to a DRA. The requirement for a 30-day exposure, as defined for the research definition of TD in DSM IV-TR, is arbitrary, although reasonable. The cutoff at age 60 years for a 1-month exposure versus a 3-month exposure is also arbitrary and reflects the fact that elderly individuals are more likely to develop the tardive syndromes.

The terminology for tardive disorders is confusing. Although many writers discuss *EPS*, *TD*, *tardive dyskinesia*, or *tardive* as if they are interchangeable terms, they are not. *EPS* refers to *extrapyramidal syndromes* or *extrapyramidal signs*, which include the acute syndromes (akathisia and dystonic reactions), the intermediate/late-onset syndrome of parkinsonism, and the late-onset tardive syndromes. The tardive syndromes encompass several types of movements that have historically been referred to collectively as *TD*. However, TD can also refer specifically to the classic oro–buccal–lingual (OBL) choreoathetoid movement in which patients look like they are chewing gum. In this article, TD refers to choreic or choreoathetoid movements that occur after exposure to a DRA.

The classic form of TD is the most common tardive syndrome, with choreoathetoid movements involving the mouth, but the choreoathetoid movements may affect the limbs, trunk, or upper face in addition to, or instead of, the mouth. Some disagreement exists as to whether the classic OBL movements are truly choreic, because choreic movements are random and the OBL movements are fairly stereotypical. The chewing movements of edentulous people are stereotypic, and OBL dyskinesias certainly resemble that. Much of the literature, however, considers these classic mouth movements choreic, and they behave pharmacologically like the choreic movements elsewhere, being suppressible by dopamine antagonists. Other tardive syndromes include dystonia, akathisia, tics, and stereotypy. The existence of tardive tremor and tardive parkinsonism is the subject of case reports and is, in the authors' opinion, questionable.

One further term requiring explanation is *atypical antipsychotic*. Although much discussed, no consensus definition exists for this term. Probably the one definition most embraced by psychiatrists is that it is an antipsychotic that is "relatively free" of extrapyramidal side effects. Others may consider an antipsychotic "atypical" if it (1) provides improved treatment of the negative symptoms of schizophrenia compared with first-generation antipsychotics, (2) has a relatively higher serotonin (5HT2a)-to-dopamine (D_2) receptor–blocking ratio or (3) does not cause catalepsy in animal models when therapeutic doses are used. The terms *atypical* or *second generation* antipsychotic have been used to describe every antipsychotic drug introduced in the United States since clozapine [4].

Does tardive dyskinesia exist?

Occasionally the question is raised whether the tardive syndromes really exist [5]. The question is not whether the movement disorders exist, but whether they are related to the DRA. Several convincing arguments have been made. The reasons for doubting their existence are discussed first.

Early texts on psychotic disorders frequently described patients who had abnormal movements and postures. These reports have been used to suggest that the same movement disorders currently ascribed to a tardive syndrome were present before antipsychotic drugs were developed. Bleuler [6] and Kraeplin [7] each provided descriptions and interpretations of the movements they encountered. Kraeplin, for example, reported "wrinkling of the forehead, distortion of the corners of the mouth, irregular movements of the tongue and lips, twisting of the eyes...in short grimacing; they remind one of the corresponding disorders of choreic patients...Connected with these are...smacking and clicking with the tongue, sudden sighing, sniffing, laughing, and clearing the throat" [7]. He invented a term *athetoid ataxia* to encompass some of these movements, but it did not catch on. Both Bleuler and Kraeplin, however, viewed these movements as reflective of the psychosis as opposed to an independent involuntary movement disorder. Bleuler stated that they were "dependent upon psychic factors for their origin as well as their disappearance. The motor symptoms which we have been able to analyze could often be explained entirely on a psychic basis" [6].

It is important to understand the severe limitations of medical diagnoses 100 years ago, when the nature of schizophrenia was first being delineated. Patients who had organic disorders, such as general paresis of the insane (tertiary syphilis), might have been included with people who had Huntington's disease, bipolar disease, thyrotoxicosis, drug intoxications, drug withdrawal syndromes, porphyria, and a myriad of other disorders. In addition, the nosology and epidemiology of psychiatric disorders has changed significantly. Disorders such as catatonia, hysteria, and hebephrenic schizophrenia are less common now.

The antipsychotics were first introduced into clinical practice in the early 1950s, and the first case of TD identified in the medical literature was published in 1957 [8]. A 1959 study that reviewed 5704 charts from a psychiatric hospital affiliated with an academic neurologic center found only 35 patients who had major choreic movements, and these were considered to always be explicable by a second neurologic disorder, not the psychosis [9]. Thus, in 1959, chorea was fairly rare among psychiatric patients.

Although some modern reports from India describing movement disorders in untreated schizophrenics and their families were intended to support the theory that the movement disorders were part of the psychosis, they do not [10,11]. These reports observed parkinsonism in both patients and families—a non-TD syndrome—and also described significant fluctuation over time, with the movements being present at some points but not others. This observation is inconsistent with what occurs in tardive syndromes when the drug dose is kept constant.

The main arguments favoring tardive syndromes as a drug-related phenomenon and not an intrinsic part of psychiatric disease involve the epidemiology and the fact that when antipsychotic drugs were introduced, the doctors who had been treating these patients for decades noted entirely new movement disorder syndromes. Other observations supporting this argument include that (1) involuntary movements are seen abundantly in people taking DRAs, but only rarely in those not taking DRAs, (2) some tardive movement disorders are so stereotypic that the diagnosis can be made without any history, (3) animals treated with DRAs develop similar movements, and (4) patients treated with DRAs who never experienced psychotic symptoms or psychiatric abnormalities also develop the stereotypical involuntary movements. In fact, some movement disorder experts have reported anecdotally that the bulk of the tardive cases they see now are patients placed on prolonged regimens of prochlorperazine (Compazine) or metoclopramide (Reglan) who had never been psychotic and took the drug for gastroenterologic symptoms.

Clinical phenomenology

Terminology

Chorea is a Greek word meaning "dance." Its technical meaning is a random, sudden, purposeless, jerking movement. Patients who suffer from chorea frequently incorporate these movements into purposeful or semipurposeful movements, such as touching their face as if to scratch when the movement of the arm begins as a choreic jerk. In this manner, the movements often look less than they really are, and, in many cases, elude detection by untrained observers.

Athetosis or *athetoid* movements are relatively slow, sinuous, and graceful movements, more like ballet movements. Like choreic movements, they are random. *Choreoathetoid* is a term that describes the combined movements of chorea and athetosis. Patient experience sudden, random, jerking movements, which are generally smoothed out as they end, producing a sudden and flowing movement. *Choreoathetoid* and *dyskinesia* are usually used interchangeably.

Dystonia means abnormal tone, and is defined as "a syndrome of sustained muscle contractions, frequently causing twisting and repetitive movements, or abnormal postures [12]." The postures are frequently associated with tremor (a regular oscillation of a body part) or spasms (sudden, irregular jerking movements). Unlike chorea, which is not sustained, spasms associated with dystonia are frequently sustained for a second or less.

Stereotypy is a habit or ritual consisting of a complex of movements to produce some ritual purpose. Chronic hair pulling, patting of a body part, and clapping are examples of stereotypies. They may also occur as tardive syndromes, although tardive stereotypies are usually without purpose. Examples include shifting position in a chair, marching in place, or moving the arms voluntarily.

Tics are brief, rapid, generally repetitive movements that can be simple (involving one group of muscles) or complex (coordinated contractions of multiple muscle groups). Tics can be motor (eg, shoulder shrugging, eye blinking) or vocal (eg, grunting, throat clearing) and are usually preceded by premonitory sensations, such as tension, burning, or itching. Expression of the tic helps relieve these sensations. Many patients can suppress tics for some length of time, although suppression generally causes the premonitory sensation to build up until the tic is performed.

Tardive dyskinesia

The different tardive syndromes are listed in Table 1. As mentioned earlier, the classic form of TD is the OBL form, in which the patient appears to be chewing something or moving the tongue as if searching for a small candy. In severe cases, the tongue may protrude beyond the teeth or lips. Patients who have classic TD frequently do not recognize that they have it or, if they do recognize it, underestimate the severity of the movement. When shown videotapes of themselves, patients often marvel at how much more pronounced the movements actually are.

Table 1
Tardive syndromes

Phenomenology	Definition
Dyskinesia	Focal, segmental, multisegmental, or generalized choreoathetoid movements
Akathisia	Subjective and observed restlessness; usually developing while on stable doses or after lowering of the dose of antipsychotic drug; it also may have developed acutely, early on in treatment, and persist on a chronic basis
Dystonia	Sustained involuntary contractions of agonist and antagonist muscles producing a sustained abnormal posture, often with twisting movements, spasms, or tremors
Tremor	Regular oscillation of a body part
Tics	Sudden, jerky movements preceded by sensations
Myoclonus	Lightning-like muscle contractions producing a very brief muscle twitch and movement (present in normal people as they fall asleep)

Patients who have classic TD often make small smacking sounds as their lips part suddenly, or as their tongues hit part of the mouth. Classic TD very rarely interferes with swallowing, and therefore patients are rarely at risk for aspiration. However, the movements may cause food to be pushed out of the mouth and interfere with eating. Some patients unfortunately develop sores from the constant movement of the tongue over teeth or from chewing inadvertently on the cheek. Because the movements are continuous throughout the waking day, the sores do not heal. Tart or salty foods may increase pain from these sores and also cause eating difficulty.

Patients who have classic TD also often have problems with their dentures. The constant tongue movements cause the dentures to become unglued and loose. Not only is this embarrassing, it impedes talking and chewing. Furthermore, the falling upper plate or the loosened lower plate needs constant repositioning and makes the involuntary movements look worse.

In TD, choreoathetoid movements may affect parts of the body other than the mouth. Commonly, the facial muscles above the mouth are involved, resulting in grimacing, eyebrow furrowing, eye closing, or smiling. The limbs, when affected, may cause the patient to look like they have a generalized form of chorea, such as Huntington's disease. The limb chorea may be symmetric or asymmetric, just as in Huntington's disease.

It is unknown why the movements induced by drugs may be asymmetric. Unless a history of brain damage is present, the two sides of the brain should be the same, and because medications are distributed evenly throughout the body, the two sides should have no difference in drug exposure. Nevertheless, asymmetric TD exists, and therefore the observation that the right side is more affected than the left or that one arm and the opposite leg are affected more does not preclude a diagnosis of a tardive syndrome.

As with most movement disorders, having the patient perform other maneuvers, such as rapid alternating hand movements, finger tapping, and toe tapping, will accentuate the involuntary movements of TD in other parts of the body. This exercise is termed a *reinforcement maneuver* and is useful for confirming the presence of a dyskinetic movement that is not always present.

Tardive dystonia

This form of dystonia may affect any part of the body and is often the most crippling tardive disorder. Tardive dystonia is distinctly less common than classic TD [13,14]. The patient may experience (1) blepharospasm (eyelid spasm), beginning with an increased blink rate and progressing to variable degrees of eyelid closure, grimacing, jaw opening, jaw closing, or sustained jaw movements to one side; (2) torticollis, with the neck turned, flexed, or extended; (3) truncal curvatures causing kyphoscoliosis, or more commonly, truncal extension, with a hyperlordosis or opisthotonic posturing; or (4) dystonia of the limbs. The dystonia may be associated with dystonic spasms, which appear to be jerky movements. Unfortunately, tardive dystonia tends to spread from one part of the body to another, regardless of the age of onset [15,16]. Tardive dystonia may be indistinguishable clinically from idiopathic dystonia, and may be improved by sensory tricks, such as touching the affected body part in a certain way to stop the dystonic movement. These movements are sometimes inferred as being indicative of a conversion disorder, but actually are supportive of the organic nature of the movement disorder.

Tardive dystonia is frequently associated with other tardive syndromes, particularly a dyskinetic syndrome, so that the patient who has tardive dystonia often appears to have a very complex movement disorder, with choreoathetoid movements in one part of the body and dystonic posturing and spasms in another. These complex movement disorders, particularly when OBL dyskinesias are present, are highly suggestive of antipsychotic drug-induced movement disorders, and may be diagnosed by experienced clinicians even without a history.

Tardive akathisia

The term *akathisia* was coined in 1902 by a psychiatrist who was caring for two young women he believed suffered from hysteria [17]. He believed his patients were unusual because they were unable to remain seated. He therefore took his history and administered his therapy while walking with them around the sanatorium. The term comes from the Greek, meaning "not to sit." By definition, tardive akathisia must develop after a 1-month exposure to an antipsychotic drug in someone older than age 60, and must persist for 1 month or more [18]. It should not have developed during the first month of treatment. When it does, it is often called *acute persistent akathisia*, but the clinical phenomenology and the response to therapy are the same as in tardive akathisia.

Tardive akathisia is an uncomfortable sensation of restlessness, and patients obtain relief by moving. While seated, they may rock back and forth, cross and uncross their legs, rub their arms, or wring their hands. When standing, they have difficulty remaining still. They shift weight or march in place. They may rub their hands or their arms, sway, or walk back and forth. They may do seemingly senseless activities to keep moving. In one study, the legs were the body part most frequently moved [19]. Less commonly, patients rubbed their face, scratched their head, folded and unfolded their arms and hands, or picked at clothing.

Recognizing tardive akathisia can be challenging when the patient is poorly communicative. Patients who are psychotic may report feeling restless at one time and deny it at another, or report that they are pacing because the devil is making them. Patients who have dementia may be unable to express themselves at all. Clinicians often wonder if these patients have somatic discomfort, such as constipation, that is making them irritable and restless, or perhaps an overextended bladder, or other type of nonpsychiatric explanation for the restlessness. Because some patients who have dementia pace, even never having taken DRAs, it may never be clear in a particular patient if the restlessness is drug-related or disease-related. In addition, a psychiatric component may be present, such as an irrational anxiety over some misperception of the environment. The important clinical point is to consider the possibility of akathisia when assessing patients taking a DRA who appear anxious, jittery, or restless. When akathisia is suspected, obtaining input from several observers who see the patient at different times in different contexts may be helpful. Tardive akathisia tends to be present all the time and interferes with activities that are usually enjoyed, such as a game of bingo or a favorite television show. When patients can sit still for some activities but not others, akathisia is a less likely explanation for the restlessness.

Tardive myoclonus, tics, tremor, and parkinsonism

These syndromes are considerably less common. Little literature is available on treating either tardive myoclonus or tics. These syndromes presumably should behave like other tardive syndromes, showing some benefit when a DRA is given, or initially worsening then improving and hopefully resolving when the offending medications are stopped. The tardive parkinsonism and tremor disorders are considered extremely rare, and the one clinical observation that supports the existence of tardive tremor is that it worsens when the DRA is stopped and improves (by being masked) when the DRA is increased [20]. Drug-induced parkinsonism, on the other hand, should improve when the patient is not taking the offending agent, and should worsen as the DRA is increased.

Differential diagnosis

Tardive dyskinesia and classic tardive dyskinesia

The differential diagnosis of classic TD in elderly patients is listed in Box 1. The main differential diagnostic point is distinguishing the stereotypic jaw movements of edentulous patients, who rub their gums together and appear to be chewing gum, from those of patients who have classic TD. These movements can only be distinguished by having the patients insert their dentures. When proper fitting dentures are in place, the stereotypic chewing movements should resolve if the movements are not caused by classic TD. Another syndrome that may not be distinguishable from classic TD is the spontaneous facial dyskinesias seen in elderly individuals. This syndrome is believed to occur in as many as 6% of elderly patients who were never exposed to antipsychotic drugs [21].

In patients who have Parkinson's disease (PD) who are taking L-dopa or any of the dopaminergic drugs, dyskinesias may be present that are indistinguishable from TD. Although L-dopa–induced dyskinesias may resemble TD, they vary during the day as the serum levels of the anti-PD drugs

---

Box 1. Differential diagnosis of classic tardive dyskinesia in elderly patients

Spontaneous oral–facial dyskinesias
Stereotypies (edentulousness)
Huntington's disease
L-dopa-induced dyskinesias Senile chorea
Stroke-induced chorea, dystonia, ballism
Lithium toxicity
Dilantin toxicity
Recrudescent Sydenham's chorea
Chorea associated with cerebral lupus
Chorea associated with lupus anticoagulant

---

rise and fall, and will cease entirely if the PD medications are stopped. Some patients who have dementia may have stereotypies, which are voluntary movement disorders such as rocking, hand clapping, and picking, that may overlap with TD phenomenology. Finally, certain uncommon or even rare movement disorders, such as senile chorea or even late-onset Huntington's disease, may look exactly like generalized forms of TD, either with choreoathetoid movements or even dystonia.

Tardive dystonia

Few syndromes cause dystonia in elderly individuals, because the inherited forms affect the young or middle-aged population. Obviously, a reliable history is required to determine when the dystonia began. Wilson's disease, a rare inherited disorder, may cause dystonia and psychiatric problems, but does not begin in elderly individuals. Huntington's disease may cause dystonia and parkinsonism, in addition to dementia and behavioral disturbances, and was once a difficult disorder to distinguish from TD or tardive dystonia until the gene test for Huntington's disease became available. On rare occasions dystonia may result from a brain or even peripheral injury. L-Dopa–induced dyskinesias in PD can be dystonic, and patients who have PD can have off-period dystonia. However, dystonic symptoms in PD usually vary with medications, whereas tardive dystonia is a persistent problem and poorly responsive to medications.

Tardive akathisia

Tardive akathisia is the most difficult clinical syndrome to recognize when the patient is not a reliable reporter. Anxiety, somatic disturbances (eg, constipation, abdominal or renal colic, bladder infection, sore throat, arthritis), frustration, and anger or anything else that might cause someone to pace, fret, or move about because they cannot figure out how to ease their distress should be considered part of the differential diagnosis. Restless legs syndrome (RLS) may also be confused with akathisia, although RLS generally has a diurnal pattern, worsens with rest, and is relieved with movement. One also must consider the problem of "pseudo-akathisia," a syndrome in which patients look restless but don't feel restless [22]. This syndrome can only be considered in patients who are able to communicate. These patients probably have tardive stereotypy [23], spontaneous stereotypy (which occurs in more than 30% of patients who have a frontotemporal dementia) [24], or TD. In patients who cannot communicate, external signs of restlessness should be considered evidence of internal distress, whether from akathisia, a somatic problem, or psychic rumination.

Pathophysiology

For many years, TD has been assumed to reflect dopamine receptor supersensitivity caused by the up-regulation of the dopamine receptors [25]. Circumstantial data support this hypothesis, but it remains unproven. Nevertheless, it is a valuable heuristic model, deriving from clinical observations in humans. It is generally very predictive of how movements will be altered by various pharmacologic interventions.

Perhaps the central problem for the supersensitive dopamine receptor hypothesis is that postmortem studies have never shown humans to have increased dopamine receptors or any sort of supersensitivity [26]. In animal models, dopamine receptor supersensitivity can be demonstrated, usually within a few weeks of starting a neuroleptic, and resolves within a few weeks of stopping. Rodents develop an increased response to dopamine agonists [27] and an increased number of dopamine D_2 receptors [27,28]. In humans, the increased motor sensitivity develops over a longer period and resolves considerably more slowly than in the animal model.

The hypothesis that neuroleptics cause direct toxicity to the basal ganglia has been explored. Unfortunately, the data in both animals and humans with long-term exposures have conflicted [29]. Damage to basal ganglia circuits is highly likely, but the damage may be biochemical as opposed to structural [30,31].

γ-Amino butyric acid (GABA) is the most widely spread inhibitory neurotransmitter in the central nervous system. Evidence exists that chronic exposure to neuroleptics alter normal GABA physiology, reducing GABA turnover or increasing binding to GABA binding sites in the basal ganglia. The reduced turnover is greatest in animals with dyskinesias [32]. A small human study found decreased activity of glutamic acid decarboxylase (GAD) in the subthalamic nucleus of humans who had PD [33]. GAD is the rate-limiting enzyme for producing GABA, and the subthalamic nucleus is the usual structure targeted for deep brain stimulation in PD, making this a plausible theory.

Genetic explanations for the variable development of TD have been explored [26]. One group found a possible aberration in a dopamine receptor gene in cases of tardive dystonia [34], but this finding was not confirmed [26].

The pharmacologically opposite disorder, L-dopa–induced dyskinesia in PD, also has no confirmed explanation, with similar hypotheses advanced. These include dopamine receptor supersensitivity, changes in other neurotransmitters, and genetic predispositions. One interesting observation, not yet confirmed, is that chronic exposure to L-dopa alters dopamine receptor gene regulation, possibly altering other neurotransmitter systems also. An analogous explanation may also be true in the tardive disorders.

The second-generation antipsychotics should undoubtedly help experts understand the basic pathophysiology of TD, because these drugs are similar to, yet different from, the first generation of antipsychotics and cause some, but not all, of the extrapyramidal side effects seen with the first generation. For example, risperidone behaves like a low-potency first-generation antipsychotic, causing acute dystonia, acute akathisia, prolactin elevation, parkinsonism, and tardive syndromes [35]. The other atypicals do not cause prolactin elevation or acute dystonic reactions. Furthermore, when used as the only antipsychotics, they either have not, or only in extremely rare circumstances, caused TD, yet all, with the exception of clozapine and quetiapine, cause parkinsonism, whereas some, but not all, cause akathisia. No one has fully explained how the different pharmacologies of these drugs cause the different extrapyramidal profiles.

Epidemiology

Prevalence and incidence

Two reviews on the prevalence of TD estimate that, overall, approximately 20% to 25% of the general population taking conventional neuroleptics are affected with TD [36,37]. Among elderly patients, this figure is higher. Yassa and Jeste [37] estimated the prevalence of TD among elderly patients to be approximately 50%. The prevalence varies depending on the population studied, but can range from approximately 35% for elderly outpatient psychiatric admissions to more than 80% for institutionalized patients [38].

Incidence studies of TD vary considerably in their rate estimates depending on the study design, population, and criteria used, but the incidence of TD is along the magnitude of 5 to 6 times greater in older patients compared with younger patients [39]. In studies using conventional neuroleptics, the cumulative incidence of TD in younger patients was 5% at 1 year, 10% at 2 years, and 15% at 3 years, whereas the cumulative incidence in older patients was 29%, 50%, and 63% at 1, 2, and 3 years, respectively [40,41].

In terms of estimating the incidence of TD with the atypical or second-generation antipsychotics, one should keep in mind that many of the patients involved in these studies were previously exposed to first-generation antipsychotics. Nevertheless, TD rates appear to be lower with the atypical antipsychotics in general, even among elderly patients. Correll and colleagues [42] performed a meta-analysis of 11 long-term studies of treatment with second-generation antipsychotics (risperidone, olanzapine, quetiapine, amisulpride, and ziprasidone) that looked at new cases of TD, with an overall weighted mean annual incidence rate of 2.1% across all age groups. Among the five trials that included elderly patients, the annual rate of TD was 5.3%. Dolder and Jeste [43] examined 240 outpatients older than 45 years who were at particularly high risk for TD. Of these, 110 were prescribed an atypical antipsychotic: 64.5% were prescribed risperidone, 20.9% olanzapine, and 14.5% quetiapine. Patients taking conventional antipsychotics (haloperidol and thioridazine were the most commonly prescribed) had a mean cumulative incidence rate of 2.9%, 19.3%, and 44.9% at 1, 3, and 6 months, respectively, compared with cumulative incidence rates of 1.0%, 3.4%, and 24.1%, respectively, for those taking atypical antipsychotics. Unfortunately, in the meta-analysis performed by Correll and colleagues [41], TD risk estimates for the individual second-generation antipsychotics varied widely. In the study by Dolder and Jeste [42], the sample size was not large enough to allow comparison between the different atypical antipsychotics. Therefore, whether certain atypical antipsychotics result in lower incidence rates than others is unknown.

Prevalence rates for tardive dystonia are lower than for TD, occurring in 1% to 4% of patients treated with antipsychotics [13,44]. Tardive akathisia is observed in approximately 10% to 36% of patients treated with conventional antipsychotics [45–48]. This figure is lower with the atypical antipsychotics, with the exception of aripiprazole, in which the rate of akathisia is approximately 10% [49,50]. Both tardive dystonia and akathisia tend to occur in conjunction with TD.

Risk factors

Although patients of all ages treated with a DRA can develop a tardive movement disorder, older patients are more susceptible. Age is the most consistent risk factor for the development of TD. As discussed earlier, incidence rates of TD are higher among older patients, but lower remission rates have also been reported [36,51].

Female gender has been reported to be a possible risk factor for TD. A review of 76 prevalence studies of TD showed that TD occurs more commonly in women [37]. This meta-analysis included 39,187 patients and found that the prevalence of TD was 26.6% in women compared with 21.6% in men. Moreover, the prevalence seemed to rise with age in women, but peaked between the ages of 50 and 70 years in men and then decreased. Thus, perhaps only older women are more at risk for TD [52]. Incidence studies, however, have not supported this gender difference, sparking much debate as to whether female gender truly is predictive of TD [53].

Other risk factors have been reported, although less consistently. A few studies have found a higher incidence of TD in the African-American population as opposed to Caucasians [40,54]. Crane [55] was the first to notice an association between TD and neuroleptic-induced parkinsonism. Since then, Kane and colleagues [51] have reported a higher incidence of TD in patients who have severe preexisting EPS compared with patients who have no EPS. Other studies have noticed that the early presence of EPS from neuroleptic treatment was associated with a greater risk for TD [38,56]. Finally, some investigators reported higher rates of TD in patients who had schizophrenia and existing substance abuse disorders [57,58]. Drug dose and duration have not been established as definitive risk factors for TD and are difficult to measure because of the complex natural history of TD.

Risk factors for TD and other tardive movement disorders do not appear to differ significantly. However, tardive dystonia tends to occur more commonly in younger patients [14,59]. It does not seem to be related to the earlier development of acute dystonia, a side effect that occurs within the first few days of starting or increasing the dose of an antipsychotic drug.

Natural history

The natural history of TD is difficult to determine for several reasons. First, the agents that cause TD can also suppress movements. Furthermore, in patients who have severe psychiatric illness, drug withdrawal is difficult and relapse rates are high. Finally, most studies on the reversibility of TD have varying lengths of follow-up, which can limit estimates because some patients who have reversible TD can experience symptom recurrence, and those who have persistent TD can become symptom-free at a later time. Generally, if the offending dopamine blocking agent can be discontinued, the signs of TD generally improve [60–62], but older patients are less likely to improve than younger patients [60]. In other longitudinal studies, where some patients are able to discontinue neuroleptics but most continue to receive low doses of neuroleptics, TD rates generally remain stable or diminish slightly [63,64]. However, in a study of 53 patients who had chronic schizophrenia with the longest follow-up interval (14 years) in the literature, TD resolved in 33 (62%) patients [65] despite ongoing antipsychotic use with a high average daily neuroleptic dose. Abnormal Involuntary Movement Scale scores worsened in 10 patients and remained the same in 8 patients.

The natural history of other tardive movement disorders in elderly individuals is also difficult to determine, partly because no studies exist in which only geriatric populations are examined. Nevertheless, tardive dystonia seems to be a persistent disorder. In one study, which includes patients of all ages, only 5 of 42 patients experienced remission of their dystonia, which

928   CHOU & FRIEDMAN

occurred anywhere from 11 months to 5 years after stopping treatment with the offending agent [59]. In another study of 107 patients who had tardive dystonia who were followed-up for a mean of 8.5 years, only 14% experienced remission, which occurred a mean of 2.6 years after discontinuation of neuroleptics [16]. Tardive akathisia also seems to be persistent after stopping treatment with dopamine receptor blocking agents. One study reported that akathisia persisted for a mean of 2.7 years, with only 33% of patients experiencing complete resolution of symptoms even with treatment [19].

Treatment

No cure for the tardive syndromes exists. Thus, preventing tardive syndrome by avoiding DRAs is the best treatment. However, if a DRA must be used, simple precautions, such as maintaining the patient on the lowest possible dose to achieve a therapeutic effect, periodically reviewing the need for DRA therapy, and withdrawing the medication when no clear effect has occurred, may help decrease the risk for developing a tardive syndrome. In addition, clinicians must discuss the possibility of a tardive syndrome with patients before placing them on a DRA long-term. Unfortunately, in one survey of 520 psychiatrists, only half discussed this risk [66].

If a patient develops TD or a tardive syndrome while taking a DRA, cessation of the offending agent should be considered first. Although a recent analysis of five small studies did not support such an approach [67], data on DRA cessation as a treatment for TD are limited. Anecdotally, TD improves in many patients, especially younger ones, if they are able to remain off dopamine blocking drugs for a long period. Unfortunately this suspension is not usually possible because most reasons for requiring these drugs are permanent. If patients must continue DRA treatment, the natural history of TD suggests at least that the movements do not worsen significantly.

Treatment of tardive dyskinesia

Various agents have been tested for TD. The most effective of these are the presynaptic dopamine depleters, reserpine and tetrabenazine. Both of these agents inhibit the vesicular monoamine transporter, allowing monoamines to be broken down, effectively depleting stores in the nerve terminals. This approach masks the dyskinesias by producing a dopamine deficit. This process is analogous to masking the dyskinesias through reinstituting or increasing the dopamine receptor blockade with the neuroleptic that caused the problem. The rationale for using the dopamine-depleting drugs is that they have not been implicated in causing any of the TD syndromes.

One double-blind placebo-controlled study of reserpine placed patients on doses of 0.75 to 1.5 mg daily and found a 50% improvement in TD [68], whereas a separate literature review showed that 64% of 96 patients on reserpine experienced at least a 50% improvement in their TD symptoms

[69]. However, the use of reserpine in elderly patients is limited by its side effects, which include depression, parkinsonism, hypotension, and lethargy. In contrast, tetrabenazine has a quicker onset of action and fewer side effects. One study showed that 90% of patients undergoing long-term treatment with tetrabenazine experienced marked improvement in TD [70]. Tetrabenazine is available in Canada and Europe, but not in the United States.

Switching patients from a first-generation antipsychotic to a second-generation antipsychotic may reduce the incidence of TD because of a decreased propensity of these agents to cause extrapyramidal side effects. This strategy is the so-called "passive healing" approach. Second-generation antipsychotics presumably allow the brain to heal itself because they—particularly clozapine and quetiapine—have no clinically measurable effect on motor function. Only one case has been reported of a tardive syndrome in a patient being treated with quetiapine who had been never previously exposed to antipsychotics [71]. However, side effects of clozapine and quetiapine, mainly sedation, limit their use in elderly patients. Furthermore, clozapine requires weekly blood monitoring because of the risk for agranulocytosis.

Vitamin E, an antioxidant, allegedly decreases the toxic effect of free radical formation and has been used to treat TD with dubious benefit. A review of 10 trials for the treatment of TD showed that patients treated with vitamin E experienced no improvement in TD symptoms compared with those treated with placebo, but suggested that vitamin E might prevent TD from worsening because patients not on vitamin E showed more deterioration [72]. Because vitamin E is virtually free of side effects, it is reasonable to try in patients who have TD. Benzodiazepines, such as valium and clonazepam, are commonly used to treat TD, but a Cochrane review of two small studies did not show that they helped the outcome of TD [73]. Other agents that have been shown to be helpful in cases or small numbers of patients who had TD include alpha-methyl-paratyrosine, amantadine, calcium channel blockers, baclofen, sodium valproate, propranolol, clonidine, and levetiracetam, but all need further study.

Treatment of other tardive syndromes

Tardive dystonia may respond to some of the same agents used for TD, especially tetrabenazine and clozapine. Anticholinergic drugs, such as trihexyphenidyl, may be helpful in dystonia, although not in choreoathetoid forms of TD [59]. Their use in elderly patients is limited, because most patients will develop one or more of the side effects of confusion, memory failure, dry mouth, sedation, constipation, blurred vision, and urinary retention. Another treatment option for patients whose tardive dystonia is focal is botulinum toxin injections [74].

Tardive akathisia is difficult to treat. One study reported a good response to the presynaptic dopamine depleters, with 58% experiencing improvement on tetrabenazine and 87% experiencing improvement on reserpine [19]. Opioids and electroconvulsive therapy have also been reported to help in isolated cases.

Tardive tics may respond to clonidine or guanfacine, but these drugs may be poorly tolerated in elderly patients because of orthostatic hypotension. Myoclonus may respond to valproic acid, clonazepam, or levetiracetam.

Summary

Tardive syndromes occur with prolonged exposure to any DRA, including gastroenterologic agents such as prochlorperazine (Compazine) or metoclopramide (Reglan). Several different types of involuntary movements are associated with these syndromes, including chorea, athetosis, dystonia, akathisia, tics, and myoclonus. Because the number of elderly patients being prescribed DRAs is increasing, and older age is the most consistent risk factor for TD, the tardive disorders will continue to be a problem despite the introduction of second-generation antipsychotics, which are less likely to cause TD. Because limited treatment is available for the tardive syndromes, prevention is the best strategy. However, if a DRA is necessary, the patient should be maintained on the lowest possible dose. Withdrawal of the DRA should be the first consideration if a tardive syndrome develops. If withdrawal is not possible, various agents may be tried to help the involuntary movements.

References

[1] Snowdon J, Day S, Baker W. Why and how antipsychotic drugs are used in 40 Sydney nursing homes. Int J Geriatr Psychiatry 2005;20(12):1146–52.
[2] Bronskill SE, Anderson GM, Sykora K, et al. Neuroleptic drug therapy in older adults newly admitted to nursing homes: incidence, dose, and specialist contact. J Am Geriatr Soc 2004; 52(5):749–55.
[3] American Psychiatric Association. Diagnostic and statistical manual of mental disorders. 4th edition. Washington (DC): American Psychiatric Association; 2000.
[4] Kapur S, Remington G. Atypical antipsychotics: new directions and new challanges in the treatment of Schizophrenia. Annu Rev Med 2001;52:503–17.
[5] Owens DG, Johnstone EC, Frith CD. Spontaneous involuntary disorders of movement: their prevalence, severity, and distribution in chronic schizophrenics with and without treatment with neuroleptics. Arch Gen Psychiatry 1982;39(4):452–61.
[6] Bleuler E. Dementia praecox or the group of schizophrenias. New York: International Universities Press; 1950.
[7] Kraeplin EP. Dementia praecox and paraphrenia. Huntington (NY): Robert E. Krieger Publishing Co.Inc.; 1971.
[8] Schonecker VM. Ein eigentumliches Syndrom im oralen Bereich bei Megaphenapplikation. Nervenarzt 1957;28:35–43.
[9] Mettler FA, Crandell A. Neurologic disorders in psychiatric institutions. J Nerv Ment Dis 1959;128(2):148–59.

[10] McCreadie RG, Padmavati R, Thara R, et al. Spontaneous dyskinesia and parkinsonism in never-medicated, chronically ill patients with schizophrenia: 18-month follow-up. Br J Psychiatry 2002;181:135–7.

[11] McCreadie RG, Thara R, Srinivasan TN, et al. Spontaneous dyskinesia in first-degree relatives of chronically ill, never-treated people with schizophrenia. Br J Psychiatry 2003;183: 45–9.

[12] Fahn S. Concept and classification of dystonia. In: Fahn S, Marsden CD, Calne DB, editors. Dystonia 2. Volume 50. New York: Raven Press; 1988. p. 2–8.

[13] Friedman JH, Kucharski LT, Wagner RL. Tardive dystonia in a psychiatric hospital. J Neurol Neurosurg Psychiatry 1987;50(6):801–3.

[14] Yassa R, Nair V, Iskandar H. A comparison of severe tardive dystonia and severe tardive dyskinesia. Acta Psychiatr Scand 1989;80(2):155–9.

[15] Burke RE, Fahn S, Jankovic J, et al. Tardive dystonia: late-onset and persistent dystonia caused by antipsychotic drugs. Neurology 1982;32(12):1335–46.

[16] Kiriakakis V, Bhatia KP, Quinn NP, et al. The natural history of tardive dystonia. A long-term follow-up study of 107 cases. Brain 1998;121(Pt 11):2053–66.

[17] Haskovec L. Akathisie. Arch Behemes Med Clin 1902;193–200.

[18] Skidmore F, Weiner WJ, Burke RE. Neuroleptic-induced dyskinesia variants. In: Factor SA, Lang AE, Weiner WJ, editors. Drug induced movement disorders. 2nd edition. Atlanta (GA): Blackwell Publishers; 2005. p. 257–84.

[19] Burke RE, Kang UJ, Jankovic J, et al. Tardive akathisia: an analysis of clinical features and response to open therapeutic trials. Mov Disord 1989;4(2):157–75.

[20] Stacy M, Jankovic J. Tardive tremor. Mov Disord 1992;7(1):53–7.

[21] Weiner WJ, Klawans HL Jr. Lingual-facial-buccal movements in the elderly. I. Pathophysiology and treatment. J Am Geriatr Soc 1973;21(7):314–7.

[22] Braude WM, Barnes TR. Late-onset akathisia–an indicant of covert dyskinesia: two case reports. Am J Psychiatry 1983;140(5):611–2.

[23] Jankovic J. Tardive syndromes and other drug-induced movement disorders. Clin Neuropharmacol 1995;18(3):197–214.

[24] Nyatsanza S, Shetty T, Gregory C, et al. A study of stereotypic behaviours in Alzheimer's disease and frontal and temporal variant frontotemporal dementia. J Neurol Neurosurg Psychiatry 2003;74(10):1398–402.

[25] Klawans HL Jr, Rubovits R. An experimental model of tardive dyskinesia. J Neural Transm 1972;33(3):235–46.

[26] Casey DE. Pathophysiology of antipsychotic drug-induced movement disorders. J Clin Psychiatry 2004;65(Suppl 9):25–8.

[27] Casey DE. Tardive dyskinesia: pathophysiology. In: Bloom FE, Kupfer DJ, editors. Psychopharmacology: the fourth generation of progress. New York: Raven Press; 1995. p. 1497–502.

[28] Waddington JL, Cross AJ, Gamble SJ, et al. Spontaneous orofacial dyskinesia and dopaminergic function in rats after 6 months of neuroleptic treatment. Science 1983;220(4596): 530–2.

[29] Hyde TM, Apud JA, Fisher WC, et al. Tardive dyskinesia. In: Factor SA, Lang AE, Weiner WJ, editors. Drug induced movement disorders. Atlanta (GA): Blackwell Publishers; 2005. p. 213–56.

[30] Andreassen OA, Jorgensen HA. Neurotoxicity associated with neuroleptic-induced oral dyskinesias in rats. Implications for tardive dyskinesia? Prog Neurobiol 2000;61(5): 525–41.

[31] Pai BN, Janakiramaiah N, Gangadhar BN, et al. Depletion of glutathione and enhanced lipid peroxidation in the CSF of acute psychotics following haloperidol administration. Biol Psychiatry 1994;36(7):489–91.

[32] Gunne LM, Haggstrom JE, Sjoquist B. Association with persistent neuroleptic-induced dyskinesia of regional changes in brain GABA synthesis. Nature 1984;309(5966):347–9.

[33] Andersson U, Haggstrom JE, Levin ED, et al. Reduced glutamate decarboxylase activity in the subthalamic nucleus in patients with tardive dyskinesia. Mov Disord 1989;4(1):37–46.

[34] Mihara K, Kondo T, Higuchi H, et al. Tardive dystonia and genetic polymorphisms of cytochrome P4502D6 and dopamine D2 and D3 receptors: a preliminary finding. Am J Med Genet 2002;114(6):693–5.

[35] Fernandez HH, Trieschmann ME, Friedman JH. Treatment of psychosis in Parkinson's disease: safety considerations. Drug Saf 2003;26(9):643–59.

[36] Kane JM, Smith JM. Tardive dyskinesia: prevalence and risk factors, 1959 to 1979. Arch Gen Psychiatry 1982;39(4):473–81.

[37] Yassa R, Jeste DV. Gender differences in tardive dyskinesia: a critical review of the literature. Schizophr Bull 1992;18(4):701–15.

[38] Woerner MG, Alvir JM, Saltz BL, et al. Prospective study of tardive dyskinesia in the elderly: rates and risk factors. Am J Psychiatry 1998;155(11):1521–8.

[39] Jeste DV. Tardive dyskinesia rates with atypical antipsychotics in older adults. J Clin Psychiatry 2004;65(Suppl 9):21–4.

[40] Jeste DV, Rockwell E, Harris MJ, et al. Conventional vs. newer antipsychotics in elderly patients. Am J Geriatr Psychiatry 1999;7(1):70–6.

[41] Kane JM, Woerner M, Lieberman J. Tardive dyskinesia: prevalence, incidence, and risk factors. J Clin Psychopharmacol 1988;8(4 Suppl):52S–6S.

[42] Correll CU, Leucht S, Kane JM. Lower risk for tardive dyskinesia associated with second-generation antipsychotics: a systematic review of 1-year studies. Am J Psychiatry 2004; 161(3):414–25.

[43] Dolder CR, Jeste DV. Incidence of tardive dyskinesia with typical versus atypical antipsychotics in very high risk patients. Biol Psychiatry 2003;53(12):1142–5.

[44] Green P. Tardive dystonia. In: Yassa R, Nair NPV, Jeste DV, editors. Neuroleptic-induced movement disorders. Cambridge: Cambridge University Press; 1997. p. 395–408.

[45] Kahn EM, Munetz MR, Davies MA, et al. Akathisia: clinical phenomenology and relationship to tardive dyskinesia. Compr Psychiatry 1992;33(4):233–6.

[46] van Harten PN, Matroos GE, Hoek HW, et al. The prevalence of tardive dystonia, tardive dyskinesia, parkinsonism and akathisia The Curacao Extrapyramidal Syndromes Study: I. Schizophr Res 1996;19(2–3):195–203.

[47] Janno S, Holi M, Tuisku K, et al. Prevalence of neuroleptic-induced movement disorders in chronic schizophrenia inpatients. Am J Psychiatry 2004;161(1):160–3.

[48] Halliday J, Farrington S, Macdonald S, et al. Nithsdale Schizophrenia Surveys 23: movement disorders. 20-year review. Br J Psychiatry 2002;181:422–7.

[49] Kasper S, Lerman MN, McQuade RD, et al. Efficacy and safety of aripiprazole vs. haloperidol for long-term maintenance treatment following acute relapse of schizophrenia. Int J Neuropsychopharmacol 2003;6(4):325–37.

[50] Marder SR, McQuade RD, Stock E, et al. Aripiprazole in the treatment of schizophrenia: safety and tolerability in short-term, placebo-controlled trials. Schizophr Res 2003; 61(2–3):123–36.

[51] Kane JM, Woerner M, Borenstein M, et al. Integrating incidence and prevalence of tardive dyskinesia. Psychopharmacol Bull 1986;22(1):254–8.

[52] van Os J, Walsh E, van Horn E, et al. Tardive dyskinesia in psychosis: are women really more at risk? UK700 Group. Acta Psychiatr Scand 1999;99(4):288–93.

[53] Glazer WM. Review of incidence studies of tardive dyskinesia associated with typical antipsychotics. J Clin Psychiatry 2000;61(Suppl 4):15–20.

[54] Morgenstern H, Glazer WM. Identifying risk factors for tardive dyskinesia among long-term outpatients maintained with neuroleptic medications. Results of the Yale Tardive Dyskinesia Study. Arch Gen Psychiatry 1993;50(9):723–33.

[55] Crane GE. Pseudoparkinsonism and tardive dyskinesia. Arch Neurol 1972;27(5):426–30.

[56] Jeste DV, Caligiuri MP, Paulsen JS, et al. Risk of tardive dyskinesia in older patients. A prospective longitudinal study of 266 outpatients. Arch Gen Psychiatry 1995;52(9):756–65.

[57] Dixon L, Weiden PJ, Haas G, et al. Increased tardive dyskinesia in alcohol-abusing schizophrenic patients. Compr Psychiatry 1992;33(2):121–2.

[58] Olivera AA, Kiefer MW, Manley NK. Tardive dyskinesia in psychiatric patients with substance use disorders. Am J Drug Alcohol Abuse 1990;16(1–2):57–66.

[59] Kang UJ, Burke RE, Fahn S. Natural history and treatment of tardive dystonia. Mov Disord 1986;1(3):193–208.

[60] Glazer WM, Morgenstern H, Schooler N, et al. Predictors of improvement in tardive dyskinesia following discontinuation of neuroleptic medication. Br J Psychiatry 1990;157:585–92.

[61] Quitkin F, Rifkin A, Gochfeld L, et al. Tardive dyskinesia: are first signs reversible? Am J Psychiatry 1977;134(1):84–7.

[62] Wegner JT, Kane JM. Follow-up study on the reversibility of tardive dyskinesia. Am J Psychiatry 1982;139(3):368–9.

[63] Casey DE, Povlsen UJ, Meidahl B, et al. Neuroleptic-induced tardive dyskinesia and parkinsonism: changes during several years of continuing treatment. Psychopharmacol Bull 1986; 22(1):250–3.

[64] Gardos G, Casey DE, Cole JO, et al. Ten-year outcome of tardive dyskinesia. Am J Psychiatry 1994;151(6):836–41.

[65] Fernandez HH, Krupp B, Friedman JH. The course of tardive dyskinesia and parkinsonism in psychiatric inpatients: 14-year follow-up. Neurology 2001;56(6):805–7.

[66] Kennedy NJ, Sanborn JS. Disclosure of tardive dyskinesia: effect of written policy on risk disclosure. Psychopharmacol Bull 1992;28(1):93–100.

[67] Soares-Weiser K, Rathbone J. Neuroleptic reduction and/or cessation and neuroleptics as specific treatments for tardive dyskinesia. Cochrane Database Syst Rev 2006;1:CD000459.

[68] Huang CC, Wang RI, Hasegawa A, et al. Reserpine and alpha-methyldopa in the treatment of tardive dyskinesia. Psychopharmacology (Berl) 1981;73(4):359–62.

[69] Jeste DV, Wyatt RJ. Therapeutic strategies against tardive dyskinesia. Two decades of experience. Arch Gen Psychiatry 1982;39(7):803–16.

[70] Jankovic J, Beach J. Long-term effects of tetrabenazine in hyperkinetic movement disorders. Neurology 1997;48(2):358–62.

[71] Ghaemi SN, Ko JY. Quetiapine-related tardive dyskinesia. Am J Psychiatry 2001;158(10): 1737.

[72] Soares KV, McGrath JJ. Vitamin E for neuroleptic-induced tardive dyskinesia. Cochrane Database Syst Rev 2001;4:CD000209.

[73] Umbrich P, Soares KV. Benzodiazepines for neuroleptic-induced tardive dyskinesia. Cochrane Database Syst Rev 2003;2:CD000205.

[74] Tarsy D, Kaufman D, Sethi KD, et al. An open-label study of botulinum toxin A for treatment of tardive dystonia. Clin Neuropharmacol 1997;20(1):90–3.

ELSEVIER
SAUNDERS

Clin Geriatr Med 22 (2006) 935–951

CLINICS IN
GERIATRIC
MEDICINE

Normal Pressure Hydrocephalus

Robin K. Wilson, MD, PhD,
Michael A. Williams, MD*

*Department of Neurology, The Johns Hopkins Hospital, Adult Hydrocephalus Program,
600 North Wolfe Street, Baltimore, MD 21287, USA*

In 1964, Colombian neurosurgeon Hakim and colleagues [1–3] described a syndrome of progressive cognitive decline, gait difficulties, and urinary incontinence in the context of ventricular dilatation and normal cerebrospinal fluid (CSF) pressure during lumbar puncture. Hakim named this condition *normal pressure hydrocephalus* (NPH) and it has since been identified as a disorder affecting elderly individuals and one of the few causes of reversible dementia. During the decade after the initial description of NPH, many elderly patients who had ventriculomegaly and dementia were treated with shunts; however, early enthusiasm waned as studies showed disappointing success rates and significant complication rates [4–6]. Experts now commonly believe that many patients who were considered "treatment failures" had Alzheimer's disease or other dementias. Fortunately, in the past 5 to 10 years, new diagnostic techniques, better shunt design, and recognition of prognostic factors have improved patient selection and outcomes [7–14]. An international independent study group published guidelines for the diagnosis and management of idiopathic NPH in 2005 [15–18].

Public awareness of NPH has increased, partly because of a television advertising campaign [6,19–22]. Patients and families are more frequently asking their physicians to be evaluated for NPH. Because gait impairment, urinary incontinence, and dementia are among the most common disorders of the geriatric population, only a small percentage of patients who have these symptoms will have NPH and experience response to shunt surgery. Thus, geriatricians should understand the symptoms and signs of NPH and the diagnostic methods with the highest likelihood of correctly identifying patients who will experience response to shunts.

---
* Corresponding author.
E-mail address: michael.a.williams@jhmi.edu (M.A. Williams).

0749-0690/06/$ - see front matter © 2006 Elsevier Inc. All rights reserved.
doi:10.1016/j.cger.2006.06.010   *geriatric.theclinics.com*

Normal pressure hydrocephalus signs and symptoms

Although NPH is thought of as a treatable dementia, the symptom most likely to appear first and to improve after shunt surgery is gait impairment. Our experience is that patients and families are more likely to seek consultation for impaired mobility and falling than they are for dementia. In NPH, gait and balance difficulties typically appear before urinary incontinence and cognitive decline, but patients do not necessarily need to have the complete triad of symptoms before proceeding with evaluation. In fact, only a few patients have the complete triad [13,17]. Most patients who have NPH have had symptoms for several years, and although longstanding symptoms may make recovery less likely [8,9,23], the duration of symptoms alone should not be used to exclude the possibility of treatable hydrocephalus [13,14].

Many common disorders of aging cause the individual components of the NPH triad of cognitive, gait, and urinary problems. Because these symptoms are ubiquitous in elderly individuals, evaluation of suspected NPH also requires consideration of the differential diagnosis of all three symptoms simultaneously. Patients who have NPH commonly have multifactorial causes of dementia, gait impairment, or incontinence, such as vascular or degenerative dementia, cervical or lumbar stenosis, peripheral neuropathy, arthritis, bladder instability, or prostate enlargement. Careful screening for these conditions is important because shunt surgery will only improve symptoms related NPH. The presence of coexisting conditions does not preclude the possibility of NPH; it only means that the degree of response to shunt surgery may be limited. The goal of assessment is to determine the proportion of impairment attributable to NPH and potentially treatable with shunt surgery.

Gait impairment

The gait abnormality of NPH may be considered a higher-level gait disorder, which is impairment not explained by musculoskeletal, upper motor neuron, lower motor neuron, cerebellar, or extrapyramidal syndromes [30]. The term *gait apraxia* is often used to describe the loss of ability to produce normal walking movements despite intact strength and sensation [26,31]. Although gait apraxia and gait ataxia are distinct terms, the term gait ataxia is also commonly used to describe the gait of NPH, from a neurologic perspective ataxic gait should be a feature only of cerebellar disorders and not NPH. Although physical therapy is often ordered for patients who have NPH, our experience has shown that impaired memory may limit its effectiveness before shunt surgery, because patients cannot remember instructions from one day to the next.

In taking a gait history, we ask about walking speed, difficulty navigating obstacles, falls, and reliance on walking aids or need for assistance. For clinical examination, we have found the Tinetti Assessment Tool to be useful [32,33]. This semiquantitative scale assesses gait and balance, takes less than 5 minutes to complete, and can be performed by a physician, therapist, or nurse.

The characteristics of a patient's gait disturbance depend on coexisting disorders. Common findings include reduced gait velocity, shorter stride length, broad base, difficulty turning, decreased foot clearance, external rotation of the feet, and poor dynamic equilibrium [24,25]. Some patients present with the classic "magnetic gait," consisting of a wide base, tiny steps, and shuffling with minimal clearance, as though the floor maintained a magnetic pull [26]. Severely impaired patients may be unable to walk, stand, or move in bed.

The gait impairment seen in NPH may be reminiscent of that seen in Parkinson's disease (PD), but the conditions can be distinguished [25]. Both disorders may have bradykinesia, short stride length, and freezing. Patients who have NPH often have a widened base compared with the narrow base of those who have PD. Patients who have NPH are more likely to demonstrate normal arm swing, although careful testing reveals subtle impairment of arm movement when walking [27,28]. In NPH, gait rarely improves with verbal or environmental cueing to the extent seen in PD [25]. Occasionally patients who have NPH may have tremor that improves after shunt surgery, although the relationship of tremor to NPH is unclear [29]. Except in the rare circumstance of coexisting PD and NPH, patients who have NPH will not experience response to a trial of levodopa.

Urinary urgency and incontinence

Urinary symptoms include urgency, frequency, and incontinence, and seem to be associated with a hyperreflexic bladder [34,35]. Although some patients experience overt incontinence, others experience urgency ("When I gotta go, I gotta go") or near-incontinence, such as losing a few drops of urine just as they get to the toilet. Very few studies of urinary function have been performed for NPH, although detrusor hyperreflexia has been reported to improve after removal of CSF [35].

Many elderly patients have additional causes of urinary dysfunction, including prostatic enlargement, urethral stricture, diuretic use, detrusor instability, or pelvic floor weakness [36]. Asking whether current symptoms differ from those associated with a previous disorder and its treatment is helpful, particularly for patients who have undergone previous surgery for incontinence, benign prostatic hyperplasia, or prostatic carcinoma.

Dementia

NPH causes a primarily subcortical dementia, characterized as decline in immediate and delayed recall with preserved memory storage, impaired complex information processing, and psychomotor slowing [37–40]. Visuo-spatial perception and visuoconstructive skills are also affected. As is characteristic of other dementias, careful questioning often reveals that family members have assumed tasks such as managing bank accounts, shopping, paying bills, remembering appointments, and dispensing medications. Neuropsychologic testing can be helpful in identifying the severity and potential causes of the dementia (ie, mixed dementia). Because the Mini-Mental State Examination was designed to reveal cortical dementia, patients who have subcortical dementia can have a normal score [39]. The HIV Dementia Scale has been studied as a quick screening tool for subcortical impairment caused by NPH [39,41]. The Montreal Cognitive Assessment may also be helpful in quickly detecting subtle cognitive dysfunction associated with early NPH [42]. Discovery of mild, and potentially reversible, cognitive impairment may help the patient and family decide whether to pursue workup for NPH.

Epidemiology

The prevalence of NPH is uncertain. Because diagnostic criteria used to select patients for shunting varies, most studies probably do not reveal the true incidence of NPH. In Sweden, approximately 1 per 60,000 persons (1.67 per 100,000) per year underwent shunting for presumed NPH between 1996 and 1998 [43], and a German study found that 1.8 per 100,000 citizens per year had NPH [44].

In two meta-analyses from 1988 and 2003, 1% to 1.6% of dementia was attributed to NPH [45,46]. Experts have suggested that NPH constitutes as much as 5% of the dementia population [12], and a study from Denmark suggests that 4% of patients referred for dementia were ultimately diagnosed with NPH [47]. However, a 2006 study from Olmstead County, Minnesota, covering 1990 through 1994 found no cases of NPH among the reversible dementias [48]. Because the epidemiology of NPH is poorly understood, the extent of its impact on the health of the elderly population is also poorly understood.

Etiology

Approximately two thirds of patients have idiopathic NPH, and in one third it is secondary to other conditions [44]. Secondary NPH may follow meningitis, encephalitis, head injury (including concussion), subarachnoid hemorrhage, or other processes causing an inflammatory response in the subarachnoid space [49]. Because hydrocephalus may develop years after the original injury, these risk factors should be sought in the patient's history because they may be forgotten. No difference exists in the signs, symptoms, or treatment, regardless of the cause. In addition, previously compensated and asymptomatic congenital hydrocephalus can manifest as NPH [50,51]. The presentation in older patients typically resembles NPH.

Patients between ages 18 and 55 tend to have very mild symptoms (syndrome of hydrocephalus in young and middle-aged adults), but are more likely to experience headaches [52,53].

Pathophysiology

NPH results from a disruption in the CSF circulation leading to gradual enlargement of the ventricles and emergence of symptoms. This mechanism contrasts with that of acute hydrocephalus, which is associated with increased intracranial pressure (ICP) and requires emergent treatment [54]. The treatment for acute hydrocephalus is to divert CSF by external CSF drainage through an intraventricular or spinal catheter; the treatment of chronic hydrocephalus is internal CSF diversion with a shunt, or endoscopic third ventriculostomy.

The traditional model of CSF circulation was described during the first half of the 1900s [55–57]. In this model, the choroid plexus produces CSF, which circulates through the ventricles, exits through the foramina of Magendie and Luschka into the subarachnoid space, then flows over the surface of the cerebral convexities to exit though the arachnoid granulations into the superior sagittal sinus [55–58]. Normal CSF production by the choroid plexus ranges from 0.3 to 0.6 mL/min, and minimal decrease in production occurs with normal aging [59–62]. An equilibrium between CSF production and resorption maintains CSF pressure at 6 to 20 cm H_2O [58].

Disorders of CSF circulation can arise from obstruction of CSF circulation at any point on the pathway or disruption of the balance between CSF production and resorption. Although overproduction of CSF is theoretically possible, it is rarely seen except with choroid plexus hyperplasia or choroid plexus papilloma [63–66]. Chronic hydrocephalus is typically associated with reduced CSF production [60].

Obstruction of CSF flow typically occurs at anatomic narrowings, including the foramina of Monro, third ventricle, Sylvian aqueduct, and the fourth ventricle outlets [67,68]. Causes include scarring or adhesions, tumors, cysts, or hemorrhage. Disruption of CSF flow also occurs within the subarachnoid space, leading to diminished conductance of CSF to the arachnoid granulations. Obstruction of CSF resorption may also occur at the arachnoid granulations.

In communicating forms of hydrocephalus, the reduced CSF conductance or resorption leads to accumulation of CSF in the ventricles [1,2,69]. Increased ICP occurs during the phase of active ventricular enlargement, which normalizes after initial expansion [70–72]. Several experimental models of hydrocephalus show a temporary increase in ventricular pressure and ventricular enlargement, followed by a return to normal ventricular pressure and chronic hydrocephalus. Hakim [2] invoked Pascal's law (force = pressure × area) to explain this pattern of ventricular dilation in NPH. He hypothesized that transiently increased intraventricular pressure initiates ventricular enlargement, and that if the force remains constant (force $=$ ICP $\times$ ventricular surface area), then as the ventricular surface area increases in response to increased ventricular volume, the ICP necessary to sustain the force is lower. This phenomenon explains the paradox of the "normal" pressure in NPH. Because most patients are not evaluated until after the active ventricular enlargement phase is complete, the ICP has already normalized.

Abnormalities of ICP pressure or pattern can be used to infer the presence of hydrocephalus [73] and may be measured in the clinical setting. Lundberg [73] was the first to characterize ICP waveforms in patients who had tumors, hemorrhages, and head trauma. Plateau waves, also called *A-waves*, involve acute elevation of ICP to more than 68 cm H_2O (50 mm Hg), lasting 5 to 20 minutes [58,74]. Plateau waves represent near exhaustion of intracranial compliance mechanisms [75]. Near-plateau waves are similar in timing and form, but do not reach such high pressures [74]. B-waves consist of brief rhythmic or semirhythmic pressure elevations occurring at a frequency of 0.5 to 2 cycles per minute [68,74]. In patients breathing spontaneously, B-waves are often seen with Cheyne-Stokes respirations [76,77]. Although plateau waves and B-waves are primarily associated with acute, life-threatening disorders such as traumatic brain injury, these patterns are also associated with NPH, particularly during sleep [68]. Even patients who have normal CSF circulation may experience brief periods of pressure fluctuation similar to B-waves, but prolonged occurrence suggests a pathologic condition [78].

Imaging

Because the cerebral ventricles enlarge with aging, diagnosing hydrocephalus in older patients based on imaging alone can be difficult, unless the MRI or CT reveals an obstructive cause. The ventricles can appear enlarged on neuroimaging either because of disordered CSF circulation (ie, hydrocephalus) or because of cerebral atrophy resulting from degenerative dementias or subcortical ischemia (ie, ventriculomegaly).

Supportive findings for communicating hydrocephalus include rounding of the lateral and third ventricles, upward bowing and thinning of the corpus callosum, and pulsation artifact (flow void) in the Sylvian aqueduct (Fig. 1) [79–81]. Although NPH is commonly described as being associated with "ventricular enlargement out of proportion to cortical atrophy," [82] the literature actually contains no support for this criterion. Volumetric assessment has not been useful in distinguishing between patients who have possible NPH who will respond to shunt surgery and those who will not [83]. Sagittal views of obstructive hydrocephalus may show narrowing at the Sylvian aqueduct. Periventricular hyperintensities (PVH) can be seen on MRI with either subcortical ischemia or NPH [84–88]. These disorders have similar symptoms, and MRI only reveals the presence of PVH, not the

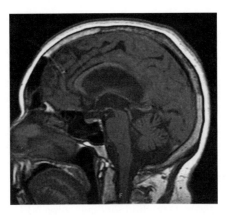

Fig. 1. Pre-shunted sagittal T1-weighted MRI of a 76 year old woman who presented with two years of progressive gait impairment, cognitive decline, and urinary urgency. This view reveals upward bowing and thinning of corpus callosum and pulsation artifact (flow void) in the Sylvian aqueduct. All symptoms gradually improved following insertion of a ventriculoperitoneal shunt.

cause. Patients who have PVH caused by small vessel disease may also have NPH. Although experts have said that NPH combined with subcortical ischemia tends to respond minimally to shunting [84], we have found that the presence of PVH has no influence on the outcome of shunt surgery [13].

Occasionally ventriculomegaly is incidentally discovered on an imaging study obtained for other indications. If no neurologic deficits are present, the hydrocephalus may be considered compensated. Because chronic compensated hydrocephalus may later decompensate and become symptomatic [50,51], these patients should be informed about NPH and followed-up at regular intervals.

Physiologic-based tests for normal pressure hydrocephalus

Three methods that test CSF dynamics have been used to diagnose NPH: (1) measurement of CSF outflow resistance (R_{out}), (2) CSF pressure monitoring, and (3) response to CSF removal.

R_{out} measurement involves infusing artificial CSF into the lumbar subarachnoid space through a spinal needle while simultaneously recording CSF pressure at a second site [89]. This test allows plateau pressure to be measured and resistance to CSF outflow to be calculated. The prospective Dutch NPH Study found that R_{out} more than 18 mm Hg/mL/min predicted shunt responsiveness, although some patients who had lower R_{out} also improved significantly after shunting [84]. Plateau pressure may be a more sensitive criterion for predicting shunt responsiveness than R_{out} [90,91]. R_{out} is more commonly performed in Europe, and is used at very few centers in the United States.

The same CSF pressure waveform abnormalities seen with brain tumor or traumatic brain injury can be seen in NPH [92,93]. Most patients who have NPH have normal baseline CSF pressure punctuated by B-waves and plateau waves, particularly during sleep, even if the opening pressure recorded during lumbar puncture is normal [94,95]. The presence of unstable waveforms can be helpful in diagnosing NPH, particularly if the symptoms are mild and the ICP is definitely abnormal, but this technique is not as accurate as assessing response to CSF drainage [17,95]. CSF pressure monitoring can be accomplished through intraventricular or lumbar catheter, or through ventricular, subdural, or intraparenchymal solid-state transducers. As with R_{out} testing, ICP monitoring for NPH is performed at very few centers in the United States.

The clinical response to CSF removal through large-volume lumbar puncture or continuous CSF drainage through spinal catheter is currently recommended as the most accurate method for diagnosing NPH [17]. Each approach has advantages and disadvantages. One advantage of the large-volume lumbar puncture is that it can be performed in the outpatient setting and does not require special equipment or expertise, except for the ability to carefully evaluate the clinical examination before and after [9,10,14,96,97]. We use an 18- or 20-gauge spinal needle to remove 40 to 50 mL of CSF, and then cause a temporary CSF leak by puncturing the dura deliberately two or three times to approximate the effect of continuous CSF drainage. Patients are kept flat for no longer than 15 to 20 minutes afterwards because their response to CSF removal cannot be assessed if they remain supine. Patients who develop low-pressure symptoms should lie down for relief, but in our experience, this occurrence is rare in NPH. We recommend that the physician evaluate the patient before and after the lumbar puncture, and not rely solely on the assessment of the patient's or family's, which can be biased by their desire for the patient to improve. Although it is widely believed that patients are better immediately after the lumbar puncture, our experience is that a response is often better observed 4 to 6 hours after the procedure. Advantages of large-volume lumbar puncture in diagnosing NPH are its relative ease of completion and that a positive response can be documented for recommending shunt surgery. A disadvantage of the procedure is that test sensitivity is not high and the procedure may identify only patients who will experience rapid response, therefore missing patients who have NPH. The absence of a response to large-volume lumbar puncture does not exclude the possibility of shunt-responsive hydrocephalus [17].

Continuous drainage of CSF through spinal catheter creates a more sustained and controlled simulation of the effects of a shunt on the brain, essentially a test-drive of shunt-like conditions without undergoing shunt surgery [13,14,98]. Controlled CSF drainage is more sensitive than a lumbar puncture (50%–100%, compared with 26%–61%) and has a high positive predictive value (80%–100%) [17]. Gait dysfunction is the symptom most likely to improve after temporary CSF drainage through lumbar puncture or spinal catheter [11,14,95]. Improved Tinetti score, increased speed of ambulation over a defined distance, or reduced need for walking aids in response to

CSF drainage are similarly useful in predicting improvement after shunt surgery [9,99]. Change in bladder control after lumbar puncture is difficult to assess, but patients may report a significant change during a CSF drainage trial. In patients who have coexisting disorders that may contribute to deficits in cognition, gait, or urinary control, CSF drainage can help identify the proportional contribution of hydrocephalus to the symptoms [13,14]. Lack of improvement after a controlled CSF drainage trial is an indication that shunt surgery is unlikely to benefit the patient. Several centers specializing in NPH throughout the United States conduct CSF drainage using a spinal catheter. Hospitalization is required and the risk for catheter-associated infection is 2% to 4% [13,14].

Outcome after shunt surgery

The likelihood of symptom improvement after shunt surgery depends on the criteria used to select patients. A 2001 meta-analysis found that 59% of patients experienced improvement immediately after shunting (range, 24%–100%), 29% experienced prolonged improvement (range, 10%–100%), 38% experienced shunt complications (range, 5%–100%), 22% required surgical revision (range, 0%–47%), and 6% experienced permanent neurologic deficit or death (range, 0%–35%) [96]. More recently, Marmarou and colleagues [14] found that 90% of patients selected based on response to controlled CSF drainage experienced improvement after shunt surgery. In our 10-year experience with 132 patients diagnosed using a protocol of ICP monitoring and controlled CSF drainage, 33% of patients experienced improvement in at least one symptom 3 months after shunt surgery, 60% at 6 months, and 75% at 18 ± 13 months [13]. All NPH symptoms improved in 46% of patients at 18 ± 13 months. Gait was the earliest and most common clinical improvement, occurring in 93% of patients. In our series, complications requiring shunt revision occurred in 33% of patients and 2% developed subdural hematomas.

Urinary symptoms improve in a substantial percentage of patients [11,13,14]. When urinary symptoms persist after shunt surgery, patients should be evaluated for a coexisting urinary disorder.

Despite its characterization as a reversible dementia, studies of cognitive improvement in treated NPH show mixed results. Some reports show little or no change even in patients who experience gains in gait and continence [12,100,101]. We observed cognitive improvements in our series. Specifically, approximately 50% of study patients experienced significant improvement defined as at least one standard-deviation increase in score in verbal memory and recall, psychomotor speed, and motor precision 3 months after shunt surgery [37,38]. By 3 to 9 months, 80% experienced significantly improved scores on the Rey Auditory Verbal Learning Test, raising the possibility of positive long-term gains in cognition. Frontal lobe executive functions do not usually improve after shunt surgery [40,102,103]. Cognitive function improvement in NPH surpasses that seen in Alzheimer's dementia treated with anticholinesterases [104].

Few studies exist of long-term outcome in NPH. In one study of 25 patients who underwent shunt surgery, 17 were still living after 5 years, of whom 45% still experienced improvement in gait and 30% in memory [101]. Many patients who have NPH have concomitant age-related diseases and will experience morbidity and mortality unrelated to hydrocephalus. Nevertheless, even temporarily enhanced mobility can prolong independent living and increase quality of life [105,106].

Care of patients who have shunts

Little has been written about the practical aspects of caring for patients with NPH who have shunts. Our impression is that many physicians are apprehensive about shunts, but by applying basic evaluation and treatment principles, we believe that most physicians can safely care for their patients who have NPH.

Patients who have NPH generally experience improvement after shunt surgery; however, recovery time varies, ranging from immediate to several months. Patients who haven't experienced recovery by 6 months deserve further treatment or evaluation. The size of the ventricles observed on imaging studies is an unreliable indicator of recovery, as they rarely change size even in the face of dramatic symptom resolution. Improvement or worsening is best determined through clinical evaluation. The extent of recovery is difficult to predict, and depends on the proportional contribution of NPH to the patient's symptoms versus that caused by coexisting disorders.

In patients who have undergone shunting, NPH symptoms tend to resolve simultaneously, although cognitive recovery takes longer than gait or urinary recovery. Therefore, if only two NPH symptoms improve and the third symptom does not, then a second cause (other than NPH) is likely contributing to the symptom that isn't recovering. If this pattern of recovery is observed, an alternative explanation for the symptoms that have not improved should be sought.

Two basic types of shunts are widely used: so-called "programmable shunts" (variable resistance) and shunts with a single valve setting (fixed resistance). The setting of programmable shunts can be changed noninvasively with a magnetic mechanism to permit either more CSF flow (lower pressure setting) for patients who aren't improving as anticipated, or less CSF flow (higher pressure setting) for patients who have evidence of overdrainage. Evidence of overdrainage includes postural headaches or presence of subdural hygroma or hematoma on neuroimaging.

Adjustment of the shunt setting requires equipment supplied by the shunt manufacturer, and usually requires the patient to return to the treating neurosurgeon or hydrocephalus center. Programmable shunts are susceptible to strong external magnetic fields, such as those associated with MRI scanners, and to weak external magnetic fields that are placed very close to the shunt (eg, placing a small kitchen magnet on the scalp). Exposure to a magnetic field can alter the shunt setting, unpredictably resulting in more or less CSF flow than intended. This susceptibility does not preclude patients who have NPH from undergoing MRI scans. After an MRI scan, patients should be seen within 1 to 3 days to have the shunt setting checked and reset to the previous setting if necessary. We routinely advise our patients about the susceptibility of their shunt to magnetic fields, and routinely ask if they underwent an MRI scan since their last clinic visit. If so, the shunt setting should be checked. Readjusting the shunt to its previous setting often results in symptom improvement.

Fixed-resistance shunts cannot be adjusted after they are inserted. Most fixed-resistance shunts are not susceptible to external magnetic fields; however, if a different shunt setting becomes necessary to manage symptoms, then the shunt valve must be surgically removed and replaced with another.

The most common complication associated with shunts in NPH is obstruction of the shunt, which occurs in up to one third of patients. We routinely advise our patients how to recognize the symptoms of obstruction. Shunt obstruction manifests in one of two ways. In patients who have shown improvement after shunt surgery, gradual return of their NPH symptoms may signify shunt obstruction. In patients who never improve after shunt surgery, the shunt setting should be gradually taken to its lowest setting. Continued absence of recovery may indicate either that the shunt is obstructed or that the diagnosis of NPH was incorrect. Shunt obstruction in NPH is rarely an acute, life-threatening problem, unlike the problems encountered in obstructive hydrocephalus, which is more commonly seen in children. Less common shunt complications include subdural hematomas or subdural hygromas.

Evaluation of patients who exhibit clinical worsening or do not experience recovery after shunt surgery is straightforward and can be initiated by primary care physicians. A series of plain radiographs with images of the proximal catheter, the valve mechanism, and the distal catheter, including its tip, can show whether the shunt components have become disconnected, which occurs rarely in adults (Fig. 2). For ventriculoperitoneal shunts, obstruction nearly always results from occlusion of the distal catheter in the peritoneal cavity, typically caused by blockage of the shunt tip by the omentum or adhesions. Normally, the peritoneal catheter is freely mobile within the abdomen. Adhesions may immobilize the shunt tip, and can be shown by obtaining two abdominal radiographs a day or more apart. A plain-head CT can be obtained to show whether a subdural hygroma or hematoma has developed.

In addition to these tests, patients can be referred to a neurosurgeon or hydrocephalus center for more detailed evaluation. A nuclear medicine shunt patency study can be performed, involving the injection of a tiny amount of

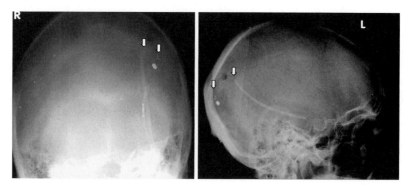

Fig. 2. 74 year old man presented with return of original NPH symptoms. Plain skull x-rays demonstrate a gap between the proximal end of the shunt valve and the ventricular catheter, as shown by the arrows.

radioisotope into the shunt reservoir followed by observation of flow through the shunt system. If the shunt is obstructed, flow is absent or significantly delayed. For ventriculoperitoneal shunts, the tracer should disperse throughout the peritoneal cavity. Evidence of loculation or restricted dispersal may indicate an obstruction. Identification and treatment of shunt obstruction results in symptom improvement for many patients [107].

Lastly, it is important to remember that many patients who have NPH have concomitant disorders that can impair their mobility, cognition, and urinary control. Evaluation of symptom worsening in a patient who has NPH should include evaluation for comorbidities and investigation into possible shunt obstruction. In patients who have NPH and a properly functioning shunt, diseases such as neuropathy, arthritis, cardiopulmonary disease, or other common disorders associated with aging should be considered. Optimal care of these patients is accomplished by cooperation and coordination of care among primary care physicians and the specialists treating the patient for NPH.

Patient and family resources

The Hydrocephalus Association is the largest patient advocacy group in the United States, offering support for patients of all ages and their families. Their Web site (www.hydroassoc.org) contains helpful information and links.

References

[1] Hakim S, Adams RD. The special clinical problem of symptomatic hydrocephalus with normal cerebrospinal fluid pressure. Observations on cerebrospinal fluid hydrodynamics. J Neurol Sci 1965;2(4):307–27.

[2] Hakim S, Venegas JG, Burton JD. The physics of the cranial cavity, hydrocephalus and normal pressure hydrocephalus: mechanical interpretation and mathematical model. Surg Neurol 1976;5(3):187–210.

[3] Adams RD, Fisher CM, Hakim S, et al. Symptomatic occult hydrocephalus with "normal" cerebrospinal-fluid pressure. A treatable syndrome. N Engl J Med 1965;273:117–26.

[4] Hughes CP, Siegel BA, Coxe WS, et al. Adult idiopathic communicating hydrocephalus with and without shunting. J Neurol Neurosurg Psychiatry 1978;41(11):961–71.

[5] Udvarhelyi GB, Wood JH, James AE Jr, et al. Results and complications in 55 shunted patients with normal pressure hydrocephalus. Surg Neurol 1975;3(5):271–5.

[6] Vanneste J, Augustijn P, Dirven C, et al. Shunting normal-pressure hydrocephalus: do the benefits outweigh the risks? A multicenter study and literature review. Neurology 1992; 42(1):54–9.

[7] Black PM, Ojemann RG, Tzouras A. CSF shunts for dementia, incontinence, and gait disturbance. Clin Neurosurg 1985;32:632–51.

[8] Graff-Radford NR, Godersky JC, Jones MP. Variables predicting surgical outcome in symptomatic hydrocephalus in the elderly. Neurology 1989;39(12):1601–4.

[9] Meier U, Konig A, Miethke C. Predictors of outcome in patients with normal-pressure hydrocephalus. Eur Neurol 2004;51(2):59–67.

[10] Mori K. Management of idiopathic normal-pressure hydrocephalus: a multiinstitutional study conducted in Japan. J Neurosurg 2001;95(6):970–3.

[11] Poca MA, Mataro M, Del Mar Matarin M, et al. Is the placement of shunts in patients with idiopathic normal-pressure hydrocephalus worth the risk? Results of a study based on continuous monitoring of intracranial pressure. J Neurosurg 2004;100(5):855–66.

[12] Vanneste JA. Diagnosis and management of normal-pressure hydrocephalus. J Neurol 2000;247(1):5–14.

[13] McGirt MJ, Woodworth G, Coon AL, et al. Diagnosis, treatment, and analysis of long-term outcomes in idiopathic normal-pressure hydrocephalus. Neurosurgery 2005;57(4): 699–705 [discussion 699–705].

[14] Marmarou A, Young HF, Aygok GA, et al. Diagnosis and management of idiopathic normal-pressure hydrocephalus: a prospective study in 151 patients. J Neurosurg 2005; 102(6):987–97.

[15] Relkin N, Marmarou A, Klinge P, et al. Diagnosing idiopathic normal-pressure hydrocephalus. Neurosurgery 2005;57(3 Suppl):S4–16 [discussion ii–v].

[16] Klinge P, Marmarou A, Bergsneider M, et al. Outcome of shunting in idiopathic normal-pressure hydrocephalus and the value of outcome assessment in shunted patients. Neurosurgery 2005;57(3 Suppl):S40–52 [discussion ii–v].

[17] Marmarou A, Bergsneider M, Klinge P, et al. The value of supplemental prognostic tests for the preoperative assessment of idiopathic normal-pressure hydrocephalus. Neurosurgery 2005;57(3 Suppl):S17–28 [discussion ii–v].

[18] Bergsneider M, Black PM, Klinge P, et al. Surgical management of idiopathic normal-pressure hydrocephalus. Neurosurgery 2005;57(3 Suppl):S29–39 [discussion ii–v].

[19] Sudarsky L, Simon S. Gait disorder in late-life hydrocephalus. Arch Neurol 1987;44(3): 263–7.

[20] Soelberg Sorensen P, Jansen EC, Gjerris F. Motor disturbances in normal-pressure hydrocephalus. Special reference to stance and gait. Arch Neurol 1986;43(1):34–8.

[21] Graff-Radford NR, Godersky JC. Normal-pressure hydrocephalus. Onset of gait abnormality before dementia predicts good surgical outcome. Arch Neurol 1986;43(9):940–2.

[22] Meier U, Zeilinger FS, Kintzel D. Signs, symptoms and course of normal pressure hydrocephalus in comparison with cerebral atrophy. Acta Neurochir (Wien) 1999;141(10): 1039–48.

[23] Caruso R, Cervoni L, Vitale AM, et al. Idiopathic normal-pressure hydrocephalus in adults: result of shunting correlated with clinical findings in 18 patients and review of the literature. Neurosurg Rev 1997;20(2):104–7.

[24] Stolze H, Kuhtz-Buschbeck JP, Drucke H, et al. Gait analysis in idiopathic normal pressure hydrocephalus—which parameters respond to the CSF tap test? Clin Neurophysiol 2000; 111(9):1678–86.

[25] Stolze H, Kuhtz-Buschbeck JP, Drucke H, et al. Comparative analysis of the gait disorder of normal pressure hydrocephalus and Parkinson's disease. J Neurol Neurosurg Psychiatry 2001;70(3):289–97.

[26] Thompson PD, Marsden CD. Walking disorders. In: Bradley WG, Daroff RB, Fenichel GM, et al, editors. Anonymous, editor. Neurology in clinical practice. Vol. I. Boston: Butterworth-Heinemann; 2000. p. 341–52.

[27] Nowak DA, Topka HR. Broadening a classic clinical triad: the hypokinetic motor disorder of normal pressure hydrocephalus also affects the hand. Exp Neurol 2006;198(1):81–7.

[28] Nowak DA, Gumprecht H, Topka H. CSF drainage ameliorates the motor deficit in normal pressure hydrocephalus evidence from the analysis of grasping movements. J Neurol 2006;(Feb):7.

[29] Racette BA, Esper GJ, Antenor J, et al. Pathophysiology of parkinsonism due to hydrocephalus. J Neurol Neurosurg Psychiatry 2004;75(11):1617–9.

[30] Nutt JG, Marsden CD, Thompson PD. Human walking and higher-level gait disorders, particularly in the elderly. Neurology 1993;43(2):268–79.

[31] Zadikoff C, Lang AE. Apraxia in movement disorders. Brain 2005;128(Pt 7):1480–97.

[32] Tinetti ME. Performance-oriented assessment of mobility problems in elderly patients. J Am Geriatr Soc 1986;34(2):119–26.

[33] Raiche M, Hebert R, Prince F, et al. Screening older adults at risk of falling with the Tinetti balance scale. Lancet 2000;356(9234):1001–2.

[34] DuBeau CE. Interpreting the effect of common medical conditions on voiding dysfunction in the elderly. Urol Clin North Am 1996;23(1):11–8.

[35] Ahlberg J, Norlen L, Blomstrand C, et al. Outcome of shunt operation on urinary incontinence in normal pressure hydrocephalus predicted by lumbar puncture. J Neurol Neurosurg Psychiatry 1988;51(1):105–8.

[36] Kevorkian R. Physiology of incontinence. Clin Geriatr Med 2004;20(3):409–25.

[37] Duinkerke A, Williams MA, Rigamonti D, et al. Cognitive recovery in idiopathic normal pressure hydrocephalus after shunt. Cogn Behav Neurol 2004;17(3):179–84.

[38] Thomas G, McGirt MJ, Woodworth G, et al. Baseline neuropsychological profile and cognitive response to cerebrospinal fluid shunting for idiopathic normal pressure hydrocephalus. Dement Geriatr Cogn Disord 2005;20(2–3):163–8.

[39] van Harten B, Courant MN, Scheltens P, et al. Validation of the HIV Dementia Scale in an elderly cohort of patients with subcortical cognitive impairment caused by subcortical ischaemic vascular disease or a normal pressure hydrocephalus. Dement Geriatr Cogn Disord 2004;18(1):109–14.

[40] Iddon JL, Pickard JD, Cross JJ, et al. Specific patterns of cognitive impairment in patients with idiopathic normal pressure hydrocephalus and Alzheimer's disease: a pilot study. J Neurol Neurosurg Psychiatry 1999;67(6):723–32.

[41] Davis HF, Skolasky RL Jr, Selnes OA, et al. Assessing HIV-associated dementia: modified HIV dementia scale versus the Grooved Pegboard. AIDS Read 2002;12(1): 29–31, 38.

[42] Nasreddine ZS, Phillips NA, Bedirian V, et al. The Montreal Cognitive Assessment, MoCA: a brief screening tool for mild cognitive impairment. J Am Geriatr Soc 2005; 53(4):695–9.

[43] Hoglund M, Tisell M, Wikkelso C. Incidence of surgery for hydrocephalus in adults surveyed: same number afflicted by hydrocephalus as by multiple sclerosis. Lakartidningen 2001;98(14):1681–5.

[44] Krauss JK, Halve B. Normal pressure hydrocephalus: survey on contemporary diagnostic algorithms and therapeutic decision-making in clinical practice. Acta Neurochir (Wien) 2004;146(4):379–88 [discussion 388].

[45] Clarfield AM. The reversible dementias: do they reverse? Ann Intern Med 1988;109(6): 476–86.

[46] Clarfield AM. The decreasing prevalence of reversible dementias: an updated meta-analysis. Arch Intern Med 2003;163(18):2219–29.

[47] Bech-Azeddine R, Waldemar G, Knudsen GM, et al. Idiopathic normal-pressure hydrocephalus: evaluation and findings in a multidisciplinary memory clinic. Eur J Neurol 2001;8(6):601–11.

[48] Knopman DS, Petersen RC, Cha RH, et al. Incidence and causes of nondegenerative non-vascular dementia: a population-based study. Arch Neurol 2006;63(2):218–21.

[49] Edwards RJ, Dombrowski SM, Luciano MG, et al. Chronic hydrocephalus in adults. Brain Pathol 2004;14(3):325–36.

[50] Graff-Radford NR, Godersky JC. Symptomatic congenital hydrocephalus in the elderly simulating normal pressure hydrocephalus. Neurology 1989;39(12):1596–600.

[51] Larsson A, Stephensen H, Wikkelso C. Adult patients with "asymptomatic" and "compensated" hydrocephalus benefit from surgery. Acta Neurol Scand 1999;99(2):81–90.

[52] Fukuhara T, Luciano MG. Clinical features of late-onset idiopathic aqueductal stenosis. Surg Neurol 2001;55(3):132–6 [discussion 136–7].

[53] Cowan JA, McGirt MJ, Woodworth G, et al. The syndrome of hydrocephalus in young and middle-aged adults (SHYMA). Neurol Res 2005;27(5):540–7.

[54] Williams MA, Razumovsky AY. Cerebrospinal fluid circulation, cerebral edema, and intracranial pressure. Curr Opin Neurol 1993;6(6):847–53.

[55] Dandy WE, Blackfan KD. Internal hydrocephalus. An experimental, clinical, and pathological study. Am J Dis Child 1914;8:406–82.

[56] Weed LH. The pathways of escape from the subarachnoid spaces with particular reference to the arachnoid villi. J of Med Res 1914;31:51–91.

[57] Weed LH. Certain anatomical and physiological aspects of the pressure of the cerebrospinal fluid. Brain 1935;58:383–97.

[58] Fishman JB. Cerebrospinal fluid in disease of the nervous system. 2nd edition. Philadelphia: WB Saunders; 1992.

[59] Silverberg GD, Heit G, Huhn S, et al. The cerebrospinal fluid production rate is reduced in dementia of the Alzheimer's type. Neurology 2001;57(10):1763–6.

[60] Silverberg GD, Huhn S, Jaffe RA, et al. Downregulation of cerebrospinal fluid production in patients with chronic hydrocephalus. J Neurosurg 2002;97(6):1271–5.

[61] May C, Kaye JA, Atack JR, et al. Cerebrospinal fluid production is reduced in healthy aging. Neurology 1990;40(3 Pt 1):500–3.

[62] Gideon P, Thomsen C, Stahlberg F, et al. Cerebrospinal fluid production and dynamics in normal aging: a MRI phase-mapping study. Acta Neurol Scand 1994;89(5):362–6.

[63] Fujimoto Y, Matsushita H, Plese JP, et al. Hydrocephalus due to diffuse villous hyperplasia of the choroid plexus. Case report and review of the literature. Pediatr Neurosurg 2004; 40(1):32–6.

[64] Fujimura M, Onuma T, Kameyama M, et al. Hydrocephalus due to cerebrospinal fluid overproduction by bilateral choroid plexus papillomas. Childs Nerv Syst 2004;20(7):485–8.

[65] Milhorat TH, Hammock MK, Davis DA, et al. Choroid plexus papilloma. I. Proof of cerebrospinal fluid overproduction. Childs Brain 1976;2(5):273–89.

[66] Aziz AA, Coleman L, Morokoff A, et al. Diffuse choroid plexus hyperplasia: an under-diagnosed cause of hydrocephalus in children? Pediatr Radiol 2005;35(8):815–8.

[67] Johnston I, Teo C. Disorders of CSF hydrodynamics. Childs Nerv Syst 2000;16(10–11): 776–99.

[68] Davson H, Welch K, Segal MB. The physiology and pathophysiology of the cerebrospinal fluid. New York: Churchill Livingstone; 1987.

[69] Hakim S. Some observations on CSF pressure. Hydrocephalic syndrome in adults with "normal" CSF pressure (recognition of a new syndrome) [dissertation/thesis]. Bogota, Colombia; Javeriana University School of Medicine: 1964.

[70] Kim DS, Oi S, Hidaka M, et al. A new experimental model of obstructive hydrocephalus in the rat: the micro-balloon technique. Childs Nerv Syst 1999;15(5):250–5.

[71] Cosan TE, Guner AI, Akcar N, et al. Progressive ventricular enlargement in the absence of high ventricular pressure in an experimental neonatal rat model. Childs Nerv Syst 2002; 18(1–2):10–4.

[72] Azzi GM, Canady AI, Ham S, et al. Kaolin-induced hydrocephalus in the hamster: temporal sequence of changes in intracranial pressure, ventriculomegaly and whole-brain specific gravity. Acta Neuropathol (Berl) 1999;98(3):245–50.

[73] Lundberg N. Continuous recording and control of ventricular fluid pressure in neurosurgical practice. Acta Psychiatr Scand 1960;36(Suppl 149):1–193.

[74] Torbey MT, Geocadin RG, Razumovsky AY, et al. Utility of CSF pressure monitoring to identify idiopathic intracranial hypertension without papilledema in patients with chronic daily headache. Cephalalgia 2004;24(6):495–502.

[75] Czosnyka M, Smielewski P, Piechnik S, et al. Hemodynamic characterization of intracranial pressure plateau waves in head-injury patients. J Neurosurg 1999;91(1):11–9.

[76] Cooper R, Hulme A. Intracranial pressure and related phenomena during sleep. J Neurol Neurosurg Psychiat 1966;29:564–70.

[77] Kjaellquist A, Lundberg N, Ponten U. Respiratory and cardiovascular changes during rapid spontaneous variations of ventricular fluid pressure in patients with intracranial hypertension. Acta Neurol Scand 1964;40:291–317.

[78] Newell DW, Aaslid R, Stooss R, et al. The relationship of blood flow velocity fluctuations to intracranial pressure B waves. J Neurosurg 1992;76(3):415–21.

[79] Grossman RI, Yousem DM. Neuroradiology, the requisites. Philadelphia: Mosby; 2003.

[80] Qureshi AI, Williams MA, Razumovsky AY, et al. Magnetic resonance imaging, unstable intracranial pressure and clinical outcome in patients with normal pressure hydrocephalus. Acta Neurochir Suppl 1998;71:354–6.

[81] Segev Y, Metser U, Beni-Adani L, et al. Morphometric study of the midsagittal MR imaging plane in cases of hydrocephalus and atrophy and in normal brains. AJNR Am J Neuroradiol 2001;22(9):1674–9.

[82] Kitagaki H, Mori E, Ishii K, et al. CSF spaces in idiopathic normal pressure hydrocephalus: morphology and volumetry. Am J Neuroradiol 1998;19(7):1277–84.

[83] Palm WM, Walchenbach R, Bruinsma B, et al. Intracranial compartment volumes in normal pressure hydrocephalus: volumetric assessment versus outcome. AJNR Am J Neuroradiol 2006;27(1):76–9.

[84] Boon AJ, Tans JT, Delwel EJ, et al. Dutch Normal-Pressure Hydrocephalus Study: the role of cerebrovascular disease. J Neurosurg 1999;90(2):221–6.

[85] Krauss JK, Regel JP, Vach W, et al. Vascular risk factors and arteriosclerotic disease in idiopathic normal-pressure hydrocephalus of the elderly. Stroke 1996;27(1):24–9.

[86] Krauss JK, Regel JP, Vach W, et al. White matter lesions in patients with idiopathic normal pressure hydrocephalus and in an age-matched control group: a comparative study. Neurosurgery 1997;40(3):491–5 [discussion 495–6].

[87] Tullberg M, Hultin L, Ekholm S, et al. White matter changes in normal pressure hydrocephalus and Binswanger disease: specificity, predictive value and correlations to axonal degeneration and demyelination. Acta Neurol Scand 2002;105(6):417–26.

[88] Tullberg M, Jensen C, Ekholm S, et al. Normal pressure hydrocephalus: vascular white matter changes on MR images must not exclude patients from shunt surgery. AJNR Am J Neuroradiol 2001;22(9):1665–73.

[89] Albeck MJ, Borgesen SE, Gjerris F, et al. Intracranial pressure and cerebrospinal fluid outflow conductance in healthy subjects. J Neurosurg 1991;74(4):597–600.

[90] Hussey F, Schanzer B, Katzman R. A simple constant-infusion manometric test for measurement of CSF absorption. II. Clinical studies. Neurology 1970;20(7):665–80.

[91] Kahlon B, Sundbarg G, Rehncrona S. Lumbar infusion test in normal pressure hydrocephalus. Acta Neurol Scand 2005;111(6):379–84.

[92] Borgesen SE, Gjerris F. The predictive value of conductance to outflow of CSF in normal pressure hydrocephalus. Brain 1982;105(Pt 1):65–86.

[93] Nornes H, Rootwelt K, Sjaastad O. Normal pressure hydrocephalus. Long-term intracranial pressure recording. Eur Neurol 1973;9(5):261–74.

[94] Pickard JD, Teasdale G, Matheson M, et al. Intraventricular pressure waves: the best predictive test for shunting in normal pressure hydrocephalus. In: Shulman K, Marmarou A, Miller JD, et al, editors. Intracranial pressure IV. Berlin: Springer-Verlag; 1980. p. 498–500.

[95] Williams MA, Razumovsky AY, Hanley DF. Comparison of Pcsf monitoring and controlled CSF drainage to diagnose normal pressure hydrocephalus. Acta Neurochir Suppl 1998;71:328–30.

[96] Sand T, Bovim G, Grimse R, et al. Idiopathic normal pressure hydrocephalus: the CSF taptest may predict the clinical response to shunting. Acta Neurol Scand 1994;89(5):311–6.

[97] Hebb AO, Cusimano MD. Idiopathic normal pressure hydrocephalus: a systematic review of diagnosis and outcome. Neurosurgery 2001;49(5):1166–84 [discussion 1184–66].

[98] Williams MA. Spinal catheter insertion via seated lumbar puncture using a massage chair. Neurology 2002;58(12):1859–60.

[99] Shore WS, deLateur BJ, Kuhlemeier KV, et al. A comparison of gait assessment methods: Tinetti and GAITRite electronic walkway. J Am Geriatr Soc 2005;53(11):2044–5.

[100] Tromp CN, Staal MJ, Kalma LE. Effects of ventricular shunt treatment of normal pressure hydrocephalus on psychological functions. Z Kinderchir 1989;44(Suppl 1):41–3.

[101] Savolainen S, Hurskainen H, Paljarvi L, et al. Five-year outcome of normal pressure hydrocephalus with or without a shunt: predictive value of the clinical signs, neuropsychological evaluation and infusion test. Acta Neurochir (Wien) 2002;144(6):515–23 [discussion 523].

[102] Caltagirone C, Gainotti G, Masullo C, et al. Neurophysiological study of normal pressure hydrocephalus. Acta Psychiatr Scand 1982;65(2):93–100.

[103] Gustafson L, Hagberg B. Recovery in hydrocephalic dementia after shunt operation. J Neurol Neurosurg Psychiatry 1978;41(10):940–7.

[104] Potyk D. Treatments for Alzheimer disease. South Med J 2005;98(6):628–35.

[105] Hope T, Keene J, Gedling K, et al. Predictors of institutionalization for people with dementia living at home with a carer. Int J Geriatr Psychiatry 1998;13(10):682–90.

[106] Gill TM, Baker DI, Gottschalk M, et al. A program to prevent functional decline in physically frail, elderly persons who live at home. N Engl J Med 2002;347(14):1068–74.

[107] Williams MA, Razumovsky AY, Hanley DF. Evaluation of shunt function in patients who are never better, or better than worse after shunt surgery for NPH. Acta Neurochir Suppl 1998;71:368–70.

ELSEVIER
SAUNDERS

CLINICS IN
GERIATRIC
MEDICINE

Clin Geriatr Med 22 (2006) 953–956

Index

Note: Page numbers of article titles are in **boldface** type.

A

Acetylcholinesterase inhibitors, in
Parkinson's disease, 784–785

Akathisia, in Parkinson's disease, 764–765
tardive, 921–922, 923–924, 929

Alprazolam, in essential tremor, 851

γ-Amino butyric acid, 924

Anxiety, in Parkinson's disease, 764–765

Ataxia(s), **859–877**
autoimmune, 871
causes of, 861–873
clinical symptoms of, 859–861
congenital, 861–863
endocrine, 871–872
infectious, 866–870
neoplastic, 870–871
nongenetic, of unknown origin,
872–873
treatment of, in elderly, 873
toxic, 872
traumatic, 863
vascular, 863–866
workup in, 864–865

B

Baclofen, in dystonia, 909

Basal ganglia, abnormalities in circuitry of,
817
organization of, 816–818

Basal ganglion mineralization, chorea in,
890–891

Botulinum toxin, in dystonia, 910

Brain stimulation, deep, 813
behavior and cognition after,
821–822
complicatitons of, 821
eligibility criteria for, 815–816
intraoperative evaluations
during, 819–820
mechanism of action of, 820
stimulator programming for, 820
targets and outcomes in, 818–819
indications and targets for, 814

C

Calcium channel blockers, in essential
tremor, 852

CALM-PD trial, 746–747

Carbidopa, 747

Carbidopa/levodopa, in Parkinson's
disease, 756

Chorea, geriatric, **879–897**
age at onset of, 880
autoimmune causes of, 887–888
causes of, 879–880, 881
investigations into,
891–892
cerebrovascular causes of,
881–882
hereditary causes of, 883–887
infectious causes of, 889
medications and toxins causing,
882–883
metabolic causes of, 888–889
movements in, 879
treatment of, 892–893
senile, 890

Chorea-acanthocytosis, 886

Clonazepam, in dystonia, 909
in essential tremor, 851

Clozapine, in essential tremor, 852
in Parkinson's disease, 787

Cognitive impairment, in Parkinson's
disease, treatment of, 783–785

Constipation, in Parkinson's disease, 767

Corticobasal degeneration, clinical
presentation of, 833–834
diagnosis of, 834–835
management and prognosis in, 835
pathophysiology of, 834

United States Postal Service

Statement of Ownership, Management, and Circulation

1. Publication Title	2. Publication Number		3. Filing Date
Clinics in Geriatric Medicine	0 0 0 - 7 0 4		9/15/06

4. Issue Frequency	5. Number of Issues Published Annually	6. Annual Subscription Price
Feb, May, Aug, Nov	4	$165.00

7. Complete Mailing Address of Known Office of Publication (Not printer) (Street, city, county, state, and ZIP+4)	Contact Person
Elsevier Inc. 360 Park Avenue South New York, NY 10010-1710	Sarah Carmichael
	Telephone
	(215) 239-3681

8. Complete Mailing Address of Headquarters or General Business Office of Publisher (Not printer)

Elsevier Inc., 360 Park Avenue South, New York, NY 10010-1710

9. Full Names and Complete Mailing Addresses of Publisher, Editor, and Managing Editor (Do not leave blank)

Publisher (Name and complete mailing address)

John Schrefer, Elsevier Inc., 1600 John F. Kennedy Blvd., Suite 1800, Philadelphia, PA 19103-2899

Editor (Name and complete mailing address)

Joanne Husovski, Elsevier Inc., 1600 John F. Kennedy Blvd., Suite 1800, Philadelphia, PA 19103-2899

Managing Editor (Name and complete mailing address)

Catherine Bewick, Elsevier Inc., 1600 John F. Kennedy Blvd., Suite 1800, Philadelphia, PA 19103-2899

10. Owner (Do not leave blank. If the publication is owned by a corporation, give the name and address of the corporation immediately followed by the names and addresses of all stockholders owning or holding 1 percent or more of the total amount of stock. If not owned by a corporation, give the names and addresses of the individual owners. If owned by a partnership or other unincorporated firm, give its name and address as well as those of each individual owner. If the publication is published by a nonprofit organization, give its name and address.)

Full Name	Complete Mailing Address
Wholly owned subsidiary of	4520 East-West Highway
Reed/Elsevier Inc, US Holdings	Bethesda, MD 20814

11. Known Bondholders, Mortgagees, and Other Security Holders Owning or Holding 1 Percent or More of Total Amount of Bonds, Mortgages, or Other Securities. If none, check box ► None

Full Name	Complete Mailing Address
N/A	

12. Tax Status (For completion by nonprofit organizations authorized to mail at nonprofit rates) (Check one)
The purpose, function, and nonprofit status of this organization and the exempt status for federal income tax purposes:
☐ Has Not Changed During Preceding 12 Months
☐ Has Changed During Preceding 12 Months (Publisher must submit explanation of change with this statement)

(See Instructions on Reverse)

PS Form 3526, October 1999

---

13. Publication Title		14. Issue Date for Circulation Data Below
Clinics in Geriatric Medicine		August, 2006

15. Extent and Nature of Circulation			Average No. Copies Each Issue During Preceding 12 Months	No. Copies of Single Issue Published Nearest to Filing Date
a.	Total Number of Copies (Net press run)		2,075	2,000
b. Paid and/or Requested Circulation	(1)	Paid/Requested Outside-County Mail Subscriptions Stated on Form 3541. (Include advertiser's proof and exchange copies)	993	913
	(2)	Paid In-County Subscriptions Stated on Form 3541 (Include advertiser's proof and exchange copies)		
	(3)	Sales Through Dealers and Carriers, Street Vendors, Counter Sales, and Other Non-USPS Paid Distribution	281	290
	(4)	Other Classes Mailed Through the USPS		
c.	Total Paid and/or Requested Circulation [Sum of 15b. (1), (2), (3), and (4)]	►	1,274	1,203
d. Free Distribution by Mail (Samples, complimentary, and other free)	(1)	Outside-County as Stated on Form 3541	121	122
	(2)	In-County as Stated on Form 3541		
	(3)	Other Classes Mailed Through the USPS		
e.	Free Distribution Outside the Mail (Carriers or other means)			
f.	Total Free Distribution (Sum of 15d. and 15e.)	►	121	122
g.	Total Distribution (Sum of 15c. and 15f.)	►	1,395	1,325
h.	Copies not Distributed		680	675
i.	Total (Sum of 15g. and h.)	►	2,075	2,000
j.	Percent Paid and/or Requested Circulation (15c. divided by 15g. times 100)		91.33%	90.79%

16. Publication of Statement of Ownership

☑ Publication required. Will be printed in the **November 2006** issue of this publication. ☐ Publication not required

17. Signature and Title of Editor, Publisher, Business Manager, or Owner

[signature] — Date 9/15/06
John Panucci - Executive Director of Subscription Services

I certify that all information furnished on this form is true and complete. I understand that anyone who furnishes false or misleading information on this form or who omits material or information requested on the form may be subject to criminal sanctions (including fines and imprisonment) and/or civil sanctions (including civil penalties).

Instructions to Publishers

1. Complete and file one copy of this form with your postmaster annually on or before October 1. Keep a copy of the completed form for your records.
2. In cases where the stockholder or security holder is a trustee, include in items 10 and 11 the name of the person or corporation for whom the trustee is acting. Also include the names and addresses of individuals who are stockholders who own or hold 1 percent or more of the total amount of bonds, mortgages, or other securities of the publishing corporation. In item 11, if none, check the box. Use blank sheets if more space is required.
3. Be sure to furnish all circulation information called for in item 15. Free circulation must be shown in items 15d, e, and f.
4. Item 15h., Copies not Distributed, must include (1) newsstand copies originally stated on Form 3541, and returned to the publisher, (2) estimated returns from news agents, and (3), copies for office use, leftovers, spoiled, and all other copies not distributed.
5. If the publication had Periodicals authorization as a general or requester publication, this Statement of Ownership, Management, and Circulation must be published; it must be printed in any issue in October or, if the publication is not published during October, the first issue printed after October.
6. In item 16, indicate the date of the issue in which this Statement of Ownership will be published.
7. Item 17 must be signed.

Failure to file or publish a statement of ownership may lead to suspension of Periodicals authorization.

PS Form 3526, October 1999 (Reverse)

Moving?

Make sure your subscription moves with you!

To notify us of your new address, find your **Clinics Account Number** (located on your mailing label above your name), and contact customer service at:

E-mail: elspcs@elsevier.com

800-654-2452 (subscribers in the U.S. & Canada)
407-345-4000 (subscribers outside of the U.S. & Canada)

Fax number: 407-363-9661

Elsevier Periodicals Customer Service
6277 Sea Harbor Drive
Orlando, FL 32887-4800

*To ensure uninterrupted delivery of your subscription, please notify us at least 4 weeks in advance of move.